THE ELEMENTS *OF* SET THEORY

THE ELEMENTS
OF
SET THEORY

K.K. VERMA
Retired Lecturer in Mathematics
D.L.W. College, Varanasi
DEEPAK KUMAR
Lecturer, Faculty of Engineering
Multimedia University
Cyberjaya, Malyaysia

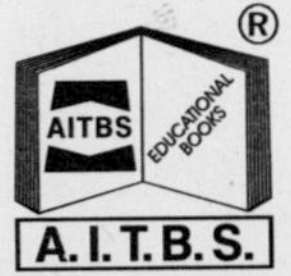

AITBS PUBLISHERS, INDIA
J-5/6, Krishan Nagar, Delhi-110051 (INDIA)
Phone: 011-40167052, 49067602; Fax: 011-22009074
E-mail: aitbsindia@gmail.com & aitbsindia@hotmail.com

First Edition : 2009
Second Edition : 2023

ISBN: 978-93-7473-504-6

Published by:
Virender Kumar Arya for
AITBS Publishers, India
J-5/6 Krishan Nagar, Delhi-110051 (INDIA)
Phone: 011-40167052, 49067602; Fax: 011-22009074
E-mail: aitbsindia@gmail.com & aitbsindia@hotmail.com

Printed by AITBS, Delhi

Preface

This book on "The Elements of Set Theory" is the result of my experience in the area of graduated level mathematics. The materials in the book have been carefully arranged to help the students of degree level and also for students who wish to appear at the various Engineering Entranc~ Examinations.

For preparing the book I have extensively consulted the relevant authoritative works by various Indian as well as foreign authors.

If this book enormously help the students and meet their requirements in tackling problems related to set-theory, I shall deem my effort to have its true justification.

Authors

Contents

CHAPTER

Set Theory, Set-Operations and Venn Diagrams

1.1 THE CONCEPT OF A SET AND ITS NOTATION

The basic concept of Mathematics is a set. A set is any well defined collection or class of definite distinguishable objects of arbitrary nature. The objects may be anything: books, cars, students, radios etc.

These objects are known as the member or elements of the set. Thus, the objects characterise the set. The words collection, system, family and class are synonyms of the word set.

Usually sets are denoted by capital letters A, B, C, X, Y, Z ..., small letters $a, b, c,$ .... are generally used to denote the elements of the sets, we enclose them in brackets { } and separate them by commas, for example, $A = \{a, e, i, o, u\}$ means A is a set and a, e, i, o, u are its elements. The elements are enclosed in the brackets { } and are separated by commas in it.

There are two basic ways of representing or describing a set

1. *Tabular method:* Here a set is defined by listing its members as shown above $A = \{a, e, i, o, u\}$. This method is also known as Roster method.

2. *Set builder form:* Here we use a letter x which represents are arbitrary element of the set and state its properties is the brackets. This method is known as rule method on symbolic method. We use here a shorter notation

$$A = \{x : x < 5\}$$

Which can be described as $A = \{ x : x \in N, x < 5\}$

$\Rightarrow$ $A = \{1, 2, 3, 4\}$

When the elements of the set are enumerated.

We can also describe the set

$$A = \{x \in N : (x - 5)\,(x^2 - 4) = 0, x \geq 0\}$$

as $A = \{2, 5\}$

by enumerating its elements.

1.2 DIFFERENT TYPES OF SETS

1. *Finite and infinite sets:* A set having finite number of elements is known as a finite set. A set which is not finite is an infinite set.

$A = \{1, 2, 3, \text{..........}\}$ is the example of an cnfinite set.

$B = \{a, e, i, o, u\}$ is a finite set.

2. *Membership:* If $A = \{x : x$ is even numbers$\}$ then we write $A = \{2, 4, 6, 8 \text{......}\}$.

Here 2 is in A and hence $2 \in A, 3 \notin A, 10 \in A, 11 \notin A$ etc.

3. *Equality of sets:* Two sets A and B are said to be equal if they have the same members. In the language of set if $x \in A \Rightarrow x \in B$ and $y \in B \Rightarrow y \in A$ then $A = B$.

We can write

$$A = B \Leftrightarrow (x \in A \Leftrightarrow x \in B)$$

If $A = \{4, 5, 6, 7\}$ and $B = \{6, 7, 5, 4\}$ then $A = B$ since 4, 5, 6, and 7 belonging to A also belong to B and vice versa.

4. *Null set or empty set:* For convenience we introduce the concept of null set. A set which contains no elements is known as an empty set or void set and is denoted by the symbol ϕ.

$A = \{x : x^2 = 9, x$ is even$\}$ is a void set.

5. *Singleton set:* A set which contains only one element is known as a singleton set.

$A = \{a\}, B = \{l\}$ and $C = \{n\}$ are the examples of singleton sets.

6. *Sub set:* If every element of A is a member of B then A is called a subset of B. This relation is denoted by writing $A \subseteq B$. In the language of set $A \subseteq B \Rightarrow (x \in A \Rightarrow x \in B)$.

If $A = \{x : x \text{ is even}\}$ and $B = \{2, 4, 8, 16 ......\}$ then $B \subseteq A$.

If $A \subseteq B$ and $B \subseteq A$ then $A = B$.

$A \not\subseteq B$ and $B \not\supseteq A$ denote, A is not a subset of B. ϕ is considered to be a subset of every set.

7. *Proper subset:* If $A \subseteq B$ and $A \neq B$ then A is a proper subset of B. We denote it by writing $A \subset B$. If $A \subseteq B$ and every element of the set B is also an element of A then A is said to be an improper subset of B.

8. *Comparable set:* Two set A and B are comparable if $A \subseteq B$ or $B \subseteq A$.

If $A = \{x, y\}$ and $B = \{x, y, z\}$ then A and B are comparable since A is a subset of B.

9. *Theorem* (i) Prove that the null set ϕ is a subset of every set.

Proof: Let A be any set and ϕ be *a* null set. Then there is no element in ϕ which is not in A and hence ϕ is a subset of A.

Theorem (ii) Prove that every set is a subset of itself.

Proof: If A is a subset of itself then every element of A belongs to it and hence $A \subseteq A$.

Theorem (iii) Prove that if $A \subseteq B$, $B \subseteq A$ then $A = B$

Proof: Since $A \subseteq B$ then $x \in A \Rightarrow x \in B$ ...(1)

and $B \subseteq A$ then $x \in B \Rightarrow x \in A$ ...(2)

From (1) and (2)

$$x \in A \Leftrightarrow x \in B$$

$$\therefore \quad A = B$$

Theorem (iv) If $A \subseteq B$ and $B \subseteq D$ then $A \subseteq D$.

Proof: Let $x \notin A$. Since A is a subset of B, x also belongs to B. But $B \subseteq D$ hence $x \in D$.

Thus $x \in A \Rightarrow x \in D \quad \therefore A \leq D$.

Theorem (v) Prove that the number of subsets of a set containing n elements is 2^n.

Proof: Let $A = \{a_1, a_2, a_3, ..., a_n\}$ be a set of n elements.

The null set is a subset of every set and hence the number of subsets containing no element = 1.

The number of subsets containing one element from a_1, a_2, a_3, ..., a_n is $n = {}^nC_1$.

The number of subsets containing two elements from a_1, a_2, a_3, ..., a_n is ${}^nC_2$.

Proceeding in the same way, we can obtain the number of subsets containing n elements from a_1, a_2, a_3, ..., a_n is ${}^nC_n$.

The total number of subsets is

$$1 + {}^nC_1 + {}^nC_2 + \dots\dots\dots\dots + {}^nC_n$$
$$= {}^nC_0 + {}^nC_1 + {}^nC_2 + \dots\dots\dots\dots + {}^nC_n$$
$$= \text{The sum of the binomial coefficients} = (1 + 1)^n = 2^n.$$

1.3 NUMBER SETS (REAL NUMBERS, INTEGERS, RATIONAL NUMBERS, NATURAL NUMBERS, IRRATIONAL NUMBERS AND COMPLEX NUMBERS)

The set of all real numbers is represented by R and we can write

$$R = \{-5, -4, -\pi, -3, -2, \dots\dots, 0, \frac{1}{2}, 1, \sqrt{2}, 2 \dots\dots\dots\}.$$

The set of all integers is represented by I or Z and we can write

$$I \text{ or } Z = \{\dots\dots\dots -2, -1, 0, 1, 2 \dots\dots\dots\dots\}.$$

The set of all negative integers is represented by I^+ and we can write

$$I^+ = \{1, 2, 3 \dots\dots\}.$$

The set of all negative integers is represented by I^- and we can write

$$I^- = \{-1, -2, -3 \dots\dots\}.$$

The set of all rational numbers is represented by Q and we can write

$$Q = \{x : x = p/q, \text{ where } p \in I, Q \in I \text{ and } q \neq 0\}$$

The set of all natural numbers is denoted by N. Natural numbers are the positive integers. We can write

$$N = \{1, 2, 3 \dots\dots\dots\}, \text{ where } N \subseteq Z \subseteq Q \subseteq R.$$

The set of irrational numbers is denoted by Q^1. Irrational numbers are $\sqrt{2}$, $\sqrt{3}$, π etc.

The set of complex numbers is denoted by C. A complex number is of the form $a + ib$ where $a \in R, b \in R$ and $c^2 = -1$.

We have $R \subseteq C$.

Note: I^+, I^-, I, Q and R are all infinite sets.

1.4 CLASSIFICATION OF SETS

1. Family of Sets or Class of Sets: If the members of a set are sets themselves, then that set is called a family of sets.

The set $A = [\{1\}, \{2, 3\}, \{4\}, \{5, 6\}]$ is a family of sets.

The set $B = \{2, 3, \{5, 6, 7\}]$ is not a family of sets. Few elements of B are sets and some of them are not sets.

2. Fundamental or Universal Set: If all the sets under consideration be the subsets of a set U, then this set U will be called the universal set as universe of discourse.

3. Power Set: If a set A has finite number of elements say n, then its power set has 2^n elements. The power set of A is denoted by 2^A or $P(A)$.

If $\quad A = \{x, y\}$

Then

$$2^A = P(\text{A}) = [\phi, \{x\}\{y\}\{x, y\}]$$

4. Disjoint Sets: Two sets A and B are said to be disjoint if they have no common elements. $A = \{a, b, c\}$ and $B = \{r, s, t\}$ are disjoint sets.

5. Cardinal Number of a Set: the number of elements in a set is called its conditional symbolized as $n(A)$.

If $\quad A = \{1, 2, 3, x, y, z\}$ then $n(A) = 6$.

6. Matching Sets: Two sets A and B are matching sets if corresponding to every element of the set A, there exists an element of the set B and vice verse.

If $\quad A = \{1, 2, 3\}$ and $B = \{x, y, z\}$, then $1 \leftrightarrow x, 2 \leftrightarrow y, 3 \leftrightarrow z$, i.e. A and B are matching sets.

We can also pair up the matching of the two elements is different ways viz,

$$2 \leftrightarrow x, 1 \leftrightarrow y, \text{and } 3 \leftrightarrow z.$$

EXAMPLES

Example 1: If A is an infinite set and $A \subset B$, prove that B is also an infinite set.

Solution: Since $A \subset B$, therefore every element of A is included in the set B and hence the cardinal number of A is less than the cardinal number of B, i.e. $n(A) \leq n(B)$, where A is an infinite set.

Thus $n(B)$ is also infinite which implies B is an infinite set.

Example 2: If $A = \{x : x \text{ is a square}\}$,

$B = \{x : x \text{ is a quadrilateral}\}$ and $C_1 = \{x : x \text{ is a rhombus}\}$, find which of these are the subsets of others.

Find also which sets are the proper subsets of others.

Solution: A square is a rhombus, but rhombus are not square and hence $A \subset C$.

Similarly a square is a quadrilateral but all quadrilaterals are not squares.

$\therefore A \subset B$. In a similar way we can write $C \subset B$.

Example 3: Write down the elements of the set $P(P(P(\phi)))$ where ϕ is an empty set.

Solution: The number of subsets in ϕ is $2^0 = 1$

$\therefore \qquad P(\phi) = \{\phi\}$

The number of subsets of $\{\phi\}$ is $2^1 = 2$

$\therefore$ Subsets of $\{\phi\}$ are $\{\phi\}$ and ϕ

Thus $\quad P(P(\phi)) = P(\{\phi\}) = \{\phi, \{\phi\}\}$

The number of subsets of $\{\phi, \{\phi\}\}$ are $2^2 = 4$

Hence subsets of $\{\phi, \{\phi\}\}$ can be written as $\{\phi, \{\phi\}, \{\{\phi\}\}, \{\phi, \{\phi\}\}\}$

$$\therefore \quad P(P(P(\phi))) = P\{\phi, \{\phi\}\}$$
$$= \{\phi, \{\phi\}, \{\{\phi\}\}, \{\phi, \{\phi\}\}\}$$

Example 4: There are 30 sets ($A_1, A_2, \ldots, A_{30}$) and each has 5 elements and $B_1, B_2, \ldots B_n$ are given n sets each with 3 elements.

Assume $\bigcup_{i=1}^{30} A_i = \bigcup_{j=1}^{n} B_j = \Omega$ and each element of Ω belongs exactly 15 of A_i's and 6 of B_j's then n is equal to

(a) 20 (b) 45 (c) 15 (d) none of these.

Solution: $\Omega = \bigcup_{i=1}^{30} A_i \quad \therefore n(\Omega) = \frac{5 \times 30}{15} = 10$

This is due to the fact that Ω contains elements exactly 15 of A_i's.

Similarly $\Omega = \bigcup_{j=1}^{n} B_j \quad \therefore n(\Omega) = \frac{3 \times n}{6} = \frac{n}{2}$

$\Rightarrow \quad \frac{n}{2} = 10 \quad \Rightarrow N = 20$

∴ Alternative (a) is correct.

PROBLEMS AND EXERCISES 1 (A)

1. Use the set notations for the following statements:

(i) The set of all pairs of number a and b, a being an integer and b a real number

(ii) x is a member of the set A.

(iii) n is a real number not equal to zero.

(iv) A is the set of the vowels of English alphabets.

2. Describe the following sets in words and then write them in the tabular form.

(i) $A = \{x : x + 3 = 9\}$

(ii) $B = \{x : x^2 - 15x + 56 = 0\}$

(iii) $C = \{x : 2^{\sin^2 x} + 5 \cdot 2^{\cos^2 x} - 7 = 0\}$

(iv) $D = \{x : x$ is numbers of two digits divisible by $7\}$

3. Write down the sets for which the following relations hold good.

(i) $3x + 1 = (4x - 3) - (x - 4)$

(ii) $|x - 1| = 3$

(iii) $|x - 4| + |x + 4| = 9$

Hint (iii) Solve the equation $\pm (x - 4) \pm (x + 4) = 9$

(iv) $25^{2x - x^2 + 1} + 9^{2y - x^2 + 1} = 34\ (15^{2x - x^2})$

(v) $\log_3 x + \log_9 x + \log_{27} x - 5.5 = 0$

(vi) $3 \log x - 54 + x^{\log 3} = 0.$

4. We are given $A = \{r, s, t, u, v\}$. Written down the correct or incorrect for the following statements

(a) $h \in A$ (b) $S \subseteq A$ (c) $v \in A$ (d) $\{u\} \subseteq A$.

5. Use the set builder form for the following sets:

(i) A is a set of letters a, b, c, d, e, f

(ii) B is a set of states in India

(iii) $C = \{2, 4, 6, ...\}$

(iv) $E = \{3\}$.

6. Which of the following sets are equal:

(i) $\{x : x$ is a letter is the word mathematics$\}$

(ii) A set containing m, a, t, h, e, i, c and s.

(iii) A set of letters appearing in the word manuscript.

7. Which of these sets is null set

$A = \{x : x$ is a letter after z in the alphabets$\}$

$B = \{x : x^2 = 4$ and $x = 1\}$

$C = \{x : x + 9 = 9\}$

$D = \{x : x \geq 4$ and $x < 1\}$.

8. Prove that $\{2, 3, 4\}$ is not a subset of $\{x : x$ is even, x is positive$\}$.

9. (i) Find the cardinal number of the set $\{\phi, \{\phi\}, \{\{\phi\}\}, \{\phi, \{\phi\}\}\}$

(ii) $\{a, e, i, o, u\}$

(iii) $\{+, -, \times, \div\}$

(iv) $\{\cup, \cap, >, <\}$.

10. Which sets are the proper subsets of the others:

$A = \{x : x$ is a quadrilateral$\}$; $B = \{x : x$ is a rhombus$\}$

$C = \{x : x$ is a rectangle$\}$; $D = \{x : x$ is a square$\}$.

11. If $A = \{e\}$; $B = \{d, e\}$; $X = \{b, c, d\}$;

$Y = \{b, c\}$; $Z = \{b, c, e\}$

Write true or false for the following statements:

(1) $Y \subseteq x$ (2) $B \not\supset A$ (3) $B \neq Z$ (4) $Z \supset A$

(5) $A \not\subseteq Y$ (6) $Z \not\supset X$ (7) $A \subseteq X$ (8) $Y \not\subseteq Z$.

12. State whether each of the following sets in infinite or finite:

(1) The set of lines parallel to y-axis

(2) The set of circles through the origin

(3) The set of roots of the equation

$(x-1)(x-2)(x-3)=0$

(4) The set of numbers which are multiple of 7.

13. If $X = \{2, 3, 4\}$; $Y = \{x : x^2 = 9, x \text{ is positive}\}$

$Z = \{2, 4\}$; $A = \{x : x \text{ is even}\}$

Complete the following statements by using $\subseteq$, $\supset$ or not comparable between each pair of sets.

(1) X .... Y (2) X .... Z (3) Y .... Z (4) Z .... A.

14. State whether each of the following statements is correct of incorrect.

(1) $A \in 2^A$ (2) $A \subseteq 2^A$ (3) $\{A\} \in 2^A$ (4) $\{A\} \subseteq 2A$

Marks the correct alternative(s) in each if the following questions.

15. A set contains n elements. The power set contains:

(a) n elements (b) 2^n elements

(c) n^2 elements (d) none of these.

[CET 1992]

16. Which of the following is the empty set:

(a) $\{x : x \text{ is a real number and } x^2 - 1 = 0\}$

(b) $\{x : x \text{ is real number and } x^2 + 1 = 0\}$

(c) $\{x : x \text{ is real number and } x^2 - 9 = 0\}$

(d) $\{x : x \text{ is real number and } x^2 = x + 2\}$. [CET 1990]

ANSWERS TO PROBLEMS AND EXERCISES 1 (A)

1. (i) $A = \{(a, b) : a \in I, b \in R\}$

(ii) $A = \{x\}$

(iii) $R = \{n : n \neq 0\}$

(iv) $A = \{a, e, i, o, u\}$.

2. (i) A is the set of elements x such that x plus there is equal to 9. $A = \{6\}$.

(ii) $B = \{7, 8\}$

(iii) $C = \left\{\frac{(2n+1)\pi}{2}\right\}$

(iv) $D = \{14, 21, 28, 35, 42, 49, 56, 63, 70, 77, 84, 91, 98\}$

3. (i) ϕ (ii) $\{3, 4\}$
   (iii) $\{-4.5, 4.5\}$ (iv) $\{1 - v_3, 0, 1 + v_3\}$
   (v) $\{27\}$ (vi) $\{1000\}$
4. (a) Incorrect (b) Incorrect (c) Correct (d) Correct.
5. (i) $A = \{x : x$ appears before g in the alphabets$\}$
   (ii) $B = \{x : x$ is a state in India$\}$
   (iii) $C = (x : x$ is even$)$
   (iv) $E = \{x : x - 2 = 1\}$ or $\{x : 2x = 6\}$
6. (i) and (ii)
7. *A*, *B* and *D*.
9. (i) 4 (ii) 5 (iii) 4 (iv) 4
10. *D* is a proper subset of the sets *A*, *B* and *C*.
    C is a proper subset of *A*.
    B is a proper subset of *A*.
11. (1) True (2) False (3) True (4) True (5) True (6) True (7) False (8) False.
12. (1) Infinite (2) Infinite (3) Finite (4) Infinite.
13. (1) $\supset$ (2) $\supset$ (3) $\subseteq$ (4) not comparable.
14. (1) Correct (2) Incorrect (3) Incorrect (4) Correct
15. (b)
16. (b)

1.5 VENN DIAGRAM

Geometical figures are used to understand the operations of the universal set and its subsets easily by Venn diagram. In Venn diagram the universal set is represented by a rectangle and other sets by circles in the rectangle. The following figures make everything clear.

In figure I : $A = \{1, 2, 3, 4\}$ which is contained in the universal set U represented by the rectangle.

In figure II : The set A contains the set B and $A \neq B$

$\therefore \quad B \subset A.$

In figure III : The set C contains B and B contains A and $A \neq B \neq C$.

$\therefore \quad A \subset B \subset C.$

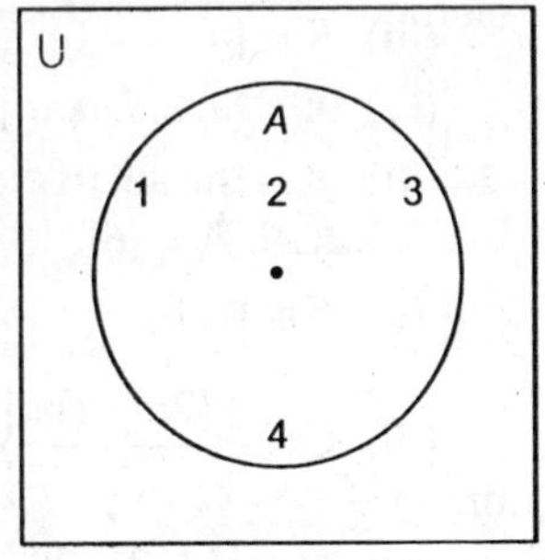

Figure I

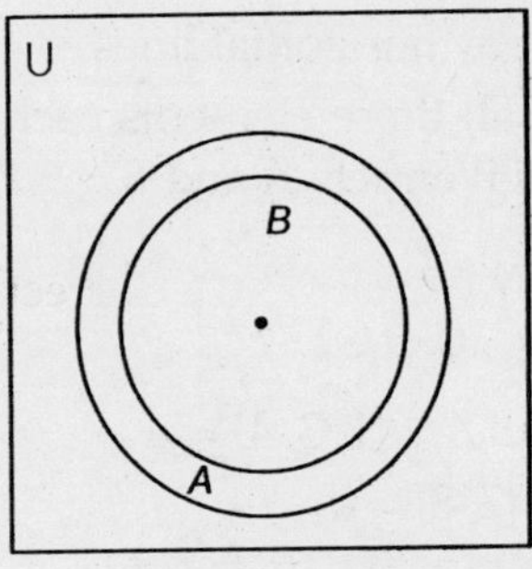

Figure II

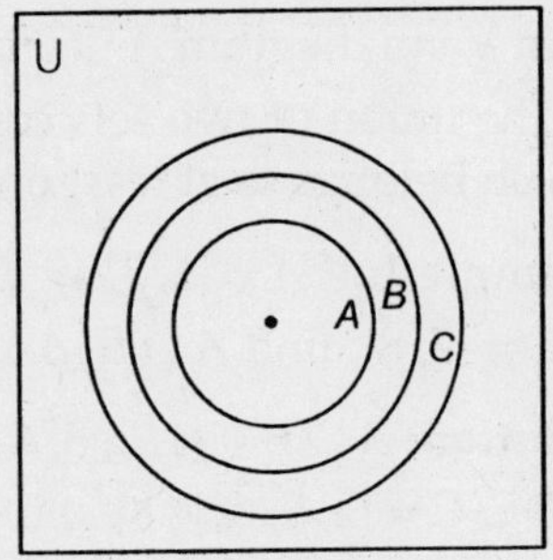

Figure III

In figure IV : A and B are disjoint sets.

In figure V : The sets A and B have common position shaded by parallel strokes.

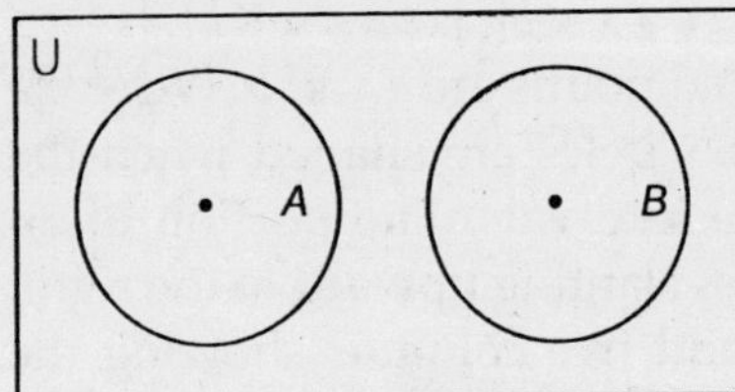

Figure IV

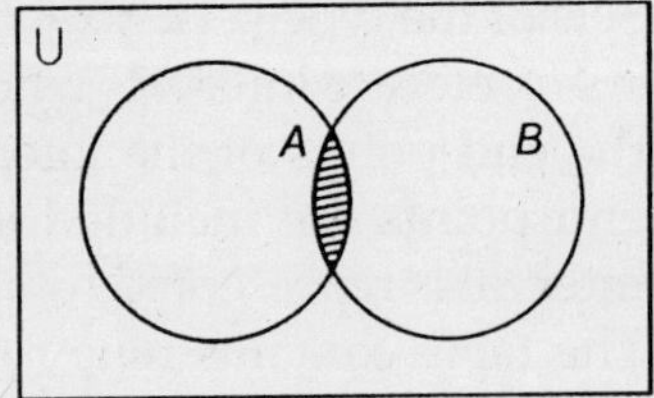

Figure V

1.6 SET OPERATIONS

New sets are obtained with the help of set operations which are (i) Union (ii) Intersection and (iii) Difference.

1. *Union of Sets:* the union of two sets A and B is the set of all elements which belong to either A or to B or to both. The symbol $\cup$ is used to denote the union of sets.

If $A = \{1, 3, 5\}$ and

$B = \{1, 2, 3, 4\}$ then

$A \cup B = \{1, 2 3, 4, 5\}$

In symbolic notation we can write

$A \cup B = \{x : x \in A \text{ or } x \in B\}$

or $x \in A \cup B \Leftrightarrow (x \in A \text{ or } x \in B)$.

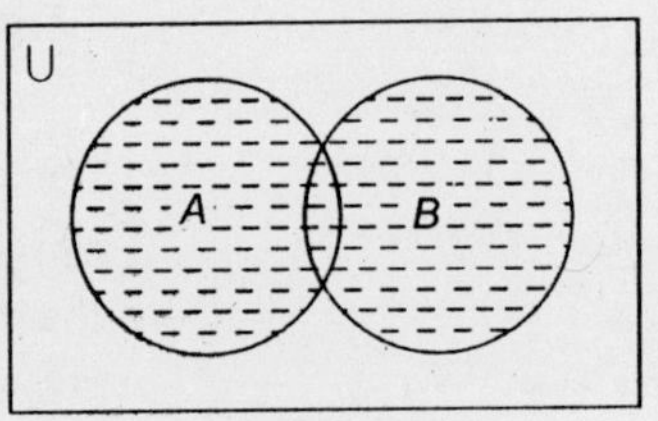

Venn Diagram A ∪ B

In Venn diagram $A \cup B$ is shaded by horizontal lines.

The union of two sets consists of all those elements each of which belongs to at least one of the given sets A and B.

Example 1: If $A = \{1, 3, 4\}$; $B = \{2, 5, 6\}$
$C = \{7, 8\}$, find $A \cup B, A \cup A, B \cup C, C \cup C$.

Solution: $A \cup B = \{1, 2, 3, 4, 5, 6\}$; $A \cup A = \{1, 3, 4\} = A$
$B \cup C = \{2, 5, 6, 7, 8\}$ and $C \cup C = \{7, 8\} = C$.

(A) *Interval in the real numbers:* The set of all real numbers x for which the two sided inequality $a < x < b$ holds good is usually designated as (a, b), and is called an open interval (a, b). By the interval (a, b) we mean the set of all points of the number line buying between the points a and b excluding these two points. The table given below describes everything related to interval. Sets of the type $\{x : a < x < b\}$, $\{x : a \leq x < b\}$, $\{x : a < x \leq b\}$, $\{x : a \leq x \leq b\}$, etc. are intervals whose end points are a and b. We circle the end points of the intervals. Circles are shaded when the end points are included in the intervals. The portion of an interval is represented by strokes slanting upward to the right. The table contains nine rows and five columns showing the names of the intervals, inequalities that define the sets. Designations, intervals in the favour of the sets and strokes slanting upward to the right that represent the set. In the table closed and open intervals have been shown clearly.

(B) *The union of number intervals:* Let these be two intervals (–1; 2) and (0; 3]. We have to determine their union. We first draw figure I which shows the interval (–1; 2) and then figure II

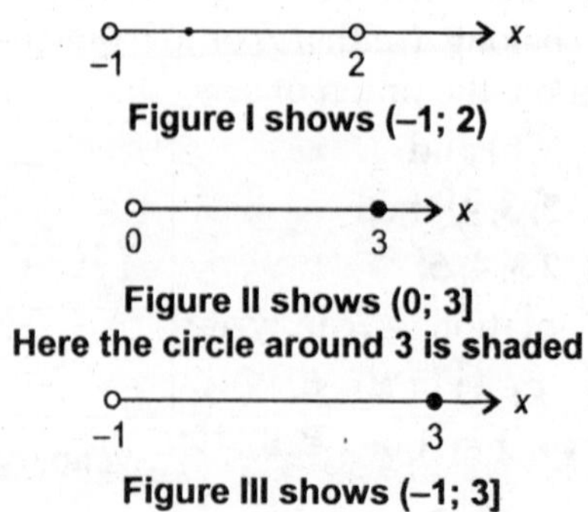

Figure I shows (–1; 2)

Figure II shows (0; 3]
Here the circle around 3 is shaded

Figure III shows (–1; 3]

Table

Names of the intervals	*Inequalities that define the set*	*Designation*	*Intervals in the form of the sets*	*Strokes slanting upward to the right that represent the sets*
Interval from a to b closed interval	$a \le x \le b$	$[a; b]$	$A = \{x : a \le x \le b\}$	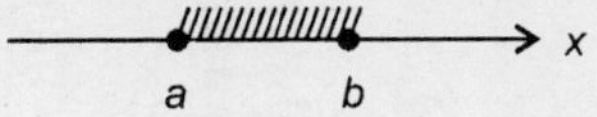 a b x
Interval from a to b open interval	$a < x < b$	$(a ;b)$	$B = \{x : a < x < b\}$	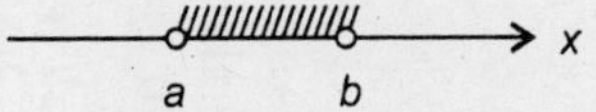 a b x
Interval from a to b open from the left	$a < x \le b$	$(a; b]$	$C = \{x : a < x \le b\}$	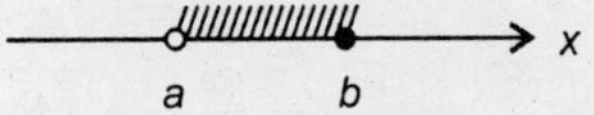 a b x
Interval from a to b open from the right	$a \le x < b$	$[a; b)$	$D = \{x : a \le x < b\}$	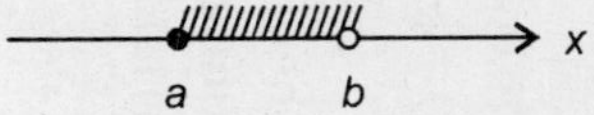 a b x
Number half line from a to $+\infty$	$a \le x$	$[a; +\infty)$	$E = \{x : x \ge a\}$	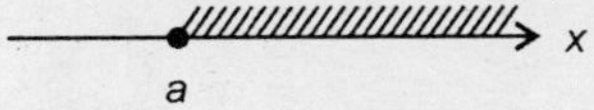 a x
Open number half line from a to $+\infty$	$a < x$	$(a; +\infty)$	$F = \{x : x > a\}$	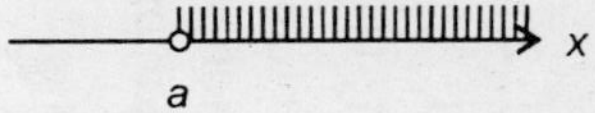 a x
Number half line from $-\infty$ to a	$x \le a$	$(-\infty; a]$	$G = \{x : x \le a\}$	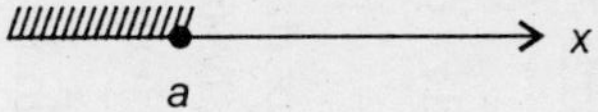 a x
Open half line from $-\infty$ to a	$x < a$	$(-\infty; a)$	$H = \{x : a < x\}$	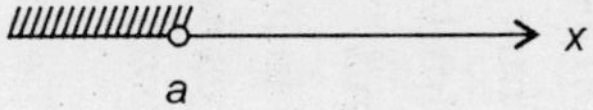 a x
Set of real numbers	—	$(-\infty; +\infty)$	$K = \{x : a \in R\}$	—

for the interval (0; 3]. We then draw figure III to obtain their union as (–1; 3]

Thus $(-1; 2) \cup (0; 3] = (-1; 3]$.

Similarly $(-1; 3) \cup [-3; 1) = [-3; 3)$.

and $[-1; 1] \cup (0; 3) = [-1; 3)$.

If in important to mention here that it is not always possible to represent the union of two number intervals by a single number is travel. The union of $(-\infty; -1)$ and $(-0.1; 0)$ is $(-\infty; -1) \cup (-0.1; 0)$

The union of $(-3; -\sqrt{6})$ and $(-\sqrt{6}; 3)$ is $(-3; -\sqrt{6}) \cup (-\sqrt{6}; 3)$.

(C) *Theorems related to union of sets:*

(i) Idempotent law: $A \cup A = A$

(ii) Commutative law: $A \cup B = B \cup A$

(iii) Associative law: $A \cup (B \cup C) = (A \cup B) \cup C$

(iv) Identity law (a) $A \cup \phi = A$ (b) $A \cup U = U$

Proofs: (i) $A \cup A = A$.

Let $x \in A \cup A$, then $x \in A \cup A \Rightarrow x \in A$ or $x \in A$

$\Rightarrow \quad x \in A \qquad \therefore A \cup A \subseteq A$ ...(1)

Again if $x \in A$, then we can write $x \in A$ or $x \in A$

$\Rightarrow \quad x \in A \cup A \qquad \therefore A \subseteq A \cup A$ ...(2)

From (1) and (2) $A \cup A = A$.

(ii) Let $x \in A \cup B \quad \therefore x \in A$ or $x \in B$

$\Rightarrow \quad x \in B$ or $x \in A \Rightarrow x \in B \cup A$

$\therefore \quad A \cup B \subseteq B \cup A$ ...(1)

Again if $x \in B \cup A$, then we can write

$x \in B$ or $x \in A \Rightarrow x \in A$ or $x \in B$

$\Rightarrow \quad x \in A \cup B$

$\therefore \quad B \cup A \subseteq A \cup B$ ...(2)

From (1) and (2) $A \cup B = B \cup A$

(iii) $x \in (A \cup B) \cup C \Rightarrow x \in (A \cup B)$ or $x \in C$

$\Rightarrow \quad x \in A$ or $x \in B$ or $x \in C$

$\Rightarrow \quad x \in A$ or $[x \in B$ or $x \in C]$

$\Rightarrow \quad x \in A$ or $x \in B \cup C \Rightarrow x \in A \cup (B \cup C)$

$\therefore \quad (A \cup B) \cup C \subseteq A \cup (B \cup C)$ ...(1)

Again if $x \in A \cup (B \cup C)$ then we can write

$x \in A$ or $x \in (B \cup C) \Rightarrow x \in A$ or ($x \in B$ or $x \in C$)

$\Rightarrow$ ($x \in A$ or $x \in B$) or $x \in C \Rightarrow$ ($x \in (A \cup B)$ or $x \in C$

$\Rightarrow$ $x \in (A \cup B) \cup C$

$\therefore$ $A \cup (B \cup C) \subseteq (A \cup B) \cup C$ ...(2)

From (1) and (2) $(A \cup B) \cup C = A \cup (B \cup C)$

(iv) (a) Let $x \in A \cup \phi$, then $x \in A \cup \phi \Rightarrow x \in A$ or $x \in \phi$

$\Rightarrow$ $x \in A$ ($\therefore x \notin \phi$)

$\therefore$ $A \cup \phi \subseteq A$ ...(1)

But $A \subseteq A \cup \phi$ ...(2)

From (1) and (2) $A \cup \phi = A$. Here ϕ is an addition identity

(b) $U \subseteq A \cup U$ ...(1)

and $A \cup U \subseteq U$ ...(2)

$\therefore$ $A \cup U = U$

(D) *Union of more than two sets:* The union of a finite number of sets $A_1, A_2, \ldots, A_n$ is denoted by $A_1 \cup A_2 \cup A_3 \ldots \cup A_n$ or

$$\bigcup_{i=1}^{n} A_i.$$

We have thus $\bigcup_{i=1}^{n} Ai = \{x : x \in A_i \text{ for at least one } i\}$

Note: $A \cup B$ is also denoted as $A + B$ and is read A plus B.

2. Intersection of Sets: The intersection of two sets A and B is a set which includes those elements which simultaneously belong to both the sets.

The intersection of two sets is known as the common part of the two sets. The symbol $\cap$ is used to represent the intersection. In Venn diagram intersection of two sets A and B is shaded in the figure I.

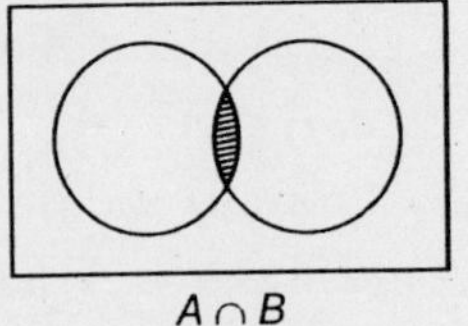

$A \cap B$

Figure I

$A \cap B$ is also denoted as AB and is read as 'A times B'.

The symbolic representation of the intersection of the sets A and B is

$$A \cap B = \{x : x \in A \text{ and } x \in B\}$$

or $x \in A \cap B \Leftrightarrow (x \in A \text{ and } x \in B)$

Example 1: If $A = \{a, b, c, d, e\}$, $B = \{c, d, f\}$ then $A \cap B = \{c, d\}$.
(A) *The intersection of intervals:* The intersection of intervals (–1; 2) and (0; 3] is (0; 2). The method to determine the intersection is as follows: We circle the end points of (–1; 2) and then shade if with strokes slanting upward to the right i.e. by ////. After tha

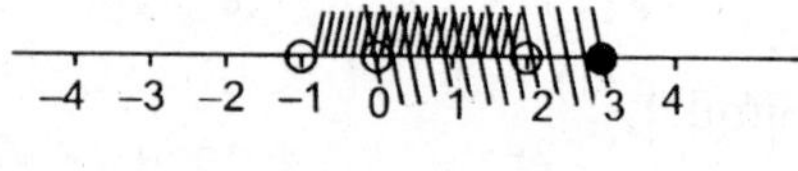

We circle the end points of (0; 3] when the circle around 3 is shaded. Now we start to shade (0; 3] with the strokes slanting down ward to the right i.e. by \\\\. Thus the cross hatchel points is $(-1; 2) \cap (0; 3]$ i.e. (0; 2) (similar the figure I the common portion).

(B) *Theorems related to the intersection of sets:* If A, B and C be three sets, then the following laws hold good:

(1) Idempotent law: $A \cap A = A$

(2) Commutative law: $A \cap B = B \cap A$

(3) Associative law: $(A \cap B) \cap C = A \cap (B \cap C)$

(4) Identity law: (a) $A \cap U = A$ (b) $A \cap \phi = \phi$

(5) Distributive law:

(a) $A \cap (B \cup C) = (A \cap B) \cup (A \cap C)$

(b) $A \cup (B \cap C) = (A \cup B) \cap (A \cup C)$

Proof: (1) Let $x \in A \cap A$

$\therefore x \in A$ and $x \in A$ i.e. $x \in A$

$\therefore A \cap A \subseteq A$ ...(i)

Again if $x \in A$ then we can write

$x \in A \Rightarrow x \in A$ and $x \in A \Rightarrow x \in A \cap A$

$\therefore A \subseteq A \cap A$ ...(ii)

From (i) and (ii) $A = A \cap A$.

(2) Let $x \in A \cap B \Rightarrow x \in A$ and $x \in B$

$\Rightarrow x \in B$ and $x \in A \Rightarrow x \in B \cap A$

$\therefore A \cap B \subseteq B \cap C$ ...(i)

Again $x \in B \cap A \Rightarrow x \in B$ and $x \in A$

$\Rightarrow x \in A$ and $x \in B \Rightarrow x \in A \cap B$

$\therefore B \cap A \subseteq A \cap B$ ...(ii)

From (i) and (ii) $A \cap B = B \cap A$.

(3) Let $x \in (A \cap B) \cap C$ then $x \in (A \cap B)$ and $x \in C$

$\Rightarrow (x \in A$ and $x \in B)$ and $x \in C$

$\Rightarrow x \in A$ and $(x \in B$ and $x \in C)$

$\Rightarrow \quad x \in A \cap (B \cap C)$

$\therefore \quad (A \cap B) \cap C \subseteq A \cap (B \cap C)$ ...(i)

Similarly assuming x to be the element of

$A \cap (B \cap C)$ we can show

$A \cap (B \cap C) \subseteq (A \cap B) \cap C$ ...(ii)

From (i) and (ii)

$$A \cap (B \cap C) = A \cap (B \cap C)$$

Proofs of (4) and (5) are left for the students.

(C) *Intersection of more than two sets:* Let $A_1, A_2, A_3, \ldots\ldots\ldots, A_n$ be the finite sets then their intersection is denoted by $A_1 \cap A_2 \cap A_3 \ldots\ldots\ldots \cap A_n$.

We can write $A_1 \cap A_2 \cap A_3 \ldots\ldots\ldots \cap A_n = \bigcap_{i=1}^{n} A_i$

$$= \{x : x \in A_i \forall\ i\}.$$

(D) *Prove the following theorems:*

(i) $A \cap B \subseteq A \subseteq A \cup B$

(ii) $A \subseteq B \Leftrightarrow A \cup A = B$

(iii) $A \cup B = A \cap B \Leftrightarrow A = B$

(iv) $A \cap B = A \Leftrightarrow A \subseteq B$.

Proofs: (i) Let $x \in A \cap B$, then $x \in A$ and $x \in B$

$\Rightarrow \quad x \in A \quad \therefore A \cap B \subseteq A$ ...(1)

Again if $x \in A \Rightarrow x \in A$ or $x \in B \Rightarrow x \in A \cup B$

$\therefore \quad A \subseteq A \cup B$ ...(2)

From (1) and (2) $A \cap B \subseteq A \subseteq A \cup B$

(ii) Let $x \in A \cup B \Rightarrow x \in A$ or $x \in B$

$\Rightarrow x \in B$ or $x \in A \Rightarrow x \in B$ or $x \in B$ ($\because A \leq B$)

$\Rightarrow x \in B \therefore A \cup B \subseteq B$ ...(1)

But $B \subseteq A \cup B$ ...(2)

From (1) and (2) $A \cup B = B$

If $A \cup B = B$, we have to show $A \subseteq B$

Let $x \in A \Rightarrow x \in A \cup B$ ($\therefore A \subseteq A \cup B$)

$\Rightarrow \quad x \in B$ ($\therefore A \cup B = B$)

$\therefore \quad A \subseteq B$

Similarly $A \cup B = B \Rightarrow A \subseteq B$.

(iii) Let $x \in A \Rightarrow x \in A$ or $x \in B \Rightarrow x \in A \cup B$

$\Rightarrow \quad x \in A \cap B \quad$ ($\therefore A \cup B = A \cap B$)

$\Rightarrow \quad x \in A$ and $x \in B \Rightarrow x \in B \quad \therefore A \subseteq B$

Similarly we can prove $B \subseteq A$

$\therefore \quad A = B$

We can also show if $A = B$ then

$$A \cup B = A \cap B$$

(iv) If $A \cap B = A$, we have to prove $A \subseteq B$.

Let $x \in A \Rightarrow x \in A \cap B \Rightarrow x \in A$ and $x \in B \Rightarrow x \in B$

$\therefore \quad A \subseteq B$

$\therefore \quad A \cap B = A \Rightarrow A \subseteq B$

Now we show if $A \subseteq B$, then $A \cap B = A$.

Let $x \in A$, then $x \in B$ ($\because A \subseteq B$)

$\Rightarrow \quad x \in A \cap B \quad \therefore A \subseteq A \cap B$

Similarly $A \cap B \subseteq A \qquad A \cap B = A$

$\therefore \quad A \subseteq B \Rightarrow A \cap B = A$.

Example: If $A = \{a, b\}$; $B = \{a, y, z\}$

Prove that (i) $P(A) \cap P(B) = P(A \cap B)$

(ii) $P(A) \cup P(B) \subseteq P(A \cup B)$

Proof: (i) We have $A \cap B = \{a\}$

$$\therefore \quad P(A \cap B) = \{\phi, \{a\}\}$$

$$P(A) = \{\{a, b\}, \{a\}, \{b\}, \phi\}$$

$$P(B) = \{\{a, y, z\}, \{a, y\}, \{a, z\}, \{y, z\}, \{a\}, \{y\}, \{z\}, \phi\}$$

$\therefore \quad P(A) \cap P(B) = \{a\}$

$\therefore \quad P(A) \cap P(B) = P(A \cap B)$

Note: $P(A) \cup P(B) = P(A \cup B)$ is not always true.

(ii) $P(A) \cup P(B)$

$$= \{\{a, b\}, \{a\}, \{b\}, \{a, y, z\}, \{a, y\}, \{a, z\}, \{y, z\}, \{y\}, \{z\}, \phi\}$$

$$A \cup B = \{a, b, y, z\}$$

$\therefore \quad P(A \cup B) = \{\{a, b, y, z\}, \{a, y, z\}, \{b, y, z\}, \{a, b, z\}, \{a, b, y\}, \{a, b\}, \{a, y\}, \{a, z\}, \{b, y\}, \{b, z\}, \{y, z\}, \{a\}, \{b\}, \{y\}, \{z\}, \phi\}$

$\therefore \quad P(A) \cup P(B) \subseteq P(A \cup B)$

(As all the elements of $P(A) \cup P(B)$ belong to $P(A \cup B)$)

(E) *Difference of two sets:* The difference of the sets A and B is the set which consists of all the members of the set A which do not belong to B and is designated as $A - B$. We write

$$A - B = \{x : x \in A \text{ and } x \notin B\}.$$

Example: (i) If $A = \{2, 3, 4\}$, $B = \{1, 2\}$, then $A - B = \{3, 4\}$.

(ii) If $A = \{1, 2\}$ and $B = \{1, 2, 4\}$, then $A - B = \phi$.

(i) *Venn Diagram for the difference of sets:* In the following diagrams the difference of two sets are shown in various circumstances. (see Figs. I and II)

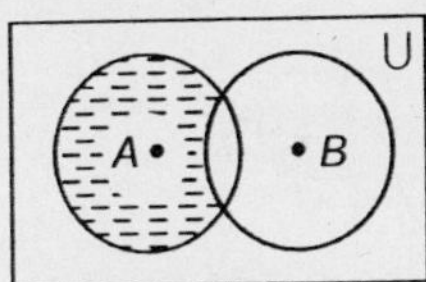

Figure I
***A* – *B* is shaded**

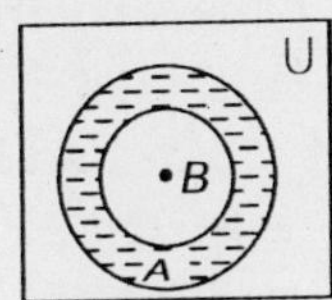

Figure II
***B* ⊂ *A* and *A* – *B* is shaded**

(F) *Compliment of a set:* If U be an universal set and A be a set then the set of all the members of U which donot belong to A is known as the compliment of the set A and is designated as A^1 or $\overline{A}$. This $A^1 = U - A$. We write

$$A^1 = U - A = \{x : x \in U \text{ and } x \notin A\}.$$

(i) *Venn diagram for the compliment of a set:* In the given figure I now we show A' by Venn diagram. The compliment of A is shaded by horizontal dotted lines.

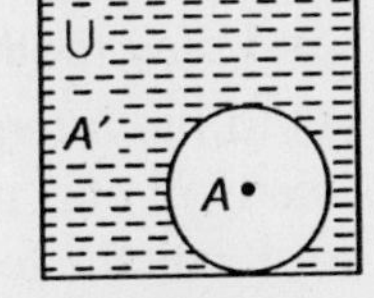

Figure 1
***A′* is shaded portion**

Example 1: If $U = \{a, b, c, d, e\}$

$A = \{b, d, e, f, g\}$

Then $A^1 = U - A = \{a, c\}$

PROBLEMS AND EXERCISES 1(B)

1. If $A = \{3, \{1, 5\}\}$. Find $P(A)$.
2. Write True and False for the following statements:
   If $A = \{1, \{4, 5\}, 4\}$, then
   (i) $\{4, 5\} \subseteq A$ (ii) $\{4, 5\} \in A$ (iii) $\{\{4, 5\}\} \subseteq A$.
3. If $A = \{x : 2x = 3 \text{ and } x \in R\}$
   $B = \{x : x/3 \text{ and } x \in N\}$
   $C = \{x : x - 3 < 5 \text{ and } x \in N\}$
   Enumerate the number fo the sets.
4. A square is inscribed into a circle. If A be the set of points of the given circle and B, the set of points of the square, find $A \cup B, A \cap B, A - B$ and $B - A$.
5. If A be the set of all possible parallalograms, B the set of rectangles, C the set of rhombuses, D the set of squares and E the set of trapezoids, find $B \cap C, B \cup C \cup D \cap A$ and $D \cap E$.
6. If $A = \{x : -1 \leq x \leq 1\}, B = \{x : -\infty < x < 0\}$
   $C = \{x : 0 \leq x < 2\}$, find
   $A \cup C, A \cap B, A \cup B \cup C, (A \cup B) \cap C$ and $B \cap C$.
7. 70 students out of 100 know Hindi, 45 know English and twenty-three know both Hindi and English. How many students know neither Hindi nor English?
8. If $A = \{x : 0 \leq x \leq 3\}; B = \{x : 1 < x < 5\}$ and $C = \{x : -2 < x \leq 0\}$, find $A \cap B \cap C$ and $(A \cup B) \cap C$.
9. If $A = \{x : -3 \leq x \leq 1\}; B = \{x : 2 \leq x < \infty\}; C = \{x : -\infty < x < -2\}$, find $B \cup C$ and $A \cap B \cap C$.
10. Out of 40 students 30 can jump, 27 can play football and only five can do neither. How many students can jump and play football.
11. Find the intersection of the number sets A and B if every element of A has the form $4n + 2, n \in N$ and every element of B has the form $3n, n \in N$.
12. What do you mean by the following notations:
    (i) $a \notin A$ (ii) $A \subset B$ (iii) $P \supset Q$.
13. Describe the set $\{x : x^2 - 5x + 6 = 0\}$ by tabulation method.

14. Write down the subsets of the following sets:
(i) $\{a, b, c\}$ (ii) $\{1, 2, 3\}$ (iii) $\{2, 4, 6\}$.

15. Are ϕ, $\{0\}$, $\{\phi\}$ equivalent? Give reasons also.

16. Express the law used in $A \cap A = A$. Write down the commutative law for the union of two sets.

17. If $A = \{x : x = 2n, n \text{ is positive integers}\}$
$B = \{x : x = 3n, n \text{ is positive integers}\}$
Find $A \cap B$.

18. Prove that $(A \cup B \cup C)' = A' \cap B' \cap C'$.

19. 50 students out of 80 obtained first class marks in mathematics, 10 students obtained first class marks in English and maths. How many students obtained first class marks in English?

ANSWERS TO PROBLEMS AND EXERCISE 1(B)

1. $\{A, \{3\}, \{\{1, 5\}\}, \phi\}$.

2. (i) False (ii) True (iii) True

3. $A = \left\{\frac{3}{2}\right\}$; $B = \{3, 6, 9, 12 \ldots..\}$

$C = \{1, 2, 3, 4, 5, 6, 7\}$

4. A; B; the set of points of the circle which do not belong to the square; ϕ.

5. D; A; ϕ.

6. $[-1; 2)$; $[-1; 0)$; $(-\infty; 2)$; $[0; 1]$ and ϕ

7. 8

8. ϕ, $\{0\}$

9. $(-\infty; -2)$, ϕ

10. 22

11. $12n + 6$ $(n = 0, 1, 2 \ldots)$

12. (i) a is not the element of A
(ii) The set A is the proper subset
(iii) P is the proper subset of Q

13. **Ans.** $\{2, 3\}$

14. (i) ϕ, $\{a\}$, $\{b\}$, $\{c\}$, $\{a, b\}$, $\{a, c\}$, $\{b, c\}$, $\{a, b, c\}$
(ii) ϕ, $\{1\}$, $\{2\}$, $\{3\}$, $\{1, 2\}$, $\{1, 3\}$, $\{2, 3\}$, $\{1, 2, 3\}$
(iii) ϕ, $\{2\}$, $\{4\}$, $\{4\}$, $\{2, 4\}$, $\{2, 6\}$, $\{4, 6\}$, $\{2, 4, 6\}$

15. Not equivalent. ϕ is an empty set.
$\{0\}$ is a singleton set and $\{\phi\}$ is a power set.

16. Indempotent law, $A \cup B = B \cup A$.

17. $\{6, 12, 18 \ldots.\}$

19. 40.

(G) *Symmetric difference fo two sets:* If A and B are two sets then their symmetric difference is $(A - B) \cup (B - A)$ and is written as $A \oplus B$ or $A \Delta B$.

In symbolic language, we write

$$A \oplus B = \{x : x \in A \text{ and } x \notin B \text{ or } x \in B \text{ and } x \notin A\}$$
$$= (A - B) \cup (B - A)$$

$A \oplus B$ contains only those elements of A and B which are not common to both A and B.

In Venn diagrams I and II the shaded portion represents $A \oplus B$.

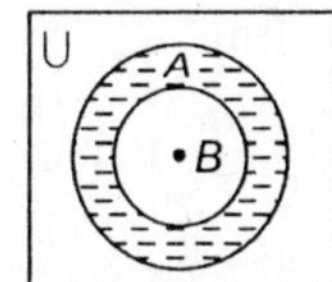

I

We have $A \oplus B = B \oplus A$.

Since the union of sets are commutative.

Also $\quad A \oplus A = \phi$

$A \oplus \phi = A$ and $(A \oplus B) \oplus C$
$= A \oplus (B \oplus C)$

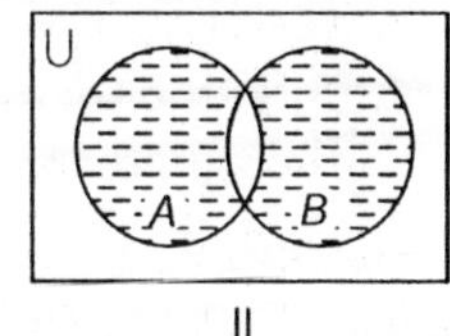

II

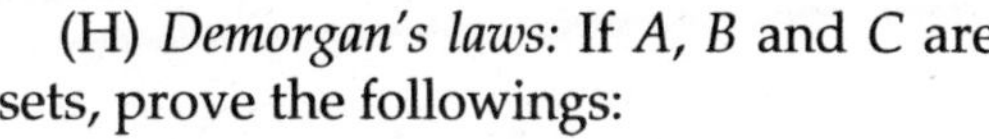

(H) *Demorgan's laws:* If A, B and C are sets, prove the followings:

(i) $(A \cup B)' = A' \cap B'$

(ii) $(A \cap B)' = A' \cup B'$

(iii) $A - (B \cup C) = (A - B) \cap (A - C)$

(iv) $A - (B \cap C) = (A - B) \cup (A - C)$.

Proof: (i) Let $x \in (A \cup B)'$, then $x \notin A \cup B$

$\Rightarrow x \notin A$ and $x \notin B$

$\Rightarrow x \notin A'$ and $x \notin B' \Rightarrow x \notin A' \cap B'$

$\therefore (A \cup B)' \subseteq A' \cap B'$ ...(1)

Again $x \in A' \cap B' \Rightarrow x \in A'$ and $x \in B'$

$\Rightarrow x \notin A$ and $x \notin B \Rightarrow x \notin A \cup B$

$\Rightarrow x \in (A \cap B)'$

$\therefore A' \cap B' \subseteq (A \cup B)'$ ...(2)

From (1) and (2) $(A \cup B)' = A' \cap B'$

(ii) Let $x \in (A \cap B)'$ then $x \notin A \cap B$

$\Rightarrow x \notin A$ or $x \notin B \Rightarrow x \notin A'$ or $x \in B'$

$\Rightarrow \quad x \in A' \cup B'$

$\therefore \quad (A \cap B)' \subseteq A' \cup B'$ ...(1)

Again $x \in A' \cup B' \Rightarrow x \in A'$ or $x \in B'$

$\Rightarrow \quad x \notin A$ or $x \notin B \Rightarrow x \notin A \cup B$

$\Rightarrow \quad x \in (A \cap B)'$

$\therefore \quad A' \cup B' \subseteq (A \cup B)'$ ...(2)

From (1) and (2) $(A \cap B)' = A' \cup B'$

Note: (i) We have $x \in A \cup B \Leftrightarrow x \in A$ or $x \in B$

But $x \notin (A \cup B) \Leftrightarrow x \notin A$ or $x \notin B$

Similarly (ii) $x \in (A \cap B) \Leftrightarrow x \in A$ and $x \in B$

But $x \notin A \cap B \Leftrightarrow x \notin A$ or $x \notin B$.

Aliter: (ii) To prove $(A \cap B)' = A' \cup B'$, we shall use the theorem $A \subseteq B \Leftrightarrow B' \subseteq A'$.

We have $A \subseteq A \cup B$ and $B \subseteq A \cup B$

$\therefore \quad (A \cup B)' = A'$ and $(A \cup B)' = B'$

$\therefore \quad (A \cup B)' \subseteq (A' \cap B)'$ ...(1)

Again $\quad A' \cap B' \subseteq A'$ and $A' \cap B' \subseteq B'$

$\Rightarrow \quad (A')' \subseteq (A' \cap B')'$ and $(B')' \subseteq A' \cap B'$

$\Rightarrow \quad A \subseteq (A' \cap B')'$ and $B \subseteq (A' \cap B')'$

$\therefore \quad A \cup B \subseteq (A' \cap B')'$

$\Rightarrow \quad (A' \cap B')' \subseteq (A \cup B)'$ ...(2)

From (1) and (2), we have

$$(A \cup B)' = A' \cap B'$$

(iii) Let $x \in A - (B \cup C)$

then $x \in A$ and $x \notin B \cup C$

$\Rightarrow x \in A$ and ($x \notin B$ and $x \notin C$)

$\Rightarrow$ ($x \in A$ and $x \notin B$) and ($x \in A$ and $x \notin C$)

$\Rightarrow x \in (A - B)$ and $x \in (A - C)$

$\Rightarrow \quad x \in (A - B) \cap (A - C)$

$\therefore \quad A - (B \cup C) \subseteq (A - B) \cap (A - C)$ ...(1)

Again $x \in (A - B) \cap (A - C)$

$\Rightarrow x \in (A - B)$ and $x \in (A - C)$

$\Rightarrow (x \in A \text{ and } x \notin B) \text{ and } (x \in A \text{ and } x \notin C)$

$\Rightarrow x \in A \text{ and } (x \notin B \text{ and } x \notin C)$

$\Rightarrow x \in A \text{ and } x \notin B \cup C$

$\Rightarrow x \in A - (B \cup C)$

$\therefore \qquad (A - B) \cap (A - C) \subseteq A - (B \cup C) \qquad ...(2)$

From (1) and (2)

$$A - (B \cup C) = (A - B) \cap (A - C)$$

(iv) Let $x \in A - (B \cap C)$

$\therefore x \in A \text{ and } x \notin B \cap C$

$\Rightarrow x \in A \text{ and } x \notin B \text{ or } x \in C.$

$\Rightarrow (x \in A \text{ and } x \notin B) \text{ or } (x \in A \text{ and } x \notin C)$

$\Rightarrow x \in (A - B) \text{ or } x \in (A - C)$

$\Rightarrow x \in (A - B) \cup (A - C)$

$\Rightarrow A - (B \cap C) \subseteq (A - B) \cup (A - C) \qquad ...(1)$

Similarly we can prove

$(A - B) \cup (A - C) \subseteq A - (B \cap C) \qquad ...(2)$

From (1) and (2)

$$A - (B \cap C) = (A - B) \cup (A - C)$$

(I) *To prove Demorgan's law with the help of Venn diagram:*

(i) $(A \cup B)' = A' \cap B'$

First shade $A \cup B$ as shown in Fig. I by horizontal parallel lines, then shade $(A \cup B)'$ out side $A \cup B$ as shown in Fig. II by

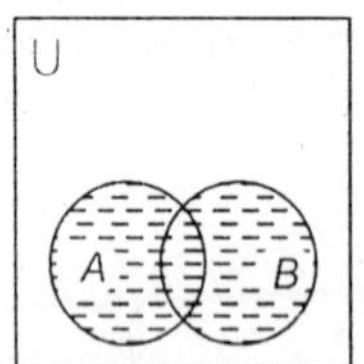

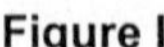
Figure I

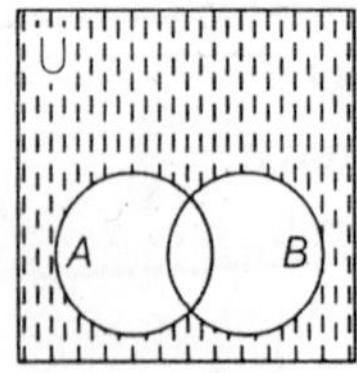

Figure II

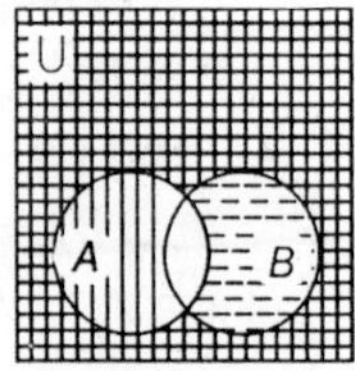

Figure III

vertical parallel lines. Now shade A′ by horizontal lines and B′ by vertical lines. The cross hatched area showing $A' \cup B'$ is shown in figure III.

(ii) $(A \cap B)' = A' \cup B'$

First shade $A \cap B$ as shown Fig. I

Now shade $(A \cap B)'$ as shown in Fig. II.

Shading A' by horizontal strokes and B' by vertical strokes $A' \cup B'$ is shown in figure III by shaded portion.

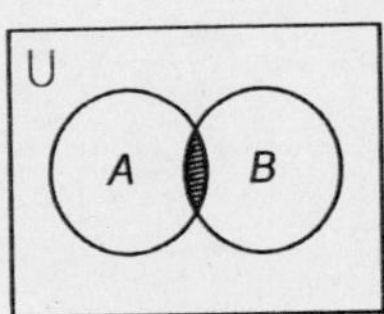

Figure I. A ∩ B

Figure II. (A ∩ B)′

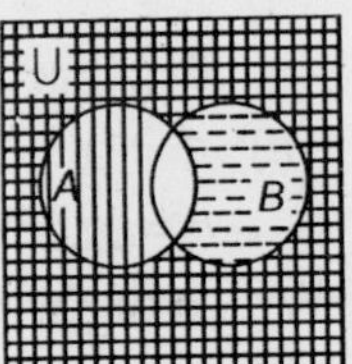

Figure III. A′ ∩ B′

(iii) The shaded portion shows $A - (B \cup C)$ in Fig. I.

The cross hatched portion shows $(A - B) \cap (A - C)$ in Fig II.

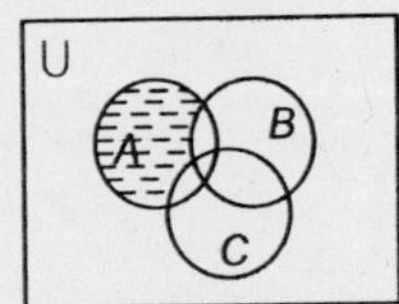

Figure I

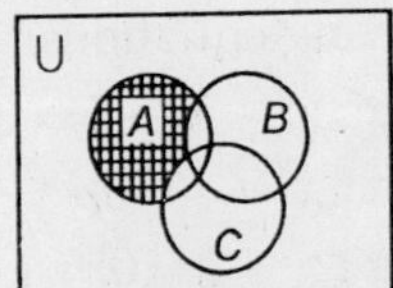

Figure II

EXERCISES 1(C) SIMPLE QUESTIONS

1. Use the symbolic method to denote the following sets:

(i) The set of all the states of India

(ii) The sets of all even numbers

(iii) The set of the roots of the equation $2x^3 - 5x^2 + 2x = 0$

(iv) The set fo all the positive integers greater than 4 and less than 7.

2. Which of the following sets are the subsets of $S = \{1, 3, 5, 7, 9, 11, 13\}$?

$A = \{2, 4, 6\}$; $B = \{3, 5, 7\}$; $C = \{5, 9, 13\}$;

$D = \{1, 3, 5, 6\}$ and $E = \{3, 5, 7, 11\}$.

3. Which of the following sets are singleton or empty?

$A = \{x : x^2 = 4, x \text{ is an odd number}\}$;

$B = \{0\}$; $C = \{x : x + 5 = 5\}$; $D = \{x : x^2 = 9, 3x = 5\}$ and

$E = \{x : x \text{ is a letter of English alphabets before } a\}$.

4. Investigate whether $A = B$ or $A \neq B$.
   (i) $A = \{3, 5, 7\}$;
   $B = \{7, 3, 5\}$
   (ii) $A = \{1, 2, 3\}$;
   $B = \{\text{Earth, Moon, Sun}\}$
   (iii) $A = \{x : 2x^2 - 5x + 2 = 0\}$
   $B = \{x : 2x^3 - 5x^2 + 2x = 0\}$.
5. Which of the following sets are finite?
   (i) $A = \{x : x^2 = 16\}$
   (ii) $B = \{x : 1 \leq x \leq 100\}$
   (iii) $C = \{x : x \text{ is an integer}\}$
   (iv) $D = \{x : x \text{ is a star fo the sky}\}$.
6. Determine the sets of real numbers which satisfy the following equations:
   (i) $\{x : x^2 - 5x + 6 = 0\}$
   (ii) $\{x : x^3 + 1 = 0\}$
   (iii) $\{x : x^2 - 2 = 0\}$.
7. If $A = \{x : x \in R \text{ and } x \geq 2\}$ and $B = \{x : x \in R \text{ and } x \geq 4\}$ then $A \cap B$ is
   (a) $\{x : x \in R, \quad 2 < x < 4\}$
   (b) $\{x : x \in R, \quad 2 \leq x < 4\}$
   (c) $\{x : x \in R, \quad 2 \leq x \leq 4\}$
   (d) none of these.
8. If A and B are two sets, then $A \cap (A \cup B)$ is
   (a) A (b) B (c) ϕ (d) none of them.
9. If A and B are two disjoint sets, then $(A \cup B) \cap B'$ is
   (a) A (b) B (c) ϕ (d) none of them.
10. Is $\{x : x^3 + 1 = 0, x \in N\} = \phi$ true?
    Where N is the set of positive integers.
11. Is the statement $A = B$ true if
    $A = \{x : x \in N, \quad 1 \leq x \leq 3\}$
    $B = \{y : 3y = 9, 2y = 2, y - 1 = 1\}$
12. Find the minimum number of elements in $A \cup B$ if A has 3 and B has 6 elements.
13. Determine the elements of the set $\{x : 3x^2 - 12x = 0\}$ if
    (i) $x \in N$ (ii) $x \in I$ and (iii) $x \in C = \{a + ib, b \neq 0, a,b \in R\}$.

14. If $A = \{1, 2, 3, 4\}$, $B = \{2, 3, 4, 5\}$ and $C = \{3, 4, 5\}$, prove that $A \cup (B \cap C) = (A \cup B) \cap (A \cup C)$.

15. If $A = \{1, 2, 3\}$, $B = \{2, 3, 4\}$ and $C = \{3, 4, 5, 6\}$ determine (i) $A - B$ (ii) $B - C$ (iii) $C - A$ (iv) $A - (B - C)$ (v) $(A - B) - C$.

16. If $A = \{1, 2, 3, 4\}$, $B = \{2, 3, 5, 6\}$ and $C = \{4, 5, 6, 7\}$

Prove that (i) $A \cup (B \cap C) = (A \cup B) \cap (A \cup C)$

(ii) $A \cap (B \cup C) = (A \cap B) \cup (A \cap C)$.

17. Write down the set of letters fo the word ALLAHABAD. How many subsets of the set of letters are there.

18. Determine which of the following sets are singleton and which are empty where x is real numbers?

(i) $\{x : x + 4 = 6\}$ (ii) $\{x : x^2 - 6x + 9 = 0\}$

(iii) $\{x : 8 < x < 9\}$ (iv) $\{x : x = x^2\}$

(v) $\{x : x \leq x\}$ (vi) $\{x : x < x\}$

(vii) $\{x : 3x = 4\}$ (viii) $\{x : 3x^2 + 2 = 0\}$.

19. If $X = \{2, 3\}$, $Y = \{3, 4, 5\}$ and $z = \{5, 2\}$

Which of the following statements are false?

(i) $X - Y \neq \phi$ (ii) $Y - Z \neq \phi$

(iii) $Z - X \neq \phi$ (iv) $(X - Y) - Z \neq \phi$

(v) $X - (Y - Z) \neq \phi$.

ANSWERS TO EXERCISE 1(C)
(Hints and Solutions)

1. (i) **Ans.** $\{x : x$ is a state of India$\}$.

Hint: Let Indian states be denoted by the letter x then the required set be $\{x : P(x)\}$.

$\therefore$ $P(x)$ = a state of India.

$\therefore$ The set is $\{x : x$ is a state of India$\}$

(ii) Ans. $\{x : x$ is an even number$\}$.

Hint: Do yourself.

(iii) **Ans.** $\left(0, \frac{1}{2}, 2\right)$.

Hint: Solving $2x^3 - 5x^2 + 2x = 0$, we get

$$x\,(2x - 1)(x - 2) = 0 \Rightarrow x = 0, \frac{1}{2} \text{ and } 2$$

$\therefore$ The required set is $\left(0, \frac{1}{2}, 2\right)$.

(iv) **Ans.** $\{5, 6\}$.

Hint: If $P(x)$ be positive integes greater than 4 and less than 7, then the required set be $\{x : P(x)\} = \{x : 4 < x < 7\} = \{5, 6\}$.

2. **Ans.** B, C and E.

Hint: The elements of A are not the elements of S

$\therefore$ $A \not\subseteq S$.

The elements of B are the elements of S

$\therefore$ $B \subseteq S$.

The elements of C are the elements of S.

$\therefore$ $C \subseteq S$.

The elements of D are not the elements of S

$\therefore$ $D \not\subseteq S$.

The elements of E are also the elements of S

$\therefore$ $E \subseteq S$.

3. **Ans.** (i) $A = \phi$, (ii) $B = \{0\}$, (iii) $C = \{0\}$,
(iv) $D = \phi$, (v) $E = \phi$.

Solution: (i) The odd numbers x do not satisfy $x^2 = 4$

$\therefore$ A is an empty set i.e. $A = \phi$.

(ii) $B = \{0\}$ is a singleton set for if has only one element 0.

(iii) $x + 5 = 5 \Rightarrow x = 0$

$\therefore$ $C = \{0\}$.

This is also a singleton set.

(iv) $3x = 5$ i.e. $x = \frac{5}{3}$ does not satisfy

$x^2 = 9$ and hence D is an empty set.

(v) There si no letter before *a* is English alphabets and hence $E = \phi$.

4. **Ans.** (i) $A = B$ (ii) $A \neq B$ (iii) $A \neq B$

Solution: (i) $A \subseteq B$ and $B \subseteq A$ and hence $A = B$

(ii) $A \not\subseteq B$ $\therefore$ $A \neq B$

(iii) Solving $2x^2 - 5x + 2 = 0$, we get $x = 0, \frac{1}{2}, 2$

$\therefore \quad A = \left\{\frac{1}{2}, 2\right\}$

Solving $2x^3 - 5x^2 + 2x = 0$ we get $x = \frac{1}{2}, 2$

$\therefore \quad B = \left\{0, \frac{1}{2}, 2\right\} \qquad \therefore \quad A \neq B$

5. Ans. (i) A (ii) B (iii) D

Solution: (i) $x^2 = 16 \Rightarrow x = \pm 4$

$\therefore A = \{4, -4\}$ = a finite set.

(ii) There are limited numbers between 1 and 100 and hence B is a finite set.

6. Ans. (i) $\{2, 3\}$ (ii) $\{-1\}$ (iii) $\{2\sqrt{3}, -2\sqrt{3}\}$

Solution: (i) $x^2 - 5x + 6 = 0 \Rightarrow (x-2)(x-3) = 0$

$\Rightarrow \quad x = 2$ or 3.

The set $\{x : x^2 - 5x + 6 = 0\}$ is $\{2, 3\}$

(ii) From $x^3 + 1 = 0$, we get

$$x = -1 \text{ or } x = \frac{1 \pm \sqrt{3}\, i}{2}$$

The real values of x is -1 and hence the set $\{x : x^3 + 1 = 0\}$ is $\{-1\}$.

(iii) Solving $x^2 - 2 = 10$, we get $x = \pm 2\sqrt{3}$

$\therefore$ The set $\{x : x^2 - 2 = 10\}$ is $\{2\sqrt{3}, -2\sqrt{3}\}$.

7. Ans. (b).

Solution: On the real line, we shade A with strokes slanting upward (///////) to the right and B with the stokes slanting downward (\\\\\\) to the right. Since the point belongs to R we shade the circle around 2, on the real line which shows A. The point 4 does not belong to R hence the circle around 4 on the line showing B is not shaded.

–4 –3 –2 –1 0 1 2 3 4

Figure Q. 7

$A \cap B$ consists only of those points which are common to both A and B.

Thus $A \cap B = [2, 4) = \{x : x \in R, 2 \leq x < 4\}$

$\therefore$ The alternative (b) is correct.

8. **Ans.** (a).

Solution: By Venn diagram we show $A \cup B$ by horizontal strokes which is the entire area of A and B.

Now $A \cap (A \cup B)$ is the common area of A and $A \cup B$ i.e. the area A shown by cross hatched area.

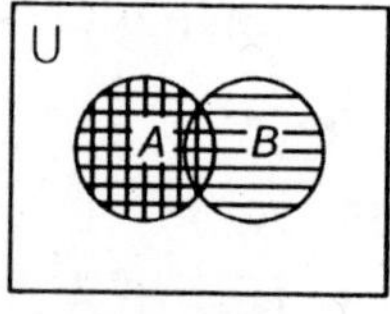

Figure Q. 8

$\therefore A \cap (A \cup B) = A.$

Hence the determinative (a) is correct.

9. **Ans.** (a)

Solution: We first shade $A \cup B$ is Venn diagram and then B'. The area $(A \cup B) \cap B'$ is the position A.

(Draw figure yourself).

The alternative (a) is correct.

10. **Ans.** True.

Solution: Solving $x^3 + 1 = 0$, we get

$x^2 - 1$ and $x = \dfrac{1 \pm \sqrt{3}\, i}{2}$

Thus, the set $\{x : x^3 + 120, x \in N\} = \phi$ is true.

11. **Ans.** True.

Solution: $1 \le x \le 3$ and $x \in N$.

$\therefore \quad A = \{1, 2, 3\}.$

$3y = 9 \Rightarrow y = 3, 2y = 2 \Rightarrow y = 1$ and $y - 1 = 1 \Rightarrow y = 2$

$\therefore \quad B = \{3, 2, 1\}$

$\therefore \quad A = B$

$\therefore$ The statement $A = B$ is true.

12. **Ans.** 6

Solution: The L.C.M. of 3 and 6 is 6 and hence the minimum number of elements in $A \cup B$ is 6.

13. **Ans.** (i) 4 (ii) 0, 4 (iii) ϕ.

Hint: The solutions of $3x^2 - 12x = 0$ are $x = 0$ and $x = 4$.

(i) Since $x \in N$

$\therefore \quad x = 4$

(ii) Since $x \in I$

$\therefore \quad x = 0, 4$

(iii) Since $x \in C$

$\therefore \quad \{x : 3x^2 - 12x = 0, \quad x \in C\} = \phi.$

14. Hint: $B \cap C = \{3, 4, 5\}$

$\therefore \quad A \cup (B \cap C) = \{1, 2, 3, 4, 5\}$

$A \cup B = \{1, 2, 3, 4, 5\}$ and $A \cup C = \{1, 2, 3, 4, 5\}$

$\therefore \quad (A \cup B) \cap (A \cup C) = \{1, 2, 3, 4, 5\}$

$\therefore \quad A \cup (B \cap C) = (A \cup B) \cap (A \cup C).$

15. Ans. (*i*) {1} (ii) {2} (iii) {4, 5, 6} (iv) {1, 3} (v) {1}.

Hint: (i) Removing the elements of B from A, we obtain

$A - B = \{1\}$

(ii) Similarly $B - C = \{2\}$

(iii) $C - A = \{4, 5, 6\}$

(iv) Removing the elements of C from B, we obtain

$B - C = \{2\}$

In a similar way $A - (B - C) = \{1, 3\}$

(v) $A - B = \{1\} \quad \therefore (A - B) - C = \{1\}$.

16. Hint: (i) Show that

$A \cup (B \cap C) = (A \cup B) \cap (A \cup C) = \{1, 2, 3, 4, 5, 6\}$.

(ii) Show that $A \cap (B \cup C) = \{2, 3, 4\} = (A \cap B) \cup (A \cap C)$.

17. Ans. 32.

Hint: The required set is $\{A, B, D, H, L\}$.

$\therefore$ The number of subsets is $2^5 = 32$.

18. Ans. (i) A singleton set. (ii) Singleton set.

(iii) Neither empty nor singleton set.

(iv) Neither empty nor singleton set.

(v) Neither empty nor singleton set.

(vi) An empty set.

(vii) A singleton set.

(viii) An empty set.

Hint: (i) $x + 4 = 6 \Rightarrow x = 2 \quad \therefore$ The set is {2}.

This is a singleton set.

(ii) $x^2 - 6x + 9 = 0 \Rightarrow (x - 3)^2 = 0 \Rightarrow x = 3$

$\therefore$ The set is {3}. This is a singleton set.

(iii) $8 < x < 9 \Rightarrow$ all real numbers is between 8, 9 and hence the set is neither empty nor singleton.

(iv) $x = x^2 \Rightarrow x(x - 1) = 0 \Rightarrow x = 0$ or $x = 1$

$\therefore$ The set is {0, 1} which is neither empty nor singleton.

(v) The set $\{x : x \le x\}$ is neither empty nor singleton as all the real numbers satisfy the relation.

(vi) The set is empty as the inequality $x < x$ does not hold good for real numbers.

(vii) The set is singleton as $3x = 4 \Rightarrow x = \frac{4}{3}$.

(viii) The set is an empty set as $3x^2 + 2 = 0$

$\Rightarrow\ x = \pm\sqrt{2/3}\,i$.

19. Ans. (i), (ii) and (iii) are true.

(iv) is false (v) true.

Hint: (i) $X - Y = \{Z\}$; (ii) $Y - Z = \{3, 4\}$

(iii) $Z - X = \{5\}$;

(iv) $(X - Y) - Z \ne \phi$

(v) $X - (Y - Z) = \{2\}$.

EXERCISE 1 (D)

1. If $X = \{1, 2, 3, 4, 5\}$; $Y = \{1, 3, 5, 7, 9\}$, find the value of $X \cap Y$ and $(X - Y) \cup (Y - X)$
2. If $A = \{1, 2, 3, 4, 5\}$ and $B = \{2, 4, 5, 6\}$, prove that
   (i) $A = \oplus B = B \oplus A$
   (ii) $A \oplus (B \oplus C) = (A \oplus B) \oplus C$
   (iii) $A \oplus A = \phi$.
3. If $X = \{4^n - 3n - 1 : n \in N\}$
   and $Y = \{9(n - 1): n \in N\}$, prove that $X \subset Y$. (I.I.T. 1971)
4. Can the sets $A \cup B$ and $A \cap B$ be equal? If yes, give reasons.
5. If $aN = \{ax : x \in N\}$, find the value of $3N \cap 7N$. (I.I.T. 1970)
6. Show by Venn diagram
   (i) $n(A \cup B) = n(A) + n(B) - n(A \cap B)$
   Where A and B are two sets.
   (ii) If $A = \{1, 2, 3, 4, 5\}$, $B = \{4, 5, 6, 7, 8\}$
   Verify the above formula.
7. If $A = \{2, 3, 4, 8, 10\}$, $B = \{3, 4, 5, 10, 12\}$ and $C = \{4, 5, 6, 7, 12, 14\}$, find the value of $(A \cup B) \cap (A \cup C)$ and $(A \cap B) \cup (A \cap C)$.

8. Denote $A \cup (B \cap C)$ and $(A \cup B) \cap (A \cup C)$ by Venn diagrams and show that $A \cup (B \cap C) = (A \cup B) \cap (A \cup C)$.

9. Show $A \cap (B \cup C) = (A \cap B) \cup (A \cap C)$ by Venn diagram.

10. Prove by logical method

(i) $A \subseteq B \Rightarrow A \cup B = B$

(ii) $A \subseteq C$ and $B \subseteq C \Leftrightarrow A \cup B \subseteq C$.

11. Of the members fo three athletics teams in a certain school, 21 are on the basketball team, 26 on hockey team and 29 on the football team.14 play hockey and basketball, 15 play hockey and football, 12 play football and basketball and 8 play all the three games. How many members are there in all? (I.I.T 1975)

12. At a certain conference of 100 people, there are 29 Indian women and 23 Indian man of these Indian people 4 are doctors 24 are either men or doctors. There are no foreign doctors. How many foreigners are attending the conference? How many women doctors are attending the conference?

13. An analysis of 100 injured persons during an incident of an industrial institute revealed that loss or injury in respect of an eye, an arm, a leg occurred in 30, 50 and 70 cars respectively. Loss on injury in respect of two of the three [an eye, an arm and a leg] numberd 44. How many claims involved loss or injury to all the three? We must assume that one or another of the three members was mentioned in each of the 100 cases.

14. In a group of 1000 people, there are 750 who can speak Hindi and 400 who can speak Bengali. How many can speak Bengali only? How many can speak both Hindi and Bengali? (Roorkee 1978)

15. If $S = \{(x, y) : |x - 3| < 1 \text{ and } |y - 3| < 1\}$

$E = \{(x, y) : 4x^2 + 9y^2 - 32x - 54y + 109 \leq 0\}$

Show that S is a subset of E. (Roorkee 1982)

16. In a town of 10000 families it was found that 40% families buy newspaper A, 20% families buy newspaper B, and 10% families buy newspaper C, 5% families buy A and B, 3% buy B and C and 4% buy A and C. If 2% families buy all the three newspaper, find the number of families which buy (i) A Only (ii) B only (iii) none of A, B and C.

(Roorkee 1991)

ANSWERS TO EXERCISE 1 (D)
(Hints and Solutions)

1. **Ans.** $\{1, 3, 5\}, \{2, 4, 7, 9\}$

Hint: $X \cap Y$ is the set of elements common to X and Y.

$$\therefore \quad X \cap Y = \{1, 3, 5\}$$

$$X - Y = \{2, 4\} \text{ and } Y - X = \{7, 9\}$$

$\therefore (X - Y) \cup (Y - X) = \{2, 4, 7, 9\}$

2. **Hint:** (i) $A \oplus B = (A - B) \cap (B - A)$

$$= \{1, 3\} \cup \{6\} = \{1, 3, 6\}$$

$$B \oplus A = (B - A) \cup (A - B)$$

$$= \{6\} \cup \{1, 3\} = \{1, 3, 6\}$$

$$\therefore \quad A \oplus B = B \oplus A.$$

(ii) $B \oplus C = (B - C) \cup (C - B)$

$$= \{2, 4, 6\} \cup \{3, 7, 9\}$$

$$= \{2, 3, 4, 6, 7, 9\} = E \text{ (Suppose)}$$

$$A \oplus (B \oplus C) = A \oplus E$$

$$= (A - E) \cup (E - A)$$

$$= \{1, 5\} \cup \{6, 7, 9\}$$

$$= \{1, 5, 6,7, 9\}$$

Again $A \oplus B = (A - B) \cup (B - A)$

$$= \{1, 3\} \cup \{6\} = \{1, 3, 6\} = F \text{ \{Suppose\}}$$

$$A \oplus B \oplus C = F \oplus C = (F - C) \cup (C - F)$$

$$= \{1, 6\} \cup \{5, 7, 9\}$$

$$= \{1, 5, 6, 7, 9\}$$

$$\therefore \quad A \oplus (B \oplus C) = (A \oplus B) \oplus C$$

(iii) $A \oplus A = (A - A) \cup (A - A)$

$= \quad \phi \cup \phi = \phi$

$\therefore \quad A \oplus A = \phi$

3. **Hint:** Putting $n = 1, 2, 3$ ....

We have $X = \{0 , 9, 54, 243 ......\}$ and $Y = \{0, 9, 18, 27 .....\}$

We see $X \subset Y$.

4. **Ans.** Possible when $A = B$.

Hint: $A \cup B =$ The set of all elements of A and $B = A$ or B

$A \cap B =$ The set of all elements common to A and B

$= A \text{ and } B$

$\therefore \quad A \cup B = A \cap B$ only when $A = B$.

5. Ans. $21N$

Hint: $aN = \{ax : x \in N\}$ ...(1)

$\therefore \quad 3N = \{3x : x \in N\}$ when $a = 3$

$= \{3, 6, 9, 12 .....\}$ when $x = 1, 2, 3 .....$

$7N = \{7x : x \in N\}$

$= \{7, 14, 21 ......\}$ when $x = 1, 2, 3 .....$

$\therefore \quad 3N \cap 7N = \{21, 42, 63 ....\} = 21N$

$\therefore \quad 3N \cap 7N = 21N.$

6. Hint: (i) Let x, y, z be the no. of elements is A, B and $A \cap B$ repectively.

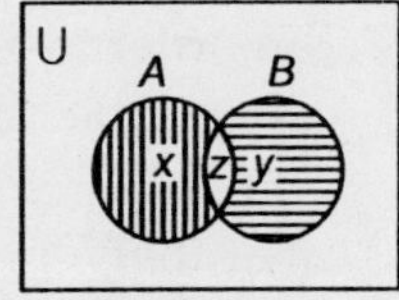

Figure Q. 6

$\therefore \quad n(A) = x + z, n(B) = y + z$ and $n(A \cap B) = z.$

$n(A \cup B)$ = no. of elements of the entire area of A and B

$= x + y + z$

$n(A) + n(B) - n(A \cap B) = x + z + y + z - z$

$= x + y + z = n(A \cup B).$

(ii) We have $n(A) = 5$ and $n(B) = 5$

$A \cup B = \{1, 2, 3, 4, 5, 6, 7, 8\}$

$\therefore \quad n(A \cup B) = 8$

$A \cap B = \{4, 5\} \therefore n(A \cap B) = 2$

R.H.S. $= n(A) + n(\text{B}) - n(A \cap B) = 5 + 5 - 2 = 8$

$= n\,(A \cup B) =$ L.H.S.

7. Ans. $\{2, 3, 4, 5, 8, 10, 12\}; \{3, 4, 10\}$.

Hint: $A \cup B = \{2, 3, 4, 5, 8, 10, 12\}$

$A \cup C = \{2, 3, 4, 5, 6, 7, 8, 10, 12, 14\}$

$\therefore (A \cup B) \cap (A \cup C) = \{2, 3, 4, 5, 8, 10, 12\}$

Similarly $(A \cap B) \cup (A \cap B) = \{3, 4, 10\}$

8. Hint: Shade the common portion of B and C by horizontal lines and A by vertical dotted lines. The set $A \cup (B \cap C)$ is represented by the entire shaded portion i.e., the portion shaded by horizontal and vertical lines is Figure I.

For the set $(A \cup B) \cap (A \cup C)$. We shade the set $A \cup B$ by horizontal lines and $A \cup C$ by vertical lines.

The set $(A \cup B) \cap (A \cup C)$ is shown by the double horizontal area i.e., the area in which horizontal and vertical lines lie in Figure II.

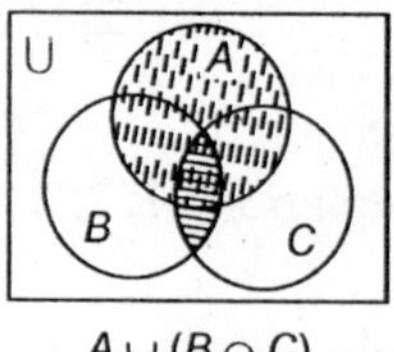

$A \cup (B \cap C)$

Figure I. Q. 8

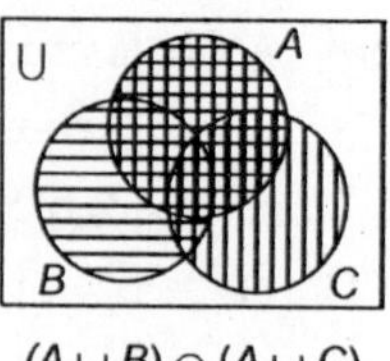

$(A \cup B) \cap (A \cup C)$

Figure II. Q. 8

9. **Hint:** The set B and C are shaded with the horizontal lines in order to get $B \cup C$. The set A is then shaded by vertical lines. The double hatched area represents $A \cap (B \cup C)$ in Fig. I

For the Venn diagram of $(A \cap B) \cup (A \cap C)$, we shade the common portion of A and B by horizontal lines which denotes $A \cap B$. Similarly the common portion of A and C is shaded by the vertical lines which denotes $A \cap C$. The entire shaded portion in Fig. II represents $(A \cap B) \cup (A \cap C)$.

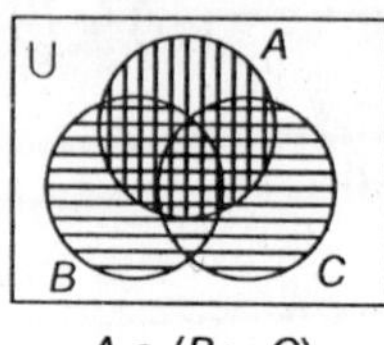

$A \cap (B \cup C)$

Figure I. Q. 9

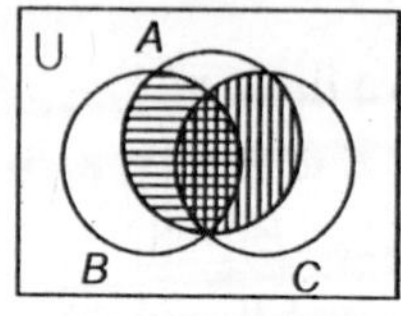

$(A \cap B) \cup (A \cap C)$

Figure II. Q. 9

10. **Solution:** (i) We have to prove $A \cup B = B$ if $A \subseteq B$.

We have $x \in A \Rightarrow x \in B \therefore A \subseteq B$

Let $x \in A \cup B$ then

$x \in A \cup B \Rightarrow x \in A$ or $x \in B$

$\Rightarrow x \in B$ or $x \in B \Rightarrow x \in B \quad \therefore A \cup B \subseteq A$ ...(1)

We can prove in a similar way $B \subseteq A \cup B$ ...(2)

$\therefore$ From (1) and (2) $A \cup B = B$.

Solution: (ii) We first of all prove that

$A \subseteq C$ and $B \subseteq C \Rightarrow A \cup B \subseteq C$

We have $x \in A \Rightarrow x \in C \quad \because A \subseteq C$

and $x \in B \Rightarrow x \in C \quad \because B \subseteq C$

Let $x \in A \cup B$, then

$x \in A \cup B \Rightarrow x \in A$ or $x \in B$

$\Rightarrow \; x \in C$ or $x \in C$

$\Rightarrow \; x \in C \quad \therefore \; A \cup B \subseteq C$ ...(1)

Now we prove its converse also , i.e.

$A \cup B \subseteq C \Rightarrow A \subseteq C$ and $B \subseteq C$

We have $A \cup B \subseteq C \quad \therefore \; x \in A \cup B \Rightarrow x \in C$

$\because \; A \cup B \subseteq C \quad \therefore A \subseteq C$

If all the elements of B are in C, then $B \subseteq C$ ...(2)

From (1) and (2)

$A \subseteq C$ and $B \subseteq C \Leftrightarrow A \cup B \subseteq C$.

11. Ans. 43

Solution: Representing the set of students playing basketball, hockey and football by the letter B, H and F. We write

$$n(B) = 21, n(H) = 26 \text{ and } n(F) = 29$$

$$n(H \cap B) = 14, n(H \cap F) = 15, n(F \cap B) = 12$$

and $\quad n(B \cap H \cap F) = 8.$

Now we have to obtain $n(B \cup H \cup F)$.

$$n(B \cup H \cup F)$$
$$= n(B) + n(H) + n(F) - n(H \cap F) - n(F \cap B)$$
$$- n(H \cap B) + n(B \cap H \cap F)$$
$$= 21 + 26 + 29 - 15 - 12 - 14 + 8$$
$$= 43.$$

Aliter: This problem can also be solved with the help of Venn diagram, also.

We write 8 for $B \cap H \cap F$. 6, 7 and 4 are written for the portion $H \cap B$, $H \cap F$ and $F \cap B$ respectively. Determining the remaining part of B, H and F respectively to be 3, 5 and 10 respectively we determine the total number of students as $3 + 6 + 5 + 4 + 8 + 7 + 10 = 43$.

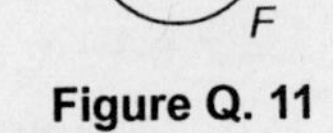

Figure Q. 11

12. Ans. 1, 48.

Solution: U = Set of all people = 100

I = set of all Indian people

I' = set of all foreigners attending the conference
W = set of Indian women
M = set of Indian men
D = set of Indian docturs.

We are given

$$n(I \cup I') = 100; n(W) = 29, n(M) = 23, n(D) = 4$$
$$n(M \cup D) = 24; \text{and } W \cup M = I;$$
$$n(I \cup I') = n(I) + n(I') - n(I \cap I')$$
$$= 100 \; (\because I \cup I' = \phi)$$
$$\Rightarrow \quad n(I') = 100 - n(I) = 100 - (29 + 23)$$
$$= 100 - 52 = 48$$

Now we find the no. of Indian doctors and for this we determine $n(W \cap D)$.

We use the formula first

$$n(M \cup D) = n(M) + n(D) - n(M \cap D)$$
$$\Rightarrow \quad 24 = 23 + 4 - n(M \cap D)$$
$$\Rightarrow n(M \cap D) = 27 - 24 = 3$$

Thus the no. of Indian male doctors is 3.

The total no. of Indian male doctors is 4.

$\therefore \; n(W \cap D) = 4 - 3 = 1$

So, the no. of Indian women doctors is one.

Aliter: Let x be the no. of Indian lady doctor attending the conference.

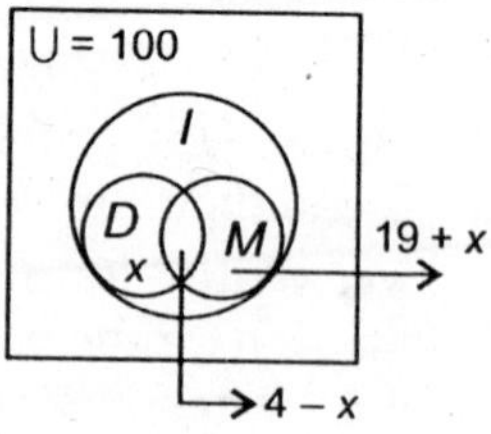

$\therefore$ The no. of remaining Indian women is $29 - x$ and the no. of remaining male doctors is $4 - x$.

$\therefore$ No. of Indian men $= 23 - (4 - x)$ $= 19 + x$.

U = 100
I
D
x
M
19 + x
4 – x

By Venn diagram $n(M \cup D) = 24$ $= x + 4 - x + 19 + x$

$\Rightarrow \; x = 1$ and $n(I') = 100 - 29 + 23 = 48$.

13. **Ans.** 3

Solution: Denoting the set of people having injuries in eyes, arms and legs by the letter E, H and L respectively, we write

$$n(E \cup H \cup L) = 100; n(E) = 30$$
$$n(H) = 50 \text{ and } n(L) = 70.$$

We are given

$n[(E \cap H \cap L') \cup (H \cap L \cap E') \cup (L \cap E \cap H')] = 44$ ...(1)

Using the formula

$$n(E \cup H \cup L) = n(E) + n(H) + n(L) - n(E \cap H) - n(H \cap L) - n(L \cap E) + n(E \cap H \cap L)$$

and substituting the value, we get

$n(E \cap H) + n(H \cap L) + n(L \cap E) - n(E \cap H \cap L) = 50$ ...(2)

The set $E \cap H \cap L'$, $H \cap L \cap E'$ and $L \cap E \cap H'$ are disjoint and therefore (1) can be replaced by

$n(E \cap H \cap L') + n(H \cap L \cap E') + n(L \cap E \cap H') = 44$

i.e. $n(E \cap H) - n(E \cap H \cap L) + n(H \cap L) - n(H \cap L \cap E) + n(L \cap E) - n(L \cap E \cap H) = 44$

$\Rightarrow$ $n(E \cap H) + n(H \cap L) + n(L \cap E) - 3n(E \cap H \cap L) = 44$ ...(3)

Subtracting (3) from (2)

$2n(E \cap H \cap L) = 6$

$\Rightarrow$ $n(E \cap H \cap L) = 3.$

Aliter: This problem can also be solved with the help of Venn diagram.

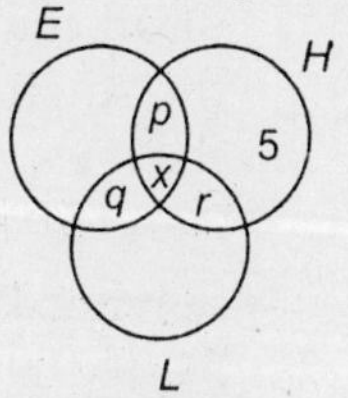

Solution: Let x be the no. of people whose eyes, arms, and legs are injured. No. of people injured inspect of eyes and legs, eyes and arms, and legs are respectively p, q and r.

E H p 5 x q r L

Figure Q. 13

$\therefore$ No. of persons whose eyes are injured is $30 - (p + q + x)$.

No. of persons whose arms are injured is $50 - (p + x + r)$ and No. of persons whose legs are injured is $70 - (q + x + r)$

$\therefore$ $30 - (p + q + x) + 50 - (p + x + r) + 70 - (q + x + r) + p + q + r + x = 100$ where $p + q + r = 44$

$\therefore$ $150 - (p + q + r) - 2x = 100$

$\therefore$ $150 - 100 - 44 = 2x \quad \therefore\ x = \frac{6}{2} = 3.$

14. Ans. (1) 600 (2) 250 (3) 150.

Solution: Let H and B be the set of persons who can speak Hindi and Bengali respectively. We are given

$$n(H \cup B) = 1000,\ n(H) = 750;\ n(B) = 400$$

Using the formula

$$n(H \cup B) = n(H) + n(B) - n\,(H \cap B). \text{ We obtain}$$

$$n\,(H \cup B) = 750 + 400 - 1000 = 150$$

Using the formula

$$n(H \cup B') = n(H) - n\,(H \cap B), \text{ we get}$$

$$n(H \cup B') = 750 - 150 = 600$$

and $\quad n(B \cup H') = n(B) - n(B \cap H)$

We get $n(B \cup H') = 400 - 150 = 250.$

Thus 150 persons speak Hindia and Bengali; 600 persons speak only Hindi and 250 persons speak only Bengali.

15. Solution: Solving the inequality $|x - 3| < 1$. We write $\pm (x - 3) < 1$

$\Rightarrow\ 2 < x < 4$

Similarly from $|y-3|<1$ we get $2 < y < 4$.

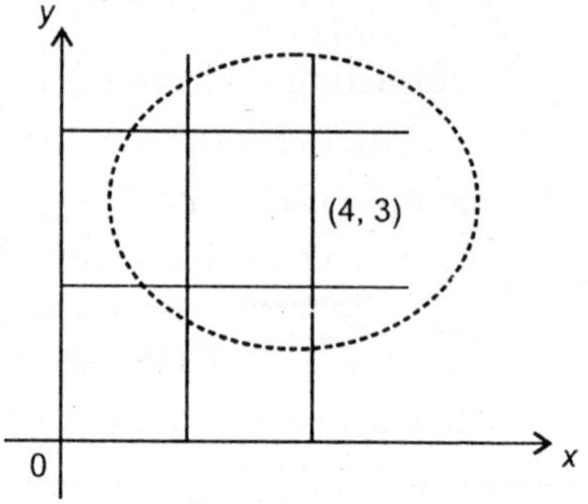

Thus, the set S consists of all the points inside the square bounded by the lines $x = 2$, $x = 4$, $y = 2$ and $y = 4$.

Solving $4x^2 + 9y^2 - 32x - 54y + 109 \le 0$

We get $4(x - 4)^2 + 9(y - 3)^2 \le 36$

$\Rightarrow \dfrac{(x-4)^2}{9} + \dfrac{(y-3)^2}{4} \le 1$ and hence the set E consists of all the points with in the ellipse whose centre is $(4, 3)$ and major and minor area are 6 and 4 respectively.

Now we proceed to show S is a subset of E.

Let (h, k) be an arbitrary element of S.

$\therefore\ \ 2 < h < 4$ and $2 < k < 4$

$\therefore\ \ 2 - 4 < h - 4 < 0$ and $2 - 3 < k - 3 < 4 - 3$

$\therefore\ \ \dfrac{(h-4)}{3} < \dfrac{2}{3} \Rightarrow \dfrac{(h-4)^2}{9} < \dfrac{4}{9}$

Similarly $\dfrac{(k-3)^2}{4} < \dfrac{1}{4}$

$$\therefore \quad \frac{(h-4)^2}{9} + \frac{(k-3)^2}{4} < \frac{4}{9} + \frac{1}{4} = \frac{25}{36} < 1$$

$\therefore$ $(h, k) \in S \Rightarrow (h, k) \in E.$

$\Rightarrow$ S is a subset of E.

16. Ans. 3300, 1400 and 4000.

Solution: Let U be the universal set. $\therefore n(U) = 10000$.

Assuming P, Q, R to be the sets of families buying newspaper A, B, C respectively. We have the following data

$n(P) = 40\%$ of $10000 = 4000$; $n(Q) = 20\%$ of $10000 = 2000$;

$n(R) = 10\%$ of $10000 = 1000$; $n(P \cap Q) = 5\%$ of $10000 = 500$;

$n(Q \cap R) = 3\%$ of $10000 = 300$; $n(R \cap P) = 4\%$ of $10000 = 400$;

$n(P \cap Q \cap R) = 2\%$ of $10000 = 200$

(i) No. of families which buy A only is

$n(P \cap Q' \cap R') = n[P \cap \{U - (Q \cup R\}]$

$= n(P) - n[(P \cap (Q \cup R)] = n(P) - n[(P \cap Q) \cup (P \cap R)]$

$= n(P) - [n(P \cap Q) + n(P \cap R) - n(P \cap Q \cap R)]$

$= 4000 - [500 + 400 - 200] = 3300$

(ii) We have to determine $n(P' \cap Q \cap R')$ which is equal to $n(Q) - [n(P \cap Q) + n(Q \cap R) - n(P \cap Q \cap R)]$

(after doing some algebra)

$= 2000 - [500 + 300 - 200] = 1400$

(iii) The required number is $n(P' \cap Q' \cap R')$

$= n[(P \cup Q \cup R)'] = n[U - (P \cup Q \cup R)]$

$= n(U) - [n(P) + n(Q) + n(R) - n(P \cap Q) - n(P \cap R)$

$- n(Q \cap R) - n(P \cap Q \cap R)]$ (After doing some algebra)

$= 10000 - [4000 + 2000 + 1000 - 500 - 300 - 400 + 200]$

$= 4000.$

CHAPTER

Ordered Pairs, Cartesian Prodcuts, Mappings and Relations

2.1 ORDERED PAIRS

If $a \in A$ and $b \in B$ then (a, b) is called an ordered pair. If consists of two elements a and b taken in definite order. An ordered pair of a and b is always denoted by (a, b), where a is the first element or number and b the second element or number. The ordered pairs (a, b) and (b, a) are different.

The points in the Cartesion plane represent ordered pairs of real numbers. The set $\{a, b\}$ can never be an ordered pair as the order of the elements a and b ae not clear here. Two ordered pairs (a, b) and (c, d) are equal iff $a = c$ and $b = d$. (a, b) is also used to denote an open interval and hence its difference from the ordered pair is defected well when we give the rigorous definition of the latter as

$$(a, b) \equiv \{\{a\}, \{a, b\}\}.$$

2.2 IMPORTANT THEOREM

Prove that $(a, b) = (c, d)$ iff $a = c$ and $b = d$.

Proof: If $a = c$ and $b = d$, then $(c, d) = \{\{c\}, \{c, d\}\} = \{\{a\}, \{a, b\}\} = (a, b)$ conversely let $(a, b) = (c, d)$

$\therefore \quad \{\{a\}, \{a, b\}\} = \{\{c\}, \{c, d\}\}$ if $a = b$ then

$$(a, b) = \{\{a\}, \{a, a\}\} = \{\{a\}\}$$
$$= \{\{c\}, \{c, d\}\}$$

By the definition of equal sets

$$\{a\} = \{c\} = \{c, d\}$$
$$\Rightarrow \quad a = c = d$$

If $a \neq b$, then $\{a, b\} \neq \{c\}$ hence $\{a, b\} = \{c, d\}$ and $\{a\} = \{c\}$

$$\Rightarrow \quad a = c \text{ and } b = d.$$

2.3 CARTESIAN PRODUCT OR DIRECT PRODUCT OF TWO SETS

The Cartesion product of two sets A and B is the set of all ordered pairs (x, y) in which the first element (component) is a member of A and the second element (component) a member of B.

The product set is denoted by

$$A \times B = \{(x, y) \mid x \in A \text{ and } y \in B\}$$

and is read as "A cross B".

Example 1: If $A = \{1, 2, 3\}$; $B = \{c, d\}$, then $A \times B = \{(1, c), (2, c)$ $(3, c), (1, d), (2, d)$ $(3, d)\}$.

Solution: If A and B are equal then their Cartesian product is called the Cartesian square and is denoted as $A \times A = A^2$.

If R is the set of real numbers, then the set of points is the Cartesian plane is a Cartesian product of the form $R \times R$ i.e. product set of real numbers with itself.

$R \times R = R^2$ represents a Cartesian plane since all the points belonging to the plane are the coordinates of the points of the same plane.

$R \times R$ is also known as "Euclidean plane".

2.4 PRODUCT SETS IN GENERAL

The Cartesian product of three sets A, B, C is denoted by the set $A \times B \times C$. Its consists of all ordered triplets (a, b, c), where $a \in A, b \in B, c \in C$.

Thus, $A \times B \times C = \{(a, b, c) \mid a \in A, b \in B, c \in C\}$.

Similarly the Cartesian product of n sets $A_1, A_2, A_3, \ldots\ldots, A_n$ can be denoted as

$A_1 \times A_2 \times ..... \times A_n$ which consists of all ordered n tuples (a_1, a_2, ..., a_n), where $a_1 \in A_1, a_2 \in A_2, ..., a_n \in A_n$.

$R \times R \times R = R^3$ denotes the Cartesian space as its elements (x, y, z) are the coordinates of a points.

R^3 is called the Euclidean space.

EXERCISE – 2. A SIMPLE QUESTIONS

1. If $A = \{1\}$ and $B = \{1, 2, 3\}$, find the value of $A \times B$.
2. If $S = \{0, 1\}$ and $T = \{0, -1\}$, find the value of $S \times T$ and $T \times S$ and show that $S \times T \neq T \times S$.
3. If $A \times B = \{(3, 3), (3, 4), (5, 2), (5, 4)\}$, find the elements of the set A and B. (U.P. 1982)
4. If $A = \{2, 6\}, B = \{1, 0, 9\}, C = \{1, 9\}$, find the value of
   (i) $A \times (B \cup C)$ (ii) $A \times (B \cap C)$
   (iii) $(A \times B) \cup (A \times C)$ (iv) $(A \times B) \cap (A \times C)$.
5. If A, B, C are the sets and $A \subseteq B$, prove that $A \times C \subseteq B \times C$.
6. If $A \subseteq B$ and $C \subseteq D$, prove that $A \times C \subseteq B \times D$.
7. Show that $A \times (B - C) = (A \times B) - (A \times C)$.
8. If $A = \{1, 2\}, B = \{2, 3\}, C = \{3, 5\}$, find the value of
   (i) $A \times (B \cup C)$ (ii) $A \times (B \cap C)$
   (iii) $(A \times B) \cup (A \times C)$ (iv) $(A \times B) \cap (A \times C)$.
   (U.P. 1984)
9. Prove that $(A \times B) \cap (S \times T) = (A \cap S) \times (B \cap T)$.
10. There are n elements common to the set A and B. How many elements are there common to $A \times B$ and $B \times A$.
11. If $A \subseteq B$, prove that $(A \times B) \cap (B \times A) = A^2$.

ANSWERS TO EXERCISE 2 (A)
(Hint and Solutions)

1. **Ans.** $\{(1, 1), (1, 2), (1, 3)\}$.

   Hint: Taking the first elements 1 of A as the first component and the elements 1, 2, 3 of B as the second component we get the ordered pair (1, 1) (1, 2) and (1, 3)

   $\therefore \quad A \times B = \{(1, 1), (1, 2) (1, 3)\}$
2. **Ans.** $\{(0, 0), (0, -1), (1, 0), (1, -1)\}$ and $\{(0, 0), (0, 1), (-1, 0), (-1, 1)\}$.

Hint: $S = \{0, 1\}, T = \{0, -1\}$

$\therefore$ $S \times T = \{(0, 0), (0, -1), (1, 0), (1, -1)\}$

$T \times S = \{(0, 0), (0, 1), (-1, 0), (-1, 1)\}$

Clearly $S \times T \neq T \times S$.

3. Ans. $A = \{3, 5\}, B = \{2, 3, 4\}$.

Hint: The set of first elements of all the ordered pairs in $A \times B$ is the set A.

$\therefore$ $A = \{3, 3, 5, 5\} = \{3, 5\}$

The set of second elements of all the ordered pairs in $A \times B$ is the set B.

$\therefore$ $B = \{3, 4, 2, 4\} = \{2, 3, 4\}$.

4. Ans. (i) $\{(2, 0), (2, 1), (2, 9), (6, 0), (6, 1), (6, 9)\}$

(ii) $\{(2, 1), (2, 9), (6, 1), (6, 9)\}$

(iii) $\{(2, 1), (2, 0), (2, 9), (6, 1), (6, 0), (6, 9)\}$

(iv) $\{(2, 1), (2, 9), (6, 1), (6, 9)\}$.

Solution: (i) We have $B \cup C = \{0, 1, 9\}$

i.e., all the elements of B and C

$$A = \{2, 6\}$$

$\therefore$ $A \times (B \cup C) = \{(2, 0)(2, 1), (2, 9), (6, 0), (6, 1)(6, 9)\}$

(ii) We have $B \cap C = \{1, 9\}$ i.e., set of elements common to B and C.

$$A = \{2, 6\}$$

$\therefore$ $A \times (B \cap C) = \{(2, 1), (2, 9), (6, 1), (6, 9)\}$

(iii) We have $(A \times B) = \{(2, 1)\ (2, 0), (2, 9), (6, 1), (6, 0), (6, 9)\}$

$$A \times C = \{(2, 1), (2, 9), (6, 1), (6, 9)\}$$

$\therefore$ $(A \times B) \cup (A \times C)$

$$= \{(2, 1)\ (2, 0), (2, 9), (6, 1), (6, 0), (6, 9)\}$$

(iv) We have $(A \times B) \cup (A \times C)$

$$= \{(2, 1), (2, 9), (6, 1), (6, 9)\}.$$

5. Solution: Let $(x, y) \in (A \times C)$, then

$(x, y) \in (A \times C) = x \in A$ and $y \in C$

$\Rightarrow x \in B$ and $y \in C$ $[\because A \leq B]$

$\Rightarrow (x, y) \in B \times C$

$\therefore A \times C \subseteq B \times C$.

6. **Solution:** Let $(x, y) \in (A \times C)$, then
$(x, y) \in (A \times C) \Rightarrow x \in A$ and $y \in C$
$\Rightarrow x \in B$ and $y \in D$ $\quad [\because A \subseteq B$ and $C \subseteq D]$
$\Rightarrow (x, y) \in (B \times D)$
$\therefore (A \times C) \subseteq (B \times D)$.
7. **Solution:** Let $(x, y) \in A \times (B - C)$, then
$(x, y) \in A \times (B - C)$
$\Rightarrow x \in A$ and $y \in B - C$
$\Rightarrow x \in A$ and $(y \in B$ and $y \notin C)$
$\Rightarrow x \in A$ and $y \in B$ and $x \in A$ and $y \notin C$
$\Rightarrow (x, y) \in A \times B$ and $(x, y) \notin A \times C$
$\Rightarrow (x, y) \in [(A \times B) - (A \times C)]$
$\therefore A \times (B - C) \leq (A \times B) - (A \times C)$ ...(1)
Now we shall prove $(A \times B) - (A \times C) \subseteq A \times (B - C)$
Let $(x, y) \in [(A \times B) - (A \times C)]$, then
$(x, y) \in [(A \times B) - (A \times C)]$
$\Rightarrow (x, y) \in [(A \times B)$ and $(x, y) \notin (A \times C)$
$\Rightarrow (x \in A$ and $x \in B)$ and $(x \in A$ and $y \notin C)$
$\Rightarrow x \in A$ and $(y \in B$ and $y \notin C)$
$\Rightarrow x \in A$ and $y \in (B - C)$
$\Rightarrow (x, y) \in A \times (B - C)$
$\therefore (A \times B) - (A \times C) \subseteq A \times (B - C)$ ...(2)
From (1) and (2), we have
$A \times (B - C) = (A \times B) - (A \times C)$.
8. **Ans.** (i) $\{(1, 2), (1, 3), (1, 5), (2, 2) (2, 3), (2, 5)\}$
(ii) $\{(1, 3), (2, 3)\}$
(iii) $\{(1, 2), (1, 3), (1, 5), (2, 2) (2, 3), (2, 5)\}$
(iv) $\{(1, 3), (2, 3)\}$
Solution: (i) We have $B \cup C$ is the set of all elements of B and C.
$\therefore \quad B \cup C = \{2, 3, 5\}$.
Now $\quad A = \{1, 2\}$
$\therefore \quad A \times (B \cup C) = \{(1, 2), (1, 3), (1, 5), (2, 2) (2, 3), (2, 5)\}$
(ii) $B \cap C$ is the set of all those elements which are common to B and C.

$\therefore \quad B \cap C = \{3\}$

Now $\quad A = \{1, 2\}$

$\therefore \; A \times (B \cap C) = \{(1, 3), (2, 3)\}$

(iii) $A = \{1, 2\}, B = \{2, 3\}$

$\therefore \quad A \times B = \{(1, 2), (1, 3), (2, 2)\ (2, 3)\}$

$A = \{1, 2\}, C = \{3, 5\}$

$\therefore \quad A \times C = \{(1, 3), (1, 5), (2, 3), (2, 5)\}$

$\therefore \; (A \times B) \cup (A \times C) = \{(1, 2), (1, 3), (1, 5), (2, 2)\ (2, 3), (2, 5)\}$

(iv) We have

$A \times B = \{(1, 2), (1, 3), (2, 2)\ (2, 3)\}$

$A \times C = \{(1, 3), (1, 5), (2, 3), (2, 5)\}$

$\therefore \; (A \times B) \cap (A \times C) = \{(1, 3), (2, 3)\}$.

9. **Solution:** Let $(x, y) \in (A \times B) \cap (S \times T)$

Then $(x, y) \in (A \times B) \cap (S \times T)$

$\Rightarrow (x, y) \in (A \times B)$ and $(x, y) \in (S \times T)$

$\Rightarrow (x \in A$ and $y \in B)$ and $(x \in S$ and $y \in T)$

$\Rightarrow (x \in A$ and $x \in S)$ and $(y \in B$ and $y \in T)$

$\Rightarrow x \in A \cap S$ and $y \in B \cap T$

$\Rightarrow (x, y) \in (A \cap S) \times (B \cap T)$

$\therefore \; (A \times B) \cap (S \times T) \subseteq (A \cap S) \times (B \cap T)$ ...(1)

Now we have to prove

$(A \cap S) \times (B \cap T) \subseteq (A \times B) \cap (S \times T)$

Let $(x, y) \in (A \cap S) \times (B \cap T)$, then

$(x, y) \in (A \cap S) \times (B \cap T)$

$\Rightarrow x \in A \cap S$ and $y \in B \cap T$

$\Rightarrow x \in A$ and $x \in S$ and $y \in B$ and $y \in T$

$\Rightarrow (x \in A$ and $y \in B)$ and $(x \in S$ and $y \in T)$

$\Rightarrow (x, y) \in A \times B$ and $(x, y) \in S \times T$

$\Rightarrow (x, y) \in (A \times B) \cap (S \times T)$

$\therefore \; (A \cap S) \times (B \cap T) \subseteq (A \times B) \cap (S \times T)$ ...(2)

From (1) and (2) the result follows.

10. **Ans.** n^2.

Solution: Let C be the set which contains those elements which are common to A and B.

$\therefore$ C $\subseteq A$ and C $\subseteq B$

The set contains n elements therefore the product set $C \times C$ has $n \times n = n^2$ elements.

Now all the n^2 elements are common to $A \times B$ and $B \times A$.

$\therefore$ The no. of common elements in n $A \times B$ and $B \times A$ is n^2.

11. Solution: Let $(x, y) \in (A \times B) \cap (B \times A)$

$\therefore (x, y) \in (A \times B)$ and $(x, y) \in (B \times A)$

$\Rightarrow x \in A$ and $y \in B$ and $x \in B$ and $y \in A$

$\Rightarrow (x \in A$ and $x \in B)$ and $(y \in A$ and $y \in B)$

$\Rightarrow x \in A \cap B$ and $y \in A \cap B$

$\Rightarrow x \in A$ and $y \in A$ $\qquad [\because A \subseteq B]$

$\Rightarrow (x, y) \in A \times A$ $\qquad$ ...(1)

Again let $(x, y) \subseteq A \times A$, then

$(x, y) \in A \times A \Rightarrow x \in A$ and $y \in A$

$\Rightarrow (x \in A$ and $x \in B)$ and $(y \in A$ and $y \in B)$ $\qquad [\because A \subseteq B]$

$\Rightarrow (x \in A$ and $y \in B)$ and $(x \in B$ and $y \in A)$

$\Rightarrow (x, y) \in (A \times B)$ and $(x, y) \in B \times A$

$\Rightarrow (x, y) \in (A \times B) \cap (B \times A)$

$\therefore A \times A \subseteq (A \times B) \cap (B \times A)$ $\qquad$ ...(2)

From (1) and (2) the result follows.

PROBLEMS AND EXERCISES 2 (B)

1. (i) If two ordered pairs $(x + y, 1)$ and $(3, x - y)$ are equal, then find the values of x and y.
   (ii) If $A = \{1, 2, 3\}$ and $B = \{4, 5, 6\}$, find $A \times B$.
2. (i) If x and y be the elements of the set $U = \{1, 2, 3, 4, 5\}$, then find the solution set of the equation $x = y - 2$ [i.e., the set of ordered pairs which satisfy the equation $x = y - 1$].
   (ii) If $A = \{a_1, a_2, a_3, ..., a_n\}$ and $B = \phi$, find $A \times B$.
3. If $A = \{1, 2, 3, 4, 5\}$, $B = \{1, 5, 6,.7, 8\}$, find the ordered pairs corresponding to the points P, Q, R, S shown the given diagram of $A \times B$ in the coordinate plane.
4. If $A = \{x, y\}$; $B = \{2, 3\}$ and $C = \{3, 4\}$, then compute
   (1) $A \times (B \cup C)$
   (2) $(A \times B) \cup (A \times C)$

(3) $A \times (B \cap C)$ and

(4) $(A \times B) \cap (A \times C)$.

5. If two ordered pairs $(b - 2, 2a + 1)$ and $(a - 1, b + 2)$ are equal, find a and b.

6. Find the ordered pairs corresponding to the points P, Q, R,

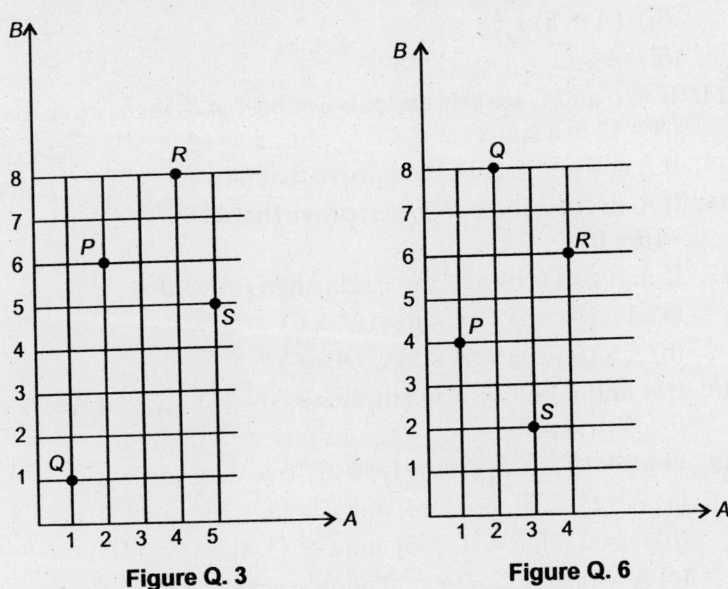

Figure Q. 3 **Figure Q. 6**

S which appear in the given diagram of $A \times B$, where $A = \{1, 2, 3, 4\}$ and $B = \{2, 4, 6, 8\}$.

7. The sets A, B and C have elements, 3, 4 and 5 respectively. How many elements are there in (1) $A \times B \times C$ (2) $C \times A \times B$ and (3) $B \times C \times A$?

8. Prove that $A \times (B \cap C) = (A \times B) \cap (A \times C)$.

9. If $A = \{1, 2, 3\}$ and $B = \{2, 3, 4\}$, then compute

(i) $\{x, y\} \mid (x, y) \in A \times B$ and $x < y\}$

(ii) $\{x, y\} \mid (x, y) \in B \times A$ and $x > y\}$

10. If $A = \{1, 2\}$, $B = \{2, 3\}$ and $C = \{3, 7\}$, then find

(i) $(A \times B) \cup (A \times C)$

(ii) $(A \times B) \cap (A \times C)$.

11. If $A = \{a, b\}$, $B = \{1, 2, 3, 4, 5\}$ and $C = \{3, 5, 7, 9\}$, thus find $(A \times B) \cap (A \times C)$.

12. If $A = \{0, 1\}, B = \{2, 3\}, C = \{1, 2, 3\}$ then verify
   (a) $A \times (B \cup C) = (A \times B) \cup (A \times C)$
   (b) $A \times (B \cap C) = (A \times B) \cap (A \times C)$.
13. If $A = \{2, 3, 4\}, B = \{3, 4\}, C = \{2, 3, 5\}$ evaluate
   (i) $A \times (B \cup C)$
   (ii) $(A \cap B) \times C$
   (iii) $A \times C$.
14. If A, B and C are sets and A is a subset of B, then prove that $(A \times C)$ is a subset of $B \times C$.
15. If $A \subseteq B$ and $C \subseteq D$, then prove that $(A \times C) \subseteq (A \times D)$.
16. If A, B, C are three sets then prove that $(A - B) \times C = (A \times C) - (B \times C)$.
17. If A, B and C be any three sets, then prove that
   (a) $A \times (B \cap C) = (A \times B) \cap (A \times C)$
   (b) $A \times (B \cup C) = (A \times B) \cup (A \times C)$.
18. If A and B be two non-empty sets then show that $A \times B = B \times A$ iff $A = B$.
19. Find $A \times B \times C$ with the help of "tree diagram"
   (a) $A = \{1, 2, 3\}, B = \{2, 4\}$ and $C = \{3, 4, 5\}$
   (b) $A = \{2, 3\}, B = \{1, 3, 5\}$ and $C = \{3, 4\}$
   (c) $A = \{a, b, c\}, B = \{b, c, d\}$ and $C = \{a, d\}$

ANSWERS TO PROBLEMS AND EXERCISES 2 (B)

1. (i) $x = 2, y = 1$
   (ii) $\{(1, 4), (1, 5), (1, 6), (2, 4), (2, 5), (2, 6), (3, 4), (3, 5), (3, 6)\}$
2. (i) $\{(1, 2), (2, 3), (3, 4), (4, 5)\}$ (ii) ϕ
3. $P = (2, 6); Q = (1, 1); R = (4, 8); S = (5, 5)$
4. (1) $\{(x, 2), (x, 3), (x, 4), (y, 2), (y, 3), (y, 4)\}$
   (2) $\{(x, 2), (x, 3), (y, 2), (y, 3), (x, 4), (y, 4)\}$
   (3) $\{(x, 3), (y, 3)\}$
   (4) $\{(x, 3), (y, 3)\}$
5. $a = 2, b = 3$
6. $P = (1, 4); Q = (2, 8); R = (4, 6); S = (3, 2)$
7. Each has 60 elements.
9. (i) $\{(1, 2), (1, 3), (1, 4), (2, 3), (2, 4), (3, 4)\}$
   (ii) $\{(2, 1), (3, 1), (3, 2), (4, 1), (4, 2), (4, 3)\}$

10. (i) $\{(1, 2), (1, 3), (1, 7), (2, 2), (2, 3), (2, 7)\}$

(ii) $\{(1, 3), (2, 3)\}$

11. $\{(a, 3), (a, 5), (b, 3), (b, 5)\}$

13. (i) $\{(2, 2), (2, 3), (2, 4), (2, 5), (3, 2), (3, 3), (3, 4), (3, 5), (4, 2), (4, 3), (4, 4), (4, 5)\}$

(ii) $\{(3, 2), (3, 3), (3, 5), (4, 2), (4, 3), (4, 5)\}$

(iii) $\{(2, 2), (2, 3), (2, 5), (3, 2), (3, 3), (3, 5), (4, 2), (4, 3), (4, 5)\}$

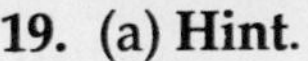

19. (a) **Hint.**

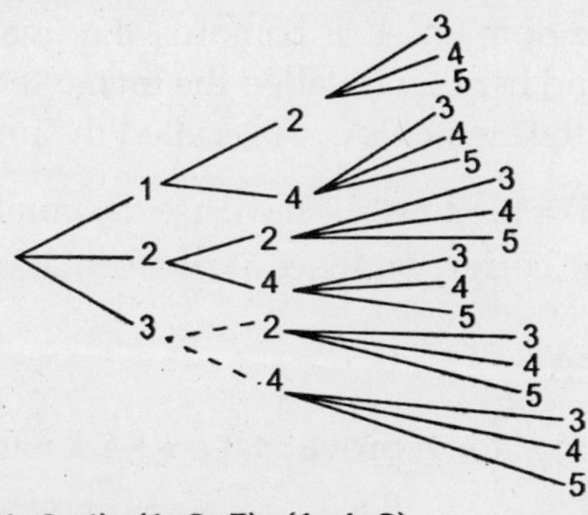

(1, 2, 3), (1, 2, 4), (1, 2, 5), (1, 4, 3)
(1, 4, 4), (1, 4, 5), (2, 2, 3), (2, 2, 4)
(2, 2, 5), (2, 4, 3), (2, 4, 4), (2, 4, 5)
(3, 2, 3), (3, 2, 4), (3, 2, 5), (3, 4, 3)
(3, 4, 4), (3, 4, 5)

Chapter 2 (A)
Function and Its Types

2.5 FUNCTION ON MAPPING

If there is some rule f which puts an unique element of the set B into correspondence with each element of the set A, then f is called a function on the set A with a set of values B. We write it $f: A \to B$. $f: A \to B$ is read as f is a function or mapping of A into B. A function is also a relationship between two sets A and B in which each element of A is associated with not more than one element of B. The set A is called the domain of definition of the function and B is called the co-domain of the function. If $a \in A$ then the element $f(a)$ in B is put into correspondence with the element a. $f(a)$ is known as the image of a and is read — "f of a"

If $f(a)$ is the image of a then we call a to be the pre-image of $f(a)$. "Each element is B appears as the image of an element is A" is not necessary. The set of those elements in B which appear as the image of at least one element is A is called the range of the function.

If the domain and the co-domain of a function f are the same set i.e., $f: A \to A$, then f is known as an operator or transformation on A. The elements of the range is B are called f image of the elements of the domain A. B contains the images of all the elements of A and hence it is called the image set. The set of all the f-images of the elements in A is called the image set and is doenoted by $f(A) = \{f(x): x \in A\}$. If we use the notation $x \xrightarrow{f} y$, this means " The correspondence f transformations x into y."

2.6 EXAMPLES

Example 1: If $f(x) = x + 4$, prove that $f: R \to R$ and $f: -1 \to 3$.

Solution: The domain and the co-domain of the functin are the sets of real numbers hence $f: R \to R$. The image of $-1 = f(-1) = -1 + 4 = 3$

$$\therefore \qquad f: -1 \to 3.$$

Example 2: The function f is defined as given in the figure. Compute $f(a), f(b), f(c)$ and $f(d)$ and the image set.

Figure Example 2

Solution: We have

$$f(a) = 2 = f(d)$$
$$f(b) = 1 \text{ and } f(c)$$

The image set is $\{1, 2, 3\}$

Example 3: Find the domain of definition of $f(x) = \dfrac{1}{\sqrt{1-x^2}}$.

Solution: The domain of difinition of the function consists of those values of x for which $f(x)$ is real. For this the cordition $1 - x^2 > 0$ must be satisfied, i.e. $1 > x^2$ i.e. $x < + 1$. Thus, the domain of difinition of the function is the set $D = \{x: |x| < 1\}$.

2.7 MAPPINGS

If A and B are two sets (not necessarily the set of numbers) then a function f of A into B is called a mapping of A into B. This is written $f: A \to B$, and we read it as — "f maps A into B". The word mapping is a synonym of the word function but we usually use the term "function" is Algebra and "mapping" in geometry. In modern mathematics the terms "function and mapping" and also transformation and "operation" are used synonymously.

2.8 CLASSIFICATION OF FUNCTIONS

1. *Equal functions:* If two functions f and g are defined on the same domain D and if $f(x) = g(x)\ \forall\ x \in D$ then f and g are equal.

Let $f: R \to R$ and $g: R \to R$, where R is the set of real number. If f is defined by $f(x) = x^2$ and g by $g(y) = y^2$, then $f = g$, where x and y are variables which define functions.

If $f(x) = x^2$, where x belongs to R and $g(z) = z^2$, where $Z \in C$ (set of complex numbers), then $f \neq g$ since they have different domains (R and C).

2. *One-one function or univalent functions on injective function:* f is called a one-one function is different elements in B are assigned to diferent elements in A. In other words, no two elements in A have the same image. Mathematically $f{:}A \to B$ is one-one function if $f(a) = f(a_1) \Rightarrow a = a_1$, where $a, a_1 \in A$.

3. *Many one functions:* The function or mapping $f: A \to B$ is said to be many one function on mapping if $f(a) = f(b) \Rightarrow a \neq b$, where $a, b \in A$.

Example (i) The domain of definition of the functions

$$f(x) = x - 1 \text{ and } g(x) = \frac{x^2 - 1}{x + 1} \text{ is } (-1, 1)$$

Prove that $f(x) = g(x)$.

Hint: Here the functions $f(x)$ and $g(x)$ are difined on the same domain (–1, 1).

Example (ii) The funtion $f: R \to R$ is defined by (A) $f(x) = x^2$ and (B) $f(x) = x^3$ find the image of two real numbers 2 and –2 and hence examine whether the function is one-one or not.

Ans. (A) f is not one-one. (B) f is one-one.

Note: Since with the help of variables we define a function hence one must know how many types of simplex funtional relations exist between the variables. We describe here some functional relations as follows:

(A) *Direct proportional relation:* $y = mx$ is the direct proportional relation between the variable x and y where m is constant.

(B) *Linear relation:* $y = mx + c$ is the linear relation between the variables x and y where m and c are constants.

(C) *Inverse proportional relation:* $y = \frac{m}{x}$ is the inverse proportional relation between the variables x and y where m is constant.

(D) *Quadratic relation:* $y = mx^2$ is the quadratic relation between the variables x and y where m is constant.

(E) *Sinusoidal relation:* $y = A \sin(\omega x+\phi)$ [where A is the amplitute, ω is the frequency and ϕ is the intial phase] is the sinusoidel relation between the variables x and y. Such functions are called Harmonic Functions.

4. *INTO and ONTO functions:* We know that the range of a function on the domain is a subset of the co-domain i.e. $f(A) \subseteq B$ if $f: A \to B$.

If each member of B is the image of at least one element of A i.e. $f(A) = B$, then f is known as an onto function. In other words we say f maps A onto B.

If there is at least one element in B, which is not the image of any element in A then f is an into function i.e. $f(A) \subseteq B$. Onto function is also called surjective mapping or surjection or epimorphisn.

The word injective mapping can also be used for one-one into mapping.

The word bijective mapping can be used for one-one onto mapping.

Example 1: If $A = \{p, q, r, s\}$; $B = \{p, q, r\}$

$$f(p) = q; f(q) = r, f(r) = r \text{ and } f(s) = q.$$

Prove that f does not map A onto B.

Solution:

We see that $B = \{p, q, r\}$ and $f(A) = \{q, r\}$

$\therefore f(A) \neq B \therefore f$ does not map A onto B.

Example 2: The mapping $f: I \rightarrow I$ defined by $f(x) = x^2\ x \in I$, where I is the set of positive intagers. Prove that f is one-one into mapping.

Solution: Every positive integers in the domain is put into correspondance with its square is the co-domain, i.e. different elements in the co-domain are assigned to different elements in the domain. Thus no two elements in the domain have the same image in the co-domain. This is why the function is one-one.

The co-domain also consists of those elements which are not the square of any positive integres and hence $f(A) \subseteq B$.

$\therefore f$ is an into function.

Example 3: If I is the set of interges and $f: I \rightarrow I$ is defined by $f(x) = x$, prove that f is a onto mapping

Hint: Do yourself.

Example 4: Test whether the following functions are indentical.
(1) $f(x) = \log_{10}x^2$ and $h(x) = 2 \log_{10}x$ in the interval $(0, \infty)$

(3) $f(x) = x$ and $h(x) = \sqrt{x^2}$ in the interval $[0, \infty)$.

Ans. Yes. **Hint:** Do yourself.

Example 5: $f, h,$ and g are functions of real numbers into function of real numbers defined by (1) $f(x) = x^2$ (2) $h(y) = y^2$ (3) $g(z) = z^2$.

Which of these functions are equal.

Ans. All are equal. Do yourself.

Example 6: $f: R \rightarrow R$ defined by $f(x) = 3x + 4$. Prove that f is one-one onto function.

Hint: Do yourself.

5. *Identity functions:* If $f: A \rightarrow A$ defined by $f(x) = x \quad \forall x \in A$ then f is called an identity function. In identity function each element is A relationship to the element itself.

Identify function is also some time known as an identitiy transformation. We denote it by I_A.

6. (i) *Constant function:* If $f: A \to B$ and each member of A is put into correspondence with the same element in B, then f is known as the constant function. If $f: R \to R$ defined by $f(x) = 3$, then f be a constant function.

(ii) *Restriction mapping:* If A_1 is the proper subset of A_2 and $f: A_1 \to B$ and $g: A_2 \to B$ are two mappings then f and g are equal on A_1. In this case $f_1: A_1 \to B$ is the restriction mapping of the extension mapping $g: A_2 \to B$.

7. *Production function:* If $f: A \to B$ and $g: B \to C$ then gof is a function from a into c and is called a product function or composition function of f and g. The product function is denoted by (gof) or (gf).

The diagram of the product funtion is

A f B g C gof

Example 1: Let $A = \{l, m, n\}$, $B = \{x, y, z\}$, $c = \{r, s, t\}$ as shown in the figures below where $f: A \to B_D$, $g: B \to C$.

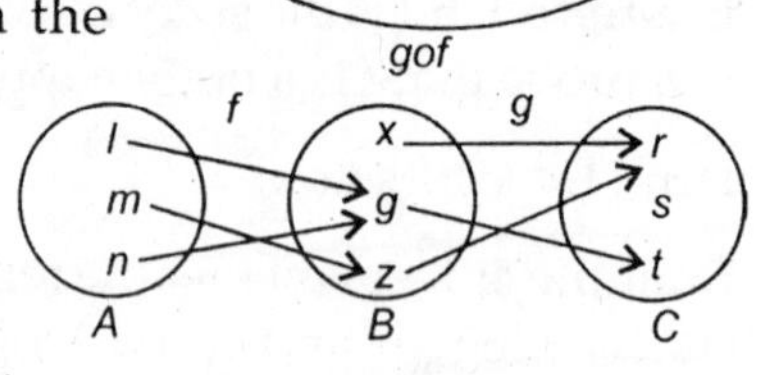

Find $gof(l)$, $gof(m)$ and $gof(n)$.

Solution: We have

$$gof(l) = g(f(l)) = g(y) = t$$
$$gof(m) = g(f(m)) = g(z) = r$$
$$gof(n) = g(f(n)) = g(y) = t$$

Example 2: If $f: A \to B$, prove that $I_B of = f$ and $fo I_A = f$.

Solution: Let $x \in A$ and $y \in B$ $\therefore$ $y = f(x)$

$$I_B of = I_B(f(x)) = I_B(y) = y = f(x)$$
$$fo I_A = f(I_A(x)) = f(x) = y$$
$$\therefore \quad I_B of = fo I_A.$$

Example 3: $f(x) = 1 - x$ and $g(x) = x^2$, find fog and gof, where $f: A \to B$ and $g: B \to C$.

Solution: $fog(x) = f(g(x)) = f(x^2) = 1 - x^2$

$$gof\,(x) = g(f(x)) = g(1 - x) = (1 - x)^2$$

Example 4: $f: A \to B$ and $g: B \to C$ defined by $f(x) = e^x$ and $g(x) = \log_e x$, find fog and gof.

Ans. $fog = gof = x$ where $x > 0$.

Hint: Do yourself.

Example 5: $f: A \to B$ and $g: B \to C$ defined by $f(x) = \sin x$ and $g(x) = \sin^{-1}x$, where $x \in [-\pi, \pi]$, find fog.

Ans. x. Do yourself.

8. *Associatively of the product function:* If $f: A \to B$, $g: B \to C$ and $h: C \to D$ then $gof: A \to C$ and $ho(gof): A \to D$

Similarly $hog: B \to D$ and $(hog)of: A \to D$.

Proof: Assume $J = gof$.

We have $gof: A \to C$

$\therefore \quad J: A \to C$

$h: C \to D$

$\therefore \quad hoJ: A \to D$

$\therefore \quad ho(gof): A \to D$

Again assume $hog = K$

$\therefore \quad K: B \to D$

$f: A \to B$

$\therefore \quad Kof: A \to D \quad \therefore (hog)of: A \to D$

$ho(gof)$ and $(hog)of$ are shown in Figure I and figure II.

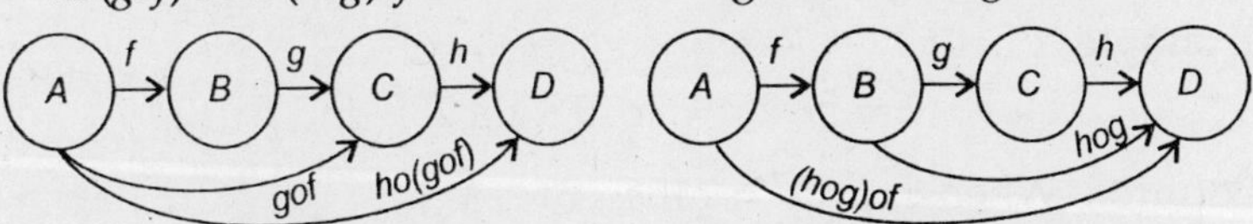

Figure I

Figure II

Example 1: If $f(x) = \dfrac{1}{1-x}$, find $fofof$.

Solution: $fofof(x) = fof\left(\dfrac{1}{1-x}\right)$

$$= f\left[\frac{1}{1-\frac{1}{x}}\right] = f\left(\frac{1-x}{1-x-1}\right) = f\left(\frac{x-1}{x}\right)$$

$$= \frac{1}{1-\frac{x-1}{x}} = \frac{x}{x-x+1} = x.$$

8. (i) *Inverse of a function:* Let $f: A \to B$ and $b \in B$ then the inverse of b consists of those elements belonging to A which are mapped onto b i.e. the elements of A whose image is b.

The inverse of b is denoted by

$$f^{-1}(b) = \{x: x \in A \text{ and } f(x) = b\}.$$

Example 1: $f: A \to B$ defined in the figure, find $f^{-1}(1), f^{-1}(2)$ and $f^{-1}(3)$.

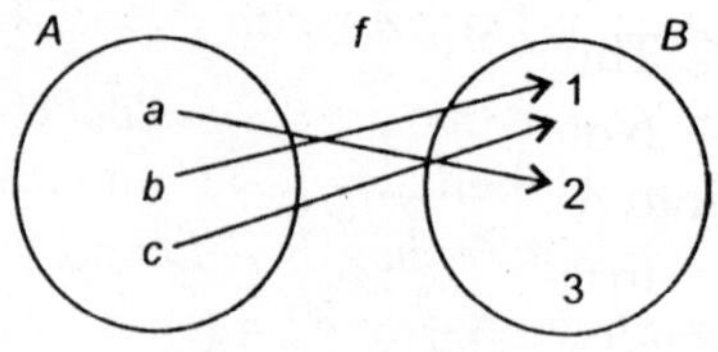

Figure Example 1

Solution: $f^{-1}(1) = \{b, c\}$

Since 1 is the image of the elements b and c in A.

$$f^{-1}(2) = \{a\}$$

and $f^{-1}(3) = \phi$. Since there is no elements in A whose image is 3.

Note: If $E \subseteq B$ and $f: A \to B$, then the inverse of E denoted by $f^{-1}(E)$ consists of those elements of A which are mapped onto some elements in E, i.e. $f^{-1}(E) = \{x: x \in A \text{ and } f(x) \in E\}$.

Thus f^{-1} has two pecularities viz.

(1) It is the inverse of an element of B

(2) It is the inverse of a subset of B.

Example 2: Let $f: R \to R$ defined by $f(x) = x^2$

$$E = [9, 25] = \{x : 9 \le x \le 25\}, \text{ find } f^{-1}(E).$$

Solution: When $f(x) = x^2 = 9$ then $x = \pm 3$

When $f(x) = x^2 = 25$ then $x = \pm 5$

$\therefore$ $f^{-1}(E) = \{x: -5 \le x \le -3 \text{ or } x \le x \le 5\}$

$= \{-3, 3, -5, 5\}$

$E = [9, 25]$ clearly indicates that $E \subseteq$ of the co-domain R.

Note 2: In the given Figure I, $f: A \to B$ is one-one as onto also.

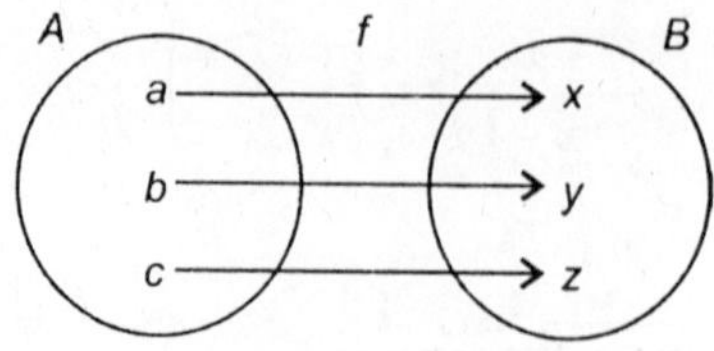

Figure I Note 2

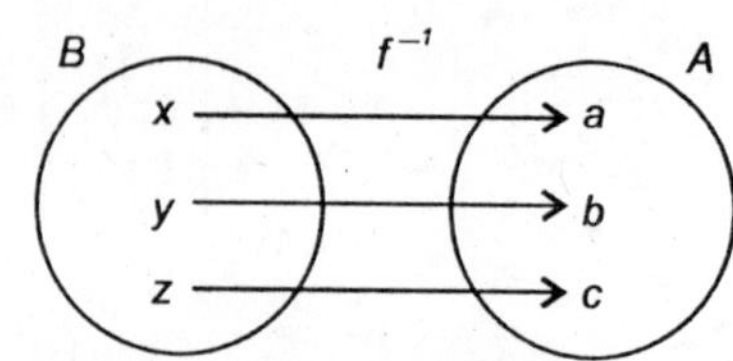

Figure II Note 2

In this case for each element belonging to B, the inverse of the elements of B will have only one element of A.

$\therefore$ $f^{-1}(x) = \{a\}$

$f^{-1}(y) = \{b\}$

$f^{-1}(z) = \{c\}$

Thus $f^{-1}: B \rightarrow A$ which is shown in Figure II.

Note 3: In the Figure I, the product function f^{-1} of maps A into A where $f: A \rightarrow B$ has an inverse $f^{-1}: B \rightarrow A$.

In the figure II, the product function fof^{-1} maps B into B, where $f^{-1}: B \rightarrow A$ and $f: A \rightarrow B$.

Thus $(f^{-1}of): A \rightarrow A$ and $(fof^{-1}): B \rightarrow B$ are respectively identity functions on A and B.

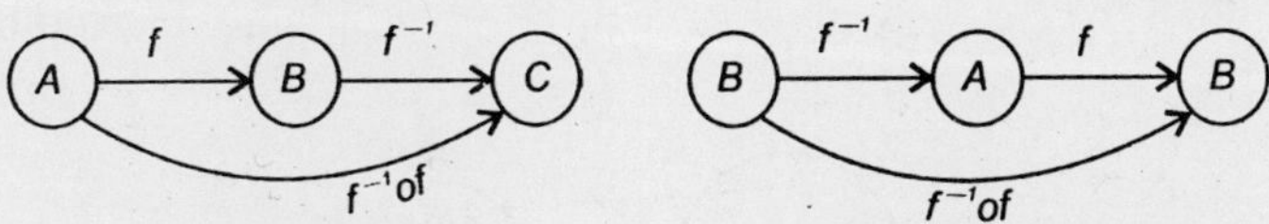

Figure I Note 3 **Figure II Note 3**

Example3: The mapping $f: R \rightarrow R$ given by $f(x) = x(x)$ is ......

(a) one to one but not onto

(b) onto but not one to one

(c) both one to one and onto

(d) neither one to one not onto. (I.S.M. Dhanbad 1994)

Solution: We have $f(x) = x^2$ if $x \geq 0$ and $f(x) = -x^2$ if $x < 0$.

Let there be two real numbers x_1 and x_2 then

$$f(x_1) = f(x_2) \Rightarrow x_1^2 = x_2^2 \Rightarrow (x_1 - x_2)(x_1 + x_2) = 0$$

If $x_1 = x_2$ then f is one-one.

If $x_1 = -x_2$ then $f(x_1) = f(-x_2)$

$\Rightarrow$ $x_1^2 \neq -x_2^2 = f(x_2)$

$\therefore f$ is also one-one. If x_1 and x_2 are negative thus

$$f(x_1) = f(x_2)$$

$\Rightarrow$ $-x_1^2 = -x_2^2$

$\Rightarrow$ $x_1^2 = x_2^2 \Rightarrow (x_1 - x_2)\,(x_1 - x_2) = 0$

If $x_1 = x_2$ then f is one-one. If $x_2 = -x_1$ then f is also one-one. For positive real numbers their pre images $\sqrt{x} \in R \ \forall \ x \in R$.

The pre image of negative real numbers are $-\sqrt{x} \in R$

$\therefore$ f is one to one and onto.

$\therefore$ alternative (*c*) is correct.

PROBLEMS AND EXERCISES 2(A)(I)

1. $f: A \rightarrow B$. Write true or false for the following diagrams.

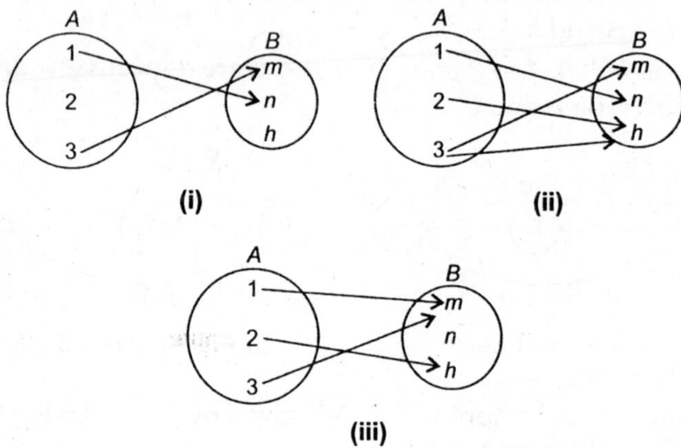

2. State whether the following three diagrams define a function of $\{a, b, c\}$ into $\{x, y, z\}$.

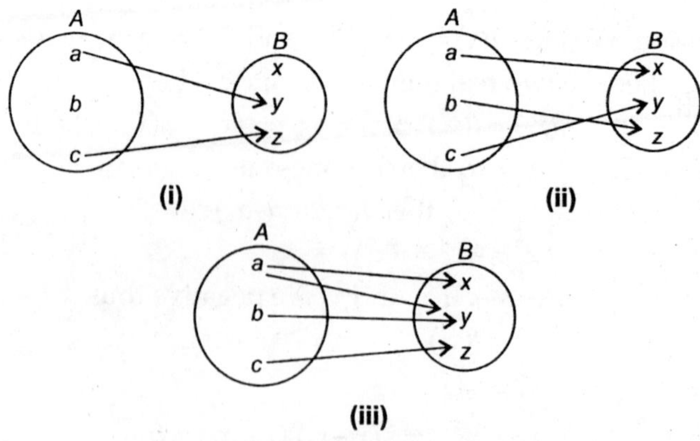

3. $g: R \to R$ defined by $g(x) = x^2 - 4x + 3$.

Compute $g(4)$, $q(-3)$, $g(y-2z)$ and $g(x-2)$.

4. $f: R \to R$ defined by $f(x) = \begin{cases} 2x^3 + 1 & x \le 2 \\ \dfrac{1}{x-2} & 2 < x \le 3 \\ 2x - 5 & x > 3 \end{cases}$ compute

$f(\sqrt{2})$, $f(\sqrt{8})$, $f(\sqrt{\log_2 1024})$

5. $f: R \to R$ defined by

$$f(x) = \begin{cases} 3^x & -1 < x < 0 \\ 4 & 0 \le x < 1 \\ 3x - 1 & 1 \le x \le 3 \end{cases}$$

compute $f(2)$, $f(0)$, $f\left(\frac{1}{2}\right)$, $f\left(-\frac{1}{2}\right)$, $f(3)$.

6. $g: R \to R$ defined by $g(x) = x^2 - 3x + 2$ compute $g(0)$, $g(1)$, $g(2)$, $g(3)$, $g(-x)$, $g\left(\frac{1}{x}\right)$, $g(x + 1)$.

7. $f: R \to R$ defined by $f(x) = \begin{cases} 1 & \text{if } x \text{ is rational} \\ 0 & \text{if } x \text{ is irrational} \end{cases}$

compute $f\left(\frac{1}{2}\right)$, $f(\sqrt{3})$, $f(\sqrt{2})$, $f\left(\frac{3}{4}\right)$, $f(\pi)$

8. If $A = \{x, y, z\}$ and $B = \{1, 0\}$ how many functions are there in the following diagrams?

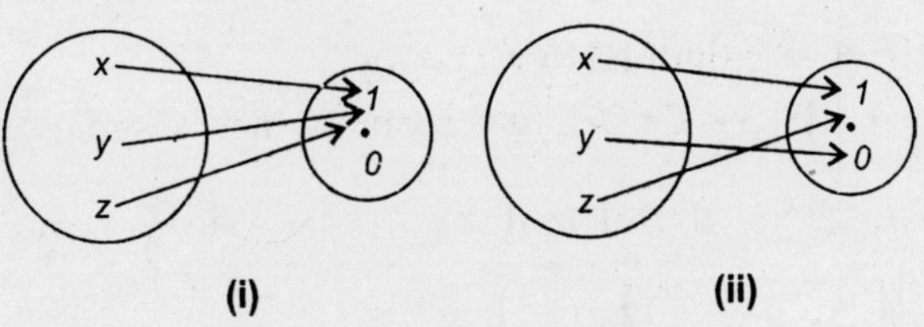

(i) (ii)

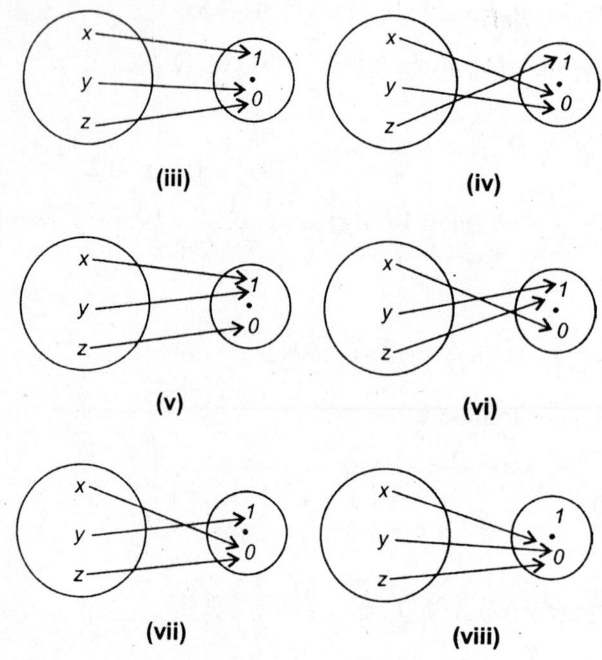

Name those functions.

9. (i) $f: A \to B$ defined by $f(x) = x^2$
$A = \{x: -1 \le x \le 2\}$, find B onto which the set A is mapped

(ii) $f: A \to B$ defined by $f(x) = |x|$.
$A = [1, 2]$, find B onto which A is mapped.

(iii) $f: A \to B$ defined by

(a) $f(x) = \dfrac{x}{2x-1}$

(b) $f(x) = \sqrt{x - x^2}$

and $A = \{x: 0 < x < 1\}$, find B on which A is mapped.

(iv) $f: A \to B$ defined by $f(x) = \log_3 x$.
$A = \{x: 3 < x < 27\}$, find B onto which a is mapped.

(v) $f: A \to B$ defined by $f(x) = \sin\dfrac{\pi x}{2}$ and $A = \left\{x: 0 \le x < \dfrac{1}{2}\right\}$, find B onto which A is mapped.

10. $A = \{1, 2, 3, 4\}$ and f, g, h are mappings from A into A is shown in the diagrams given below, find the range of f, g, h.

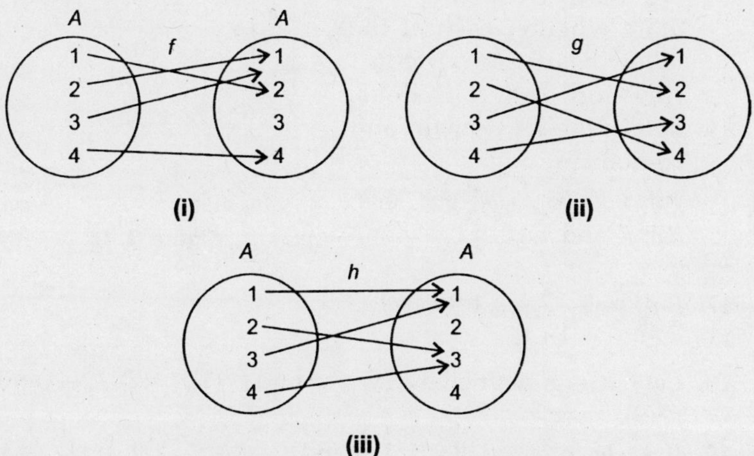

(i) (ii) (iii)

11. $A = \{-2, -1, 0, 1, 2\}$ and $f: A \rightarrow R$ defined by $f(x) = x^2 - x - 2$, find the range of f.

12. If $f: \{x: -2 \leq x \leq 2\} \rightarrow R$, $q: \{x: 0 \leq x \leq 3\} \rightarrow R$ and $h: \{x: -3 \leq x \leq 0\} \rightarrow R$ and each of these is defined by function of $x = x^3$. Find the range of f, g and h.

13. If $f: A \rightarrow B$, write Yes or No, whether each of the following defines a one-one function.

(i) $f(a) = f(b) \Rightarrow a = b$ (ii) $a = b \Rightarrow f(a) = f(b)$

(iii) $f(a) \neq f(b) \Rightarrow a \neq b$ (iv) $a \neq b \Rightarrow f(a) \neq f(b)$

14. If $f: A \rightarrow B$ is one-one, $g: B \rightarrow C$ is also one-one. Prove that $gof: A \rightarrow C$ is one-one.

(Hint: See answer sheet)

15. If $f: A \rightarrow B$. Write True or False for the following statements:

(1) $f(A)$ is a subset of B

(2) $f(A)$ is equal to B

(3) $f(A)$ is a superset of B.

16. The functions $f: A \to B$, $g: B \to A$, $h: C \to B$, $\phi: B \to C$ and $\psi: A \to C$ are shown in the adjoining figure.

State whether each of the followings defines a product function and if it does, determine its domain and co-domain.

$go f$, $ho f$, $\phi o f$, $\psi o f$, $go h$, $\phi o h$, $ho\psi o g$ and $ho\psi$.

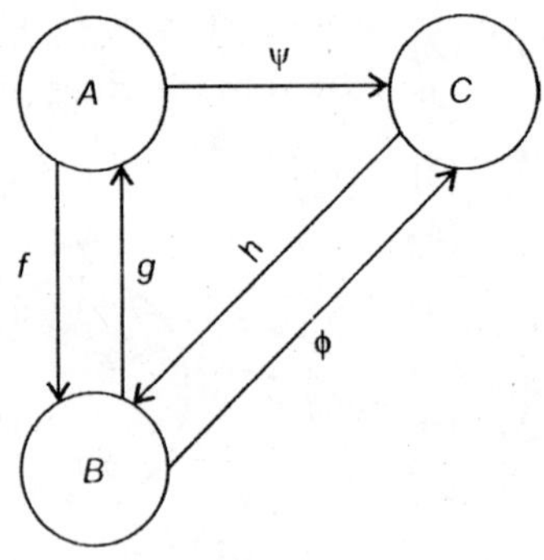

Figure Q. 16

17. If $f(x) = \dfrac{x}{\sqrt{1+x^2}}$, find $fofof$.

18. Let $f: R \to R$ defined by $f(x) = x^2$ find $f^{-1}(1), f^{-1}(2), f^{-1}(4)$ and $f^{-1}(9)$.

19. If $A = \{a_1, a_2, a_3, a_4\}$, $B = \{1, 2, 3\}$ and $a_1 \to 1, a_2 \to 2, a_3 \to 1, a_4 \to 3$, then the mapping is (a) one-one onto (b) many one and ont (c) one-one into (d) many one into.

20. If the set $A = \{x: x \in R, x \neq 0\}$, then the mapping $f: A \to A$ defined by $f(x) = \dfrac{1}{x}$ is

(a) one-one into (b) one-one onto
(c) many-one onto (d) none of the above.

21. The function $f: N \to N$ defined by $f(x) = x$ is

(a) one-one and onto (b) one-one and into
(c) many one and into (d) many one and onto.

22. The function $f: \left[-\dfrac{\pi}{2}, \dfrac{\pi}{2}\right] \to [-1, 1]$ defined by $f(x) = \sin x$ is

(a) one-one and onto (b) one-one but not onto
(c) many-one and onto (d) many-one but not onto.

23. $f: R \to R$ defined by $f(x) = x^2 + 2$, find the value of
(1) $f^{-1}(6)$ (2) $f^{-1}(0)$, (3) $f^{-1}(-6)$ (4) $f^{-1}([18, 27])$ (5) $f^{-1}([2, 6])$.

Hint: (1) For $f^{-1}(6)$, we put $x^2 + 2 = 6$

$\Rightarrow x = \pm 2 \quad \therefore \; f^{-1}(6) = \{-2, 2\}$

(2) For $f^{-1}(0)$, put $x^2 + 2 = 0 \therefore x^2 = -2$

$\therefore f^{-1}(0) = \phi$ as $x \notin R$

(3) Similarly $f^{-1}(6) = \phi$

(4) $18 \le x^2 + 2 \le 27 \Rightarrow +16 \le x^2 \le 25$

$\therefore f^{-1}([18, 27]) = \{x: -5 \le x \le -4 \text{ or } 4 \le x \le 5\}$

(5) Do yourself. **Ans.** $\{x: -2 \le x \le 0 \text{ or } 0 \le x \le 2\}$

24. In a class of 100 students, 55 students have passed in mathematics and 67 students have passed in physics. Then the number of students who have passed in physics only is (a) 22 (b) 33 (c) 10 (d) 45. [I.S.M 1994]

25. A and B are two sets containing 4 and 8 elements respectively. What is the maximum and minimum elements is A ∪ B. **(Hint:** See the answer sheet)

ANSWERS TO PROBLEMS AND EXERCISES 2A (I)

1. (i) False (ii) False (iii) True

2. (i) No (ii) Yes (iii) No.

3. 3, 24, $(y - 2z)^2 - 4y + 8z + 3$, $x^2 - 8x + 15$

4. $4\sqrt{2}+1, \dfrac{\sqrt{2}+1}{2}, 2\sqrt{10}-5$

5. $5, 4, 4, \dfrac{\sqrt{3}}{3}, 8.$

6. $2, 0, 0, 2, x^2+3x+2, \dfrac{1-3x+2x^2}{x^2}, x^2-x$

7. 1, 0, 0, 1, 0

8. (i) and (viii) constant function

(ii), (iii), (iv), (v), (vi), and (vii) onto function

9. (i) $B = \{0, 4\}$ (ii) $B = [1, 2]$ (iii) (a) $(-\infty, 0) \cup (1, +\infty)$

(b) $\left(0, \dfrac{1}{\sqrt{2}}\right]$ (iv) (1, 3) (v) $\left[0, \dfrac{1}{\sqrt{2}}\right)$.

10. (i) $\{1, 2, 4\}$ (ii) $\{1, 2, 3, 4\}$ (iii) $\{1, 3\}$

11. $\{-2, 0, 4\}$

12. [–8, 8], [0, 27], [–27, 0]

13. (i) Yes (ii) No (iii) No (iv) Yes.

14. **Hints:** If is sufficiant for us to prove

$$(gof)\,(a) = (gof)(c) \Rightarrow a = c$$

Let $\quad (gof)\,(a) = (gof)\,(c)$

$\therefore \quad g(f(a)) = g(f(c))$

Since g is one-one $\therefore f(a) = f(c)$

Since f is one-one $\therefore a = c$

$\therefore$ *gof* is one-one.

15. (1) True (2) False (3) False.

16. $gof: A \to A$; *hof* is not defined; $\phi of: A \to C$; $\psi\, of$ is not defined; $goh: c \to A$; $\phi oh: c \to c$; $ho\psi og: B \to B$; $ho\psi: A \to B$

17. $$\frac{x}{\sqrt{1+3x^2}}$$

18. {1, –1}, ϕ, {–2, 2}, {–3, 3}

19. (b) (20) (b) (21). (b) (22) (a)

24. (d)

25. 8, 12

Hint: Take the advantage of the formula

$$n(A \cup B) = n(A) + n(B) - n(A \cap B)$$

For maximum $n(A \cap B)$ we have

$$n(A \cap B) = 4 \text{ and } A \subseteq B$$

$\therefore$ $[n(A \cup B)]$ maximum $= 4 + 8 - 4 = 4$

For minimum $n(A \cup B)$ we have

$$n(A \cap B) = 0 \text{ and } A \cap B = \phi$$

$\therefore$ $[n(A \cup B)]$ minimum $= 4 + 8 - 0 = 12$

2.9 GRAPH OF THE FUNCTION

If f is a mapping of A into B i.e. $f: A \to B$, we define graph of the function f to be the set of points or set of all ordered pairs (a, b) which satisfies the following conditions:

(1) every point (a, b) where $b = f(a)$ belongs to the set.

(2) every point which belongs to the set has co-ordinates (a_1, b_1) such that $b_1 = f(a_1)$. The elements of the set A are generally

shown on the horizontal axis (abscissa axis) and the elements of the set B on the vertical axis (the axis of ordinates).

If $f: A \to B$ then its graph is

$$F = \{(a, b): a \in A, b = f(a)\}$$

The graph F is a subset of $A \times B$.

We thus see that the graph of the function f consists of all the ordered pairs in which the first element belongs to A and the image of the first element belongs is the second component of the ordered pair.

Example 1: If $A = \{1, 2, 3, 4, 5\}$ and $f: A \to R$ defined by $f(x) = x^2+2x-1$, find the graph of the function f.

Solution: We have

$$f(x) = x^2 + 2x - 1$$

$$\therefore \quad f(1) = 1^2 + 2.1 - 1 = 2$$

$$f(2) = 2^2 + 2.2 - 1 = 7$$

$$f(3) = 3^2 + 2.3 - 1 = 14$$

$$f(4) = 4^2 + 2.4 - 1 = 23$$

$$f(5) = 5^2 + 2.5 - 1 = 34$$

$\therefore$ The graph of the function f is

$$F = \{(1, 2)\ (2, 7)\ (3, 14)\ (4, 23)\ (5, 34)\}$$

2.10 CHARACTERISTICS OF THE GRAPH OF A FUNCTION

The graph of a function has the following two characteristics:

(1) For every $a \in A$ these exists an ordered pair $(a, b) \in F$ where F is the graph of the function f and $f: A \to B$.

(2) Every $a \in A$ appears as the first element in only one ordered pair in F.

$\therefore$ We can say if $(a, b) \in F$ and $(a, c) \in F$

Then $b = c$.

2.11 CHARACTERISTICS OF THE GRAPH *F* ON THE DIAGRAMS IN THE COORDINATE PLANE

Each vertical line contains at least one point of F and each vertical line contains only one point of F, where F is the graph of the function f.

Example 1: $A = \{1, 2, 3, 4\}$ and $f: A \to A$ defined by $f(1) = 3$; $f(2) = 2$; $f(3) = 4$ and $f(4) = 2$, find the graph of f. Show the graph of f on the diagram in the coordinate plane of $A \times A$.

Solution: The required graph is the set of ordered pairs,

$F = [(1, 3), (2, 2), (3, 4), (4, 2)]$

The graph is shown on the diagram in the coordinate plane.

Note: If $f: A \to A$ be one-one and onto then the inverse function f^{-1} consists of those ordered pairs which when reversed belong to f, i.e. $f^{-1} = \{(b, a) : (a, b) \in f\}$.

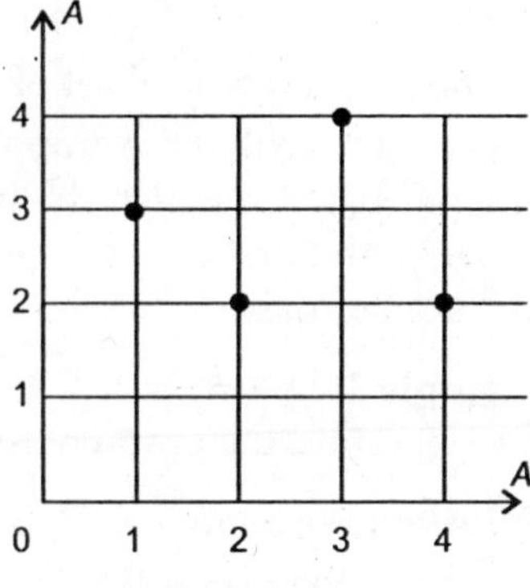

Figure Example 1

2.12 FUNCTIONS AS SETS OF ORDERED PAIRS

We know that for $a \in A$ there exists an ordered pair (a, b) which belongs to the graph of the function. Where $f: A \to B$. In addition, no two different ordered pairs in F have the same first element. Thus by a rule we assign the elemnets $b \in B$ to every element $a \in A$. This rule appears in the ordered pairs $(a, b) \in F$. We can thus say that every element in A will have an image and that image is unique and that is why F is a function of A into B.

"A function of A into B is a subset of $A \times B$ in which $a \in A$ is the first component in one and only one ordered pair belonging to the function".

This definitaion of a function does not include the word" assigns', 'rule', 'corresondence' etc.

Example 1: $A = \{1, 2, 3\}$, $B = \{a, b, c\}$ and $f = \{(1, b), (3, a), (2, b)\}$. Is f a function of A into B?

Solution: Here the function f has the characteristics.

(1) For $1 \in A$ these exists an ordered pair $(1, b) \in f$.

(2) No two different oıdered pairs in f are there whose first elements are the same.

Therefore f is a function of A into B. The figure is as follows:

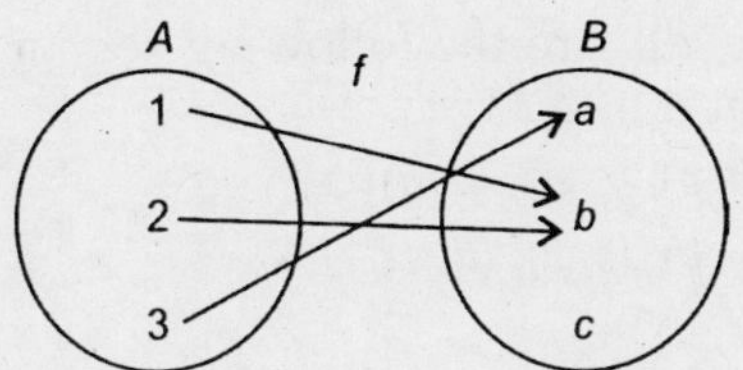

PROBLEMS AND EXERCISES 2A (II)

1. If $A = \{1, 2, 3\}$ and $f: A \to R$ defined by $f(x) = x^2$, find the graph of f.
2. $L = \{a, c, e, m\}$ and to each letter in L the function h assigns the letters which come after it in the alphabet. Find the graph of h.
3. $f: I \to R$ and $I = \{1, 2, 3, 4\}$. The function f is defined by $f(x) = x^3$. Find the graph of f.
4. Let $g: R \to R$ defined by $g(x) = x + 2$. Write Yes or No for the following ordered pairs belonging to the graph of the function g.
   (a) (2, 4) (b) (8, 10) (c) (–1, 2) and (d) (4, 6).
5. Let $A = \{a, e, i, o, u\}$. To every letter in A the function h assigns the letter which follows it is the alphabet. Find the graph of h.
6. If $A = \{1, 2, 3, 4\}$. State whether each of the following sets of ordered pairs is a function of A into A.
   (1) $f_1 = \{(2, 2), (1, 3), (2, 1), (3, 2), (4, 3)\}$
   (2) $f_2 = \{(3, 4), (1, 4), (2, 1), (4, 4), (2, 1)\}$
   (3) $f_3 = \{(2, 1), (3, 2), (4, 1)\}$
   (4) $f_4 = \{(1, 2), (2, 3), (3, 4), (4, 6)\}$.
7. If $A = \{a, b, c\}$. State whether the set of points in the folllowing diagrams of $A \times A$ represents a function from A into A.

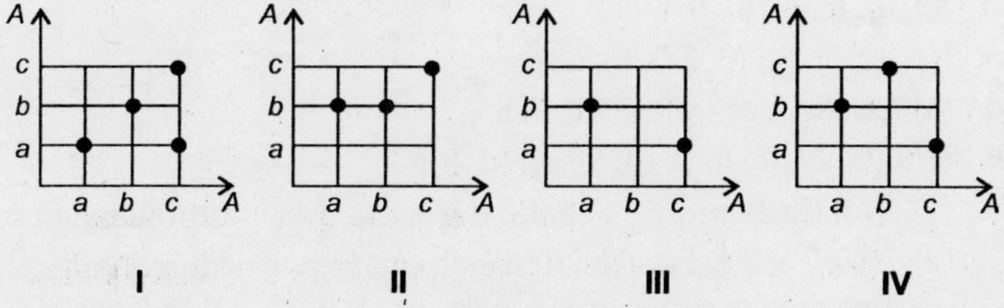

8. If $A = \{a, b, c, d\}$. Are the following sets of ordered pairs function from A into A?
   (i) $\{(a, d), (b, a), (c, d), (d, a)\}$
   (ii) $\{(a, b), (b, b), (c, b), (d, c)\}$
   (iii) $\{(d, b), (d, d), (c, a)\}$
   (iv) $\{(a, a), (a, b), (b, c), (b, d)\}$.
9. (a) If $N = \{1, 2, 3, 4, 5\}$ and $f: N \to N$. Is the set of ordered pairs $\{(1, 2), (2, 1), (3, 5), (4, 4), (5, 2)\}$ a function of N into N?
   (b) If $N = \{1, 2, 3, 4, 5\}$ and $g: N \to N$. Is the set of ordered pairs $\{(1, 1), (2, 3), (3, 5), (4, 3), (5, 1)\}$ a function of N into N?
10. Find $f(1), f(2), f^{-1}(2), f^{-1}(4)$ of Q. No. 9(a).
11. Find $g(1), g(2), g^{-1}(1)$ of Q. No. 9(b).
12. Taking the advantage of Q. No. 9 (a) and 9(b) prove that $fog \neq gof$.
13. There are three sets A, B, C such that $A = B \cap C$. Write ture or false for the following relations.
   (a) $A \times A = (B \times B) \cap (C \times C)$
   (b) $A \times A = (B \times C) \times (C \times B)$.
   Hint: Put $A = \{4, 5\}$, $B = \{3, 4, 5\}$ and $C = \{4, 5\}$ and other then obtain the result.
14. If $A = \{1, 2, 3, 4\}$ and the set $\{(1, 2), (2, 4), (3, 1), (4, 3)\}$ is a one-one and onto funtion of A into A. Find the inverse of f.
    Hint: When the function is one-one and onto then the inverse function consists of these ordered pairs which when reversed belong to the function.

ANSWERS TO PROBLEMS AND EXERCISES 2A (II)

1. $F = \{(1, 1), (2, 4), (3, 9)\}$.
2. $\{(a, b), (c, d), (e, f)\}$
3. $\{(1, 1), (2, 8), (3, 27), (4, 64)\}$
4. (a) Yes (b) Yes (c) No (d) Yes.
5. $H = \{(a, b), (e, f), (i, g), (o, p), (u, v)\}$
6. (1) No. (2, 2) and (2, 1) have the same first component.
   (2) Yes. 2 appears as the first element in two ordered pairs, but they are the same.

(3) No. $1 \in A$ does not appear as the first element in any ordered pair of f_3.

(4) No. Thougth every element of A appears as the first element in one and only one ordered pair but $f_4 \not\subseteq A \times A$. We see that $(4, 6) \in f_4 \not\Rightarrow (4, 6) \in A \times A$.

7. In Fig. I No. This diagram does not represent a function as the vertical line though C contains two points of the set.

In Fig. II Yes. This diagram represents a function from A into A. The horizontal line through b contains two points not violating the characteristics of the function. The vertical line contains one and only one point of the set.

In Fig. III No. The vertical line through b does not contain any point.

In Fig. IV Yes. Each vertical line contains one and only one point of the set.

8. (i) Yes (ii) Yes (iii) No (iv) No.

9. (a) Yes (b) Yes

10. 2, 1, {1, 5}, {4}

11. 1, 3, {1, 5}

13. (a) true (b) true.

14. {(2, 1), (4, 2), (1, 3), (3, 4)}.

Chapter 2 (B)
Relation, its Types, Domain Range and Graphs

2.13 RELATIONS

The word " Relation" means similarily connecting things or persons. *A* relation may exist between two things, objcets or persons. In the set theory we need two sets A and B and an open sentence of the type $P(x, y)$ in ordered to define a relation.

Let the open sentence $p(x, y)$ represents " x is greater than y", then $P(4, 3)$ is an open sentence which is true, but $P(1, 2)$ in this case is a false open sentence. Thus a relation consists of a set A, a set B and an open sentence $P(x, y)$ where $P(a, b)$ for any ordered pair $(a, b) \in A \times B$ is either true or false. A relation is denoted by

$$R = (A, B, P(x, y)).$$

If $P(c, d)$ is true, then we write c is related to d i.e. cRd.

If $P(c, d)$ is false, then we write c is not related to d i.e. $c \not R d$.

Example 1: $R_1 = (A, B, P(x, y))$ where A is the set of boys and B is the set of girls and $P(x, y)$ is an open surface which reads x is the brother of y. Is R_1 a relation?

Ans. Yes.

Example 2: $R_2 = (A, B, P(x, y))$. $P(x, y)$ is an open surface which reads x is the husband of y where A is the set of cars and B is the set of scooters. Is R_2 a relation?

Solution: In this case, R_2 is not a relation since $P(a, b)$ is meaningless. $P(a, b)$ has no sentence when we say car is the husband of scooter or the car is divided by scooter.

Note: If $R = (A, B\ P(x, y))$ is a relation, then we can say that the open sentence $p(x, y)$ defines a relation from A to B.

If $A = B$ then $P(x, y)$ defines a relation in A i.e. R is a relation in A.

Example 3: R is a relation from A to B defined by an open sentence " x is less than y". $A = \{5, 6, 7\}$, $B = \{8, 3, 2\}$.

Write R as an ordered pair.

Ans. $R = \{(5, 8), (6, 8), (7, 8)\}$.

2.14 GRAPHS OF RELATIONS AND SOLUTION SETS

If $R = (A, B, P(x, y))$ be a relation then the solution set J of the relation R consists of those elements (a, b) in $A \times B$ for which the open sentence $P(a, b)$ is true.

Mathematically, we can write

$$J = \{(a, b) : a \in A, b \in B, P(a, b) \text{ is true}\}.$$

Thus the solution set J of the relation R from A to B is clearly a subset of $A \times B$ and hence we cam sketch J on the diagram of $A \times B$ in the coordinate plane.

" The graph of a relation R from A to B consists of only those points on the diagram of $A \times B$ in the coordinate plane which belong to J i.e. the solution set of R."

Example 1: $R = (A, B, P(x, y))$.

$A = \{1, 3, 4\}$, $B = \{2, 3, 4, 5\}$ and the open sentence $P(x, y)$ reads – "x is less than y". What is the solution set of R? Show it on the diagram in the coordinate plan.

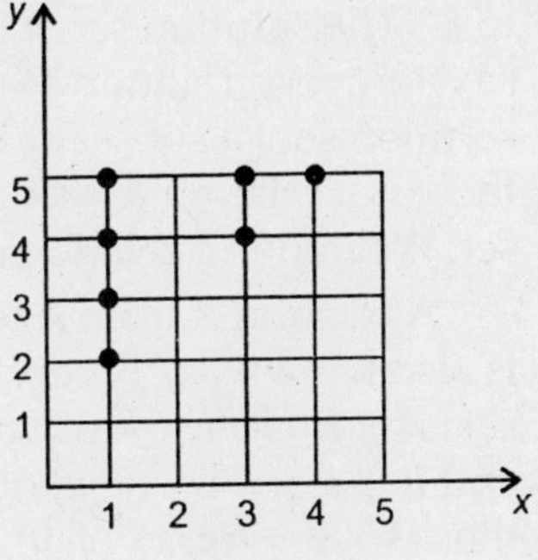

Figure I

Solution: The solution set of R will contain those ordered pairs of $A \times B$ in which first element is less than the second.

The solution set J is shown on the diagram is the coordiante plane in Fig. I.

Example 2: Let R be the relation in the real numbers defined by $y < 2 - x$. Sketch the relation on the diagram of $R \times R$ in the coordinate plane.

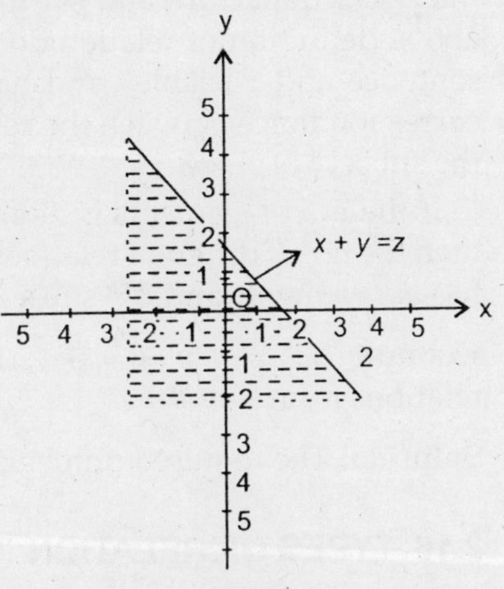

Figure II

Solution: The real numbers in the left of O are negative. Similarly real numbers below O are also negative. First of all the line $x + y = 2$ is drawn in the usual way. The shaded area (by dotted lines ...) in Fig. II consists of those points which belong to J (the solution set of R) below the line $x + y = 2$.

Note: To sketch a relation on the axis of real numbers defined by an open sentence of the form $y = f(x)$, $y > f(x)$, $y \geq f(x)$, $y < f(x)$ and $y \leq f(x)$ the readers are advised to plot first $y = f(x)$. Then the relation (the required set) will consist of points respectively on $y = f(x)$, above $y = f(x)$, above on $y = f(x)$, below $y = f(x)$ and below and on $y = f(x)$.

2.15 RELATIONS AS SETS OF ORDERED PAIRS

Let J be a subset of $A \times B$. We have $R = (A, B, P(x, y))$, where the open sentence $P(x, y)$ read,—" The ordered pair (x, y) belongs to J." The solution set of the relation R is the set J. We can thus say to every relation $R = (A, B, \ P(x, y))$ there is a unique solution set J a subset of $A \times B$ and to every subset of J of $A \times B$ there is a relation $R = (A, B, \ P(x, y))$ for which J is its solution set. We define a relation now as follows:

"A relation R from A to B is a subset of $A \times B$." This relation is also known as "Binary Relation". This relation between two sets $A \times B$ is a set R of ordered pairs (x, y) where $x \in A, y \in B$ and $R \subseteq A \times B$ i.e. $(x, y) \in R \Leftrightarrow xRy$. If $A = \{a, b, c\}$, and $B = \{x, y\}$ then $A \times B = \{(a, x), (a, y), (b, x), (b, y), (c, x), (c, y)\}$.

If R is $\{(a, x), (b, y), (c, x)\}$ then we can say $R \subseteq A \times B$ and therefore R is a relation from A to B. A and B are also known as the set of departure and set fo destination respectively. The above definition of relation does not contain the word "open sentence and variable" and has been given due to one-one correspondance between the relation $R = (A, B, \ P(x, y))$ and the subset J of $A \times B$.

If the no. of elements in A and B are respectively m and n, then the no. of different relations from A to B be 2^{mn} since $A \times B$ has mn elements and 2^{mn} subsets.

Example 1: $A = \{x, y\}$, $B = \{1, 2, 3\}$, find the number of different relations from A to B.

Solution: The required number is 2^6.

2.16 TYPES OF RELATION

Now we shall describe some relations.

(1) *Inverse relation:* The inverse relation of R from A to B is a relation from B to A defined by

$$R^{-1} = \{(b, a) : (a, b) \in R\}$$

The inverse relation R^{-1} contains those ordered pairs which when reversed belong to R.

Example 1: If $A = \{a, b, c\}$ and $B = \{1, 2\}$ and R is a relation from A to B given by $R = \{(a, 1), (b, 2), (c, 2)\}$ find R^{-1}.

Solution: Since $R = \{(a, 1), (b, 2), (c, 2)\}$

Hence $R^{-1} = \{(1, a), (2, b), (2, c)\}$

(2) *Reflexive relation:* If $R \subseteq A \times A$, then R is called a reflexive relation if every element in A is related to itself, i.e., $(a, a) \in R \ \forall \ a \in A$.

Example 1: $A = \{1, 2, 3, 4\}$, then $R = \{(1, 1), (2, 2), (3, 3), (4, 4)\}$ is a reflexive relation.

Example 2: Let A be the set of triangles. The relation R in A is given by "x is similar to y". Is R a reflexive relation?

Solution: Here R is reflective relation since every triangle is similar to itself.

(3) *Symmetric relations:* Let R be a relation is A, then $R \subseteq A \times A$. We define R to be the symmetric relations if $(a, b) \in R \Rightarrow (b, a) \in R$.

In other words, we can also say if a is related to b then b is also related to a.

Example 1: Let A be the set of equal triangles and R be the relation in A given by " x is equal to y". Is R symmetric?

Solution: Hence R is symmetric, since if the triangle a is equal to b, then be is also equal to a.

Note: If $(a, b) \in R \Rightarrow (b, a) \in R^{-1}$, then R is symmetric relation if and only if $R = R^{-1}$.

(4) *Anti-symmetric relations:* If R is a relation in a set A i.e. $R \subseteq A \times A$, then it is called an anti-symmetric relation if

$(a, b) \in R$ and $(b, a) \in R \Rightarrow a = b$

i.e. If $A \neq b$ then aRb or bRa, but not both.

Example 1: Let $A = \{1, 2, 3\}$ and R is a relation is A where $R = \{(1, 2), (1, 3), (2, 3), (3, 2)\}$. Is R anti-symmetric?

Solution: Here $(2, 3) \in R$ and $(3, 2) \in R$ but $2 \neq 3$

$\therefore$ R is not an anti-symmetric relation is A.

Example 2: R is a relation is A, and $A \subseteq B$ and $B \subseteq A$, prove that R is anti-symmetric.

Solution: Let $x \in A$ and $y \in B$ $\therefore$ $x \in B$ and $y \in A$.

$\therefore$ $(x, y) \in R$ and $(y, x) \in R \Rightarrow x = y$

$\therefore$ R is anti-symmetric.

Note: The set of all ordered pairs $(a, a) \in A \times A$ is known as the diagonal line of $A \times A$ and is denoted by H. In this case, a relation R in A is anti-symmetric if and only if $R \cap R^{-1} \subseteq H$.

(5) *Transitive relations:* If R is a relation in A then R is called a transistive relation if $(a, b) \in R$ and $(b, c) \in R \Rightarrow (a, c) \in R$.

i.e., aRb, $bRc \Rightarrow aRc$.

Example 1: $A = \{1, 2, 3, 4\}$, $R = \{(1, 2), (2, 3), (1, 3)\}$ where $R \subseteq A \times A$. Show that R is trasitive.

Solution: We have $(1, 2) \in R, (2, 3) \in R$

$\Rightarrow (1, 3) \in R$

$\therefore$ R is transitive.

(6) *Equivalence relation:* Let R is a relation in A.

$\therefore$ $R \subseteq A \times A$. R is known as an equivalance relation if R is (i) reflexive (ii) Symmetre and (iii) transitive.

Example 1: R is a relation in N defined by an open sentence $P(x, y)$ which reads $x - y$ is divisible by 5. Prove that R is an equivalence relation.

Solution: Let $a \in N$ $\therefore$ $a - a = 0$ is divisible by 5.

$\therefore$ $(a, a) \in R$ and therefore R is reflexive.

Now if $(a, b) \in R$ then $(a - b)$ is divisible by 5

$\therefore$ $(b - a) = -(a - b)$ is also divisible by 5.

$\therefore$ $(b, a) \in R$.

$\therefore$ $(a, b) \in R \Rightarrow (b, a) \in R$

$\therefore$ R is symmetric.

Again if $(a, b) \in R$ and $(b, c) \in R$, then $a - b$ and $b - c$ are divisible by 5.

Now $a - c = (a - b) + (b - c)$ is divisible by 5.

$\therefore$ $(a, c) \in R$.

$\therefore$ $(a, b) \in R, (b, c) \in R \Rightarrow (a, c)\ R$

$\therefore$ R is transitive.

$\therefore$ R is an equivalence relation.

Example 2: Write down all the equivalence relation on the set $S = \{1, 2\}$. (Utkal B.Sc. 1978)

Solution: $\because$ $R \subseteq S \times S$

$\therefore$ R may be taken as $R = \{(1, 1), (1, 2), (2, 1), (2, 2)\}$

Here $(1, 1) \in R$ and $(2, 2) \in R$

$\therefore$ $(a, a) \in R$ $\quad$ $\therefore$ R is reflexive.

Again $(1, 2) \in R \Rightarrow (2, 1) \in R$

i.e. $(a, b) \in R \Rightarrow (b, a) \in R$

$\therefore$ R is symmetric.

Also $(1, 2) \in R$ and $(2, 1) \in R \Rightarrow (1, 1) \in R$

i.e. $(a, b) \in R$ and $(b, c) \in R \Rightarrow (a, c) \in R$

$\therefore$ R is transive.

Therefore R is an equivalence relation.

(6) *Identity relations:* The identity relation in A is the set of ordered pairs $\in A \times A$ represented by I_A is defined as

$$I_A = \{(x, y): x \in A, y \in A, x = y\}$$

Thus $$I_A = \{(x, x): x \in A\}$$

Example 1: If $A = \{a, b, c\}$, then $I_A = \{(a, a), (b, b), (c, c)\}$.

The identity relation is also known as diagonal relation. In addition, $I_A = (I_A)^{-1}$.

(7) *Universal relations:* If the set R is the set $A \times A$, then the relation R in A is called the universal relation.

Let $A = \{1, 2, 3\}$, then $R = \{(1, 1), (1, 2), (1, 3), (2, 1), (2, 2), (2, 3), (3, 1), (3, 2), (3, 3)\}$ is the universal relation is A.

(8) *Composition relations:* Let R be a relation A and B and S that between B and C then the composition relation between A and C is SoR and is defined as

$SoR = \{(x, z)$: iff $\exists$ a point $y \in B$ such that $(x, y) \in R$ and $(y, z) \in S\}$

If $R = \{(2, 3)$ and $S = (3, 4)\}$ then

$SoR = \{(2, 4)\}$ since there is 3 such that $(2, 3) \in R$ and $(3, 4) \in S$ but $RoS = \phi$.

2.17 DOMAIN AND RANGE OF A RELATION

Let $R \subseteq A \times B$ then the domain D of the relation R is the set formed by all the first elements of its ordered pairs.

Thus $D = \{x : (x, y) \in R \text{ and } x \in A\}$

The range E of the relation R is the set formed by all the second elements of its ordered pairs.

We can write $E = \{y : (x, y) \in R \text{ and } y \in B\}$

Example 1: Let $A = \{a, b, c, d\}$ and $B = \{1, 2, 3\}$ and $R = \{(b, 1), (d, 1), (d, 3)\}$, then $D = \{b, d\}$ and $E = \{1, 3\}$.

Note: We see that the domain of a relation from A to B is a subset of A and its range is a subset of B.

2.18 RELATIONS AND FUNCTIONS

In the previous article we saw $f : A \rightarrow B$ is a subset of $A \times B$ where $a \in A$ is present in only one order pair which belongs to f. In addition, a subset of $A \times B$ is a relation. A function has domain and range. A relation has also domain and range. What is the difference between a relation and a function?

Let us examine it with the help some solved examples.

Example 1: A relation R on the real numbers is defined by $x + y - 3 = 0$. R is shown on the diagram of $R_1 \times R_1$ is the coordinate plane where R_1 is the set fo real number B. Is R a function?

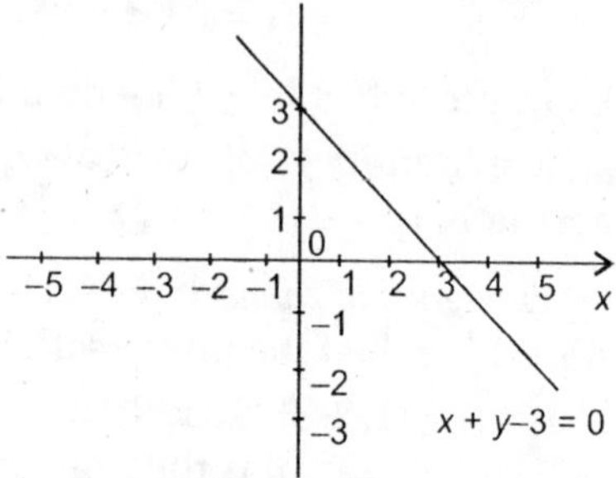

Figure Example 1

Solution: The relation is a straight line and each vertical line contains only one point of R. Thus R is a function,

$$\therefore x + y - 3 = 0 \therefore y = f(x) = -x + 3$$

i.e. we obtain a formula defining a function – R.

Example 2: *A* relation R on the real numbers is defined by $x^2 + y^2 = 16$. The relation is shown on the diagram of $R_1 \times R_1$ in the coordinate plane where R_1 is the set of real numbers. Is R a function?

Solution: We see that the relation R is a circle of radius 4. Different vertical lines contain more than one point $\in R$. This clearly shows R is not a function.

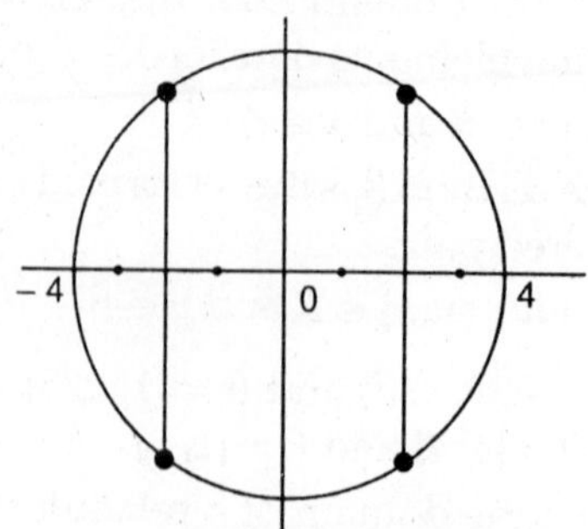

Figure Example 2

Example 3: $A = \{1, 2, 3, 4, 5\}$. The relation R is A is the set of points shown on the diagram of $A \times A$ is the coordiante plane. Find the domain, range and inverse of R. Draw R^{-1} on a diagram of $A \times A$ is the coordinate plane.

Solution: We have from figure

$$R = \{(2, 1), (2, 4), (4, 2), (4, 4), (5, 2)\}$$

The domain of R is $\{2, 4, 5\}$ and its range is $\{1, 2, 4\}$.

The inverse is

$$R^{-1} = \{(1, 2), (4, 2), (2, 4), (4, 4), (2, 5)\}$$

R^{-1} is shown on the diagram of $A \times A$ in the coordinate plane.

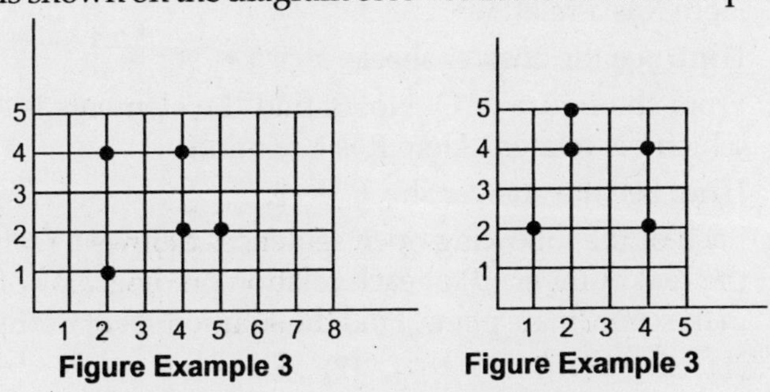

Figure Example 3 **Figure Example 3**

PROBLEMS AND EXERCISES 2B (I)

1. If R be a relation from $A = \{2, 3, 4, 5\}$ to $B = \{3, 6, 7, 10\}$ defined by an open sentence "x divides y". Express R as a set of orered pairs.
2. R is a relation from A to B defined by an open sentence "x is greater than". $A = \{3, 4\}$; $B = \{2, 3, 4, 5\}$. Express R as a set of ordered pairs.
3. R is a relation from A to B defined by an open sentence "x is equal to y".
   $A = \{3, 4\}$; $B = \{2, 3, 4, 5\}$. Express R as a set of ordered pairs.
4. R is a relation is A defined by an open sentence "x and y are prime relatively".
   $A = \{2, 3, 4, 7\}$. Express R as a set of ordered pairs.
   Hint: x and y are relatively prime if 1 is their common division.
5. R is a relation from N to N i.e. $R = (N, N, P(x, y))$. $P(x, y)$ reads "x divides y". If R a relation? Write Yes or No for the following symbolic representations $2 \not{R}\ 5, 3\, R\, 9, 5\, R\, 10, 7\, R\, 11$.

6. $A = \{a, b, c, d, e\}$ and R be a relation in A shown on the diagram of $A \times A$ is the coordinate plane.

   Write Yes or No for each of the following statements

   (i) $a\,R\,b$ (ii) $b\,R\,a$

   (iii) $c \not R\, c$ (iv) $d \not R\, b$

   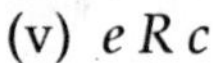

   (v) $e\,R\,c$

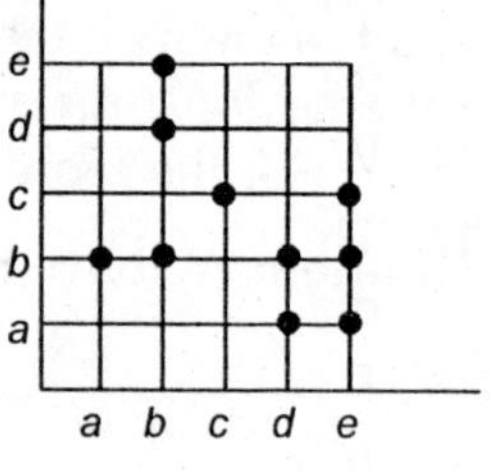

Figure Q. 6

7. From the figure of Q. No. 6, find all the elements in A which are related to c i.e. $\{x : (x, c) \in R\}$. Here R is a relation.

   Hint: See the answer sheet.

8. From the figure of Q. No. 6, find the elements is A with which e is related . Here R is a relation.

   Hint: See the answer sheet.

9. Each of the following open sentences defines a realtion in the real numbers. Plot each relation on diagrams of $R \times R$ in the coordinate plane. Find the solution set of the relation.

   (1) $x^2 + y^2 < 4$ (2) $x^2 + y^2 \geq 4$

   (3) $y^2 = x$ (4) $y \leq x^2$

   (5) $y \geq x^3$ (6) $\dfrac{x^2}{16} - \dfrac{y^2}{4} \geq 1$

   (7) $y \geq x$ (8) $x \geq |y|$

   (9) $\dfrac{x^2}{16} - \dfrac{y^2}{9} < 1$

10. Write T or F for the following definitions of a function.

    (1) We define a function by formulae of two variables. The example is $y = x^2$. This is the analytic method of defining a function.

    (2) The domain of the function is tabulated in one column. The range of the function is tabulated in the other column and then the function defined as $f = \{(1, 1), (2, 4), (3, 9), (4, 16)\}$ $\begin{bmatrix} 1 \\ 2 \\ 3 \\ 4 \end{bmatrix} \begin{bmatrix} 1 \\ 4 \\ 9 \\ 16 \end{bmatrix}$

(3) A function is defined by a graph.

(4) Every correspondence defined by a graph is a function.

11. Write the set of all non-zero numbers.

12. There are three elements in A and form in B. Find the no. of different relations from A to B.

13. R is a relation is A given by

$R = \{(x, y), (x, z), (z, z), (z, y)\}$

where $A = \{x, y, z\}$. Find R^{-1}.

14. Let R be the relation $<$ from $A = \{1, 2, 3, 4\}$ to $B = \{1, 3, 5\}$ i.e. $(a, b) \in R$ iff $a \in A, b \in B$ and $a < b$. Express R and R^{-1} as the set of ordered pairs. (Magadh B.Sc. 1976)

15. If R is a relation on A, prove that $(R^{-1})^{-1} = R$.

Hint: $R^{-1} = \{(b, a) : (a, b) \in R\}$

$\therefore \quad (R^{-1})^{-1} = \{(a, b) : (a, b) \in R\} = R$

16. Express relationships betweeen the domain and range of a relation R and its inverse.

17. Let A be the set of the first ten natural numbers from 1 to 10. R is a relation on A, defined by $x\ R\ y \Rightarrow x + 2y = 10$ $x, y \in A$. Find R^{-1}. (Agra B.Sc. 1981)

18. Let A be the set of first five natural numbers from 1 to 5. Let a relation R on A be defined by $x\ R\ y \Rightarrow x \leq y$. Find (i) R (ii) R^{-1} (iii) domain R (iv) domain R^{-1} and (v) range R^{-1}.

19. If $N = \{1, 2, 3 \,......\}$ and $R = \{(x, y) : x \in N, y \in N$ and $2x + y = 10\}$ in $N \times N$, find R^{-1}.

20. If R is a relation on A, Prove that $RoI_A = I_AoR$.

Hint: $R = \{(x, y) : x, y \in A\}$

$I_A = \{(y, y) : y \in A\}$

$\therefore \quad I_AoR = \{(x, y) : x, y \in A\} = R$

Again $I_A = \{(x, x) : x \in A\}$

$R = \{(x, y) : x, y \in A\}$

$\therefore \quad RoI_A = \{(x, y) : x, y \in A\} = R.$

21. If $R \subseteq A \times B$ and $S \subseteq B \times C$ be two relations, prove that $(SoR)^{-1} = R^{-1}\, oS^{-1}$

Hint: $R = \{(x, y) : x \in A, y \in B\}$

$S = \{(y, z) : y \in B, z \in c\}$

$\therefore \quad SoR = \{(x, z) :$ if and only if there exists a point $y \in B$ such that $(x, y) \in R$ and $(y, z) \in S\}$

$(SoR)^{-1} = \{(z, x) : z \in c, x \in A\}$

$S^{-1} = \{(z, y) : z \in c, y \in B\}$

$R^{-1} = \{(y, x) : y \in B, x \in A\}$

$\therefore \quad R^{-1}\, S^{-1}\, \{(z, x) : z \in c, x \in A\}$

22. Write Yes or No.

(i) Let A be the set of lives in a plane and R be a relation which reads "parallel to". Is R reflexive?

(ii) Let A be the set of member of a family and R be a relation which reads "is the follow of". Is R reflexive?

(iii) Let A be the set of all natural numbers and be a rational which reads "is equal to". Is R reflexive?

(iv) If R be a relation in N defined by "x is greater theory". Is R symmetric?

(v) If P is a family of sets and R is a relation in P which reads "x is a subset of y". Is R reflexive?

(vi) R is a relation is N defined by "a divides b". Is R anti-symmetric?

(vii) $A = \{a, b, c, d\}$ and R is a relative in a defined by $R = \{(a, b), (b, a)\}$. Is R anti-symmetric?

(viii) P is a family of sets and R is the relative in P defined by "x is a subset of y". Is R anti-symmetic and transitive?

23. (i) Is $R = \{(3, 3), (3, 4), (4, 3), (4, 4)\}$ an equivalence relation on the set $\{3, 4\}$?

(ii) Is R^{-1} symmetric if R is symmetric?

(iii) Is R^{-1} anti-symmetric if R is anti-symmetirc?

24. If (i) $R \cap R^{-1} = f$ and (ii) $R = R^{-1}$. What type of realtion in R?

25. Write the correct alternatives.

If R be a relation < from $A = \{1, 2, 3, 4\}$ to $B = \{1, 3, 5\}$ i.e. $(a, b) \in R$ if $A < b$ then R^{-1} is

(a) $\{(1, 3), (1, 5), (2, 3), (2, 5), (3, 5), (4, 5)\}$

(b) $\{(3, 1), (5, 1), (3, 2), (5, 2), (5, 3), (5, 4)\}$

(c) $\{(3, 3), (3, 5), (5, 3), (5, 5)\}$

(d) $\{(3, 3), (3, 4), (4, 5)\}$ (MLNRE 1984)

26. What the correct alternatives. $\frac{n}{m}$ means that n is a factor of m then the relation f is

(a) Reflexive and symmetric

(b) Transitive and symmetric

(c) Reflexive, transitive and symmetric

(d) Reflexive, transitive and non-symmetric.

(MNLNE 1985)

27. A relation in integres is defined by the open sentence $x\ R\ y \Leftrightarrow x$ is the square of y, which of the following statement is incorrect?

(a) $4\ R\ (-2)$ (b) $3\ R\ 9$

(c) $9\ R\ 3$ (d) $4\ R\ (2)$.

28. In the set of real numbers, the relation "greater then" is

(a) Reflexive (b) Symmetric

(c) Transitive (d) none of these.

Write correct alternatives.

29. A relation R in real numbers defined by the open sentence $x\ R\ y \Leftrightarrow 2x + 3y = 4$.

Which of the following statements is true?

(a) $OR1$ (b) $1\ R\left(\frac{2}{3}\right)$

(c) $\frac{2}{3}\ R1$ (d) $\frac{4}{3}\ Ro$.

30. A relative is the set of natural numbers N defined by xRy if $x^2 - 4xy + 3y^2 = 0, x, y \in N$ is

(a) Reflexive (b) Symmetric

(c) Transitive (d) None of these.

Hint: $x^2 - 4xy + 3y^2 = 0 \Rightarrow x = y$.

31. R is a transitive relation in A which does not contain any of the " diagonal elements" $(x, x) \in A \times A$; prove that R is not a function in A. A is a non-empty set.

Hint: Let $a \in R$. If R is a function then $(a, b) \in R$ where $a \neq b$. Again $b \in A$ $\therefore$ $(b, c) \in R$ where $b \neq c$.

R is transitive therefore

$(a, b) \in R$ and $(b, c) \in R \Rightarrow (a, c) \in R$

Thus $(a, b) \in R$, $(a, c) \in R$, and $b \neq C$

Thus R is not a function as it contains two different ordered pairs with the same first element.

32. Let R_1 and R_2 be two relations is the real numbers R defined by $R_1 = \{(x, y): x \in R, y \in R, x^2 + y^2 \leq 16\}$ and R_2

$$= \left\{(x, y): x \in R, y \in R, y \, ^3 \frac{x^2}{6}\right\}$$

Sketch the relation $R_1 \cap R_2$ on the diagram of $R \times R$ in the coordinate plane and find the domain and range of $R_1 \cap R_2$.

33. Let R_1 and R_2 be two relations is the real numbers R defined by $R_1 = \{(x, y): x \in R, y \in R, x^2 + y^2 \leq 16\}$ and R_2

$$= \left\{(x, y): x \in R, y \in R, y \, ^3 \frac{x^2}{6}\right\}$$

Sketch each relation on the diagram of $R \times R$ in the coordinate plane and find its domain and range.

34. Let I be the set of integers and the relation R be defined over the set I by $a\ R\ b$ if $A^b = b^a$, where $a, b \in I$. Examine whether the relation R is an equivalence relation or not?

Hint: $a\ R\ b \Rightarrow A^b = b^a \therefore b\ R\ a \Rightarrow b^a = a^b$

$a\ R\ b \Rightarrow a^b = a^a$

Thus $a\ R\ a$ and $a\ R\ b \Rightarrow b\ R\ a$

$\therefore R$ is reflexive since every element in I is related to itself.

R is symmetric $\therefore a\ R\ b \Rightarrow b\ R\ a$

But $a\ R\ b, b\ R\ c \not\Rightarrow a\ R\ c$

$\because a^b = b^a$ and $b^c = c^b$

$\not\Rightarrow a^c = c^a$

$\therefore R$ is not transitive relation.

$\therefore R$ is not an equivalence relation.

35. (i) A relation R is the natural numbers N is $R = \{a, b\} : a, b \in N$ and $a - b$ is divisible *lay* 13. Show that R is an equivalence relation. (IIT 1973, Roorkee 1976)

(ii) Let S be the set of all integers. Let $m > 1$ be same fixed integers. R is a relation defined on S $a\ R\ b$ means that $a - b$

is divisible by m for all $a, b \in S$. Prove that R is an equivalence relation S. (Roorkee 1978)

36. Prove that the relation R defined by $a \; R \; b \Rightarrow |a| = |b|$, where a and b are real numbers is an equivalence relation.

Hint: $a \; R \; a \Rightarrow |a| = |a|$ hence R is reflexive.

$a \; R \; b \Rightarrow b \; R \; a$, since $|a| = |b| \Rightarrow |b| = |a|$ hence R is symmetric.

$|a| = |b|, |b| = |c| \Rightarrow |a| = |c|$, hence $aRb, bRc \Rightarrow aRc$ and hence R is transitive.

Thus R is an equivalence relation.

37. An integer m is said to be related to anotehr integer n if m is a multiple of n. Checking if the relation is reflexive, symmetric and transitive. (IIT 1974)

38. Two points P and Q in a plane are related.

If $OP = OQ$ where O is a fixed point in the plane. Show that the above relation is an equivalent relation.

Hint: $OP = OP \Rightarrow$ The relation is reflexive.

$OP = OQ \Rightarrow OQ = OP$, hence the relation is symmetric

$OP = OQ, OQ = OR \Rightarrow OP = OR$

Hence the relaion is transitive.

$\therefore$ R is an equivalence relation.

39. A relation R on the set of compex numbers is defined by z_1 R z_2 if and only if $\dfrac{z_1 - z_2}{z_1 + z_2}$ is real. Show that R is an equivalence relation. (IIT 1982)

Hint: $z_1 \; R \; z_1$ since $z_1 - z_1 = 0$ is real

$\therefore$ R is reflexive.

$$z_1 \; R \; z_2 \Rightarrow z_2 \; R \; z_1 \text{ since } \frac{z_1 - z_2}{z_1 + z_2} \text{ real}$$

$$\Rightarrow -\left(\frac{z_2 - z_1}{z_2 + z_1}\right) \text{ is also real.}$$

$\therefore$ R is symmetric.

For the transitive relation $z_1 \; R \; z_2, z_2 \; R \; z_3 \Rightarrow z_1 \; R \; z_3$

In order to test it we set

$$z_1 = x_1 + iy_1, z_2 = x_2 + iy_2 \text{ and } z_3 = x_3 + iy_3$$

$z_1 R z_2 \Rightarrow \dfrac{z_1 - z_2}{z_1 + z_2}$ is real

$\Rightarrow \dfrac{(x_1 - x_2) + i(y_1 - y_2)}{(x_1 + x_2) + i(y_1 + y_2)} \cdot \dfrac{(x_1 + x_2) - i(y_1 - y_2)}{(x_1 + x_2) - i(y_1 + y_2)}$ is real.

Equating imaginary parts to zero is the numerator we get

$\dfrac{x_1}{y_1} = \dfrac{x_2}{y_2}$

Similarly $z_2 R z_3 \Rightarrow \dfrac{x_2}{y_2} = \dfrac{x_3}{y_3}$

$\therefore \quad \dfrac{x_1}{y_1} = \dfrac{x_2}{y_2} = \dfrac{x_3}{y_3}$

i.e. $\quad \dfrac{x_1}{y_1} = \dfrac{x_3}{y_3}$

$\therefore z_1 R z_3 \therefore R$ is transitive.

Thus R is an equivalence relation.

40. If $A = \{1, 2, 3, 4\}$ define relation on A which have the properties of being (i) reflexive, transitive but not symmetric (ii) symmetric but not reflexive and not transitive (iii) reflexive, transitive and symmetric. [I.I.T 1970]

Hint: See the answersheet.

41. Is it true that every realtion which is symmetric and transitive is also reflexive? Give reasons. [I.I.T 1970]

Hint: Every relation which is symmetric and transitive is not always reflexive. Consider a relation R defined by $a R b$ iff $a + b$ is even defined on I of positive integers including zero and $a, b \in I$ is symmetric and transitive but not reflexive.

42. In a set $S = \{a, b, c, d\}$ of four men, a is younger to other three, b is younger to c only, and c is younger to d only. Is the relation "is younger to" an equivalence relation? Give reasons for your answer.

43. Consider the non-empty set consisting of children in a family. State giving reasons whether each of the following relation is

(i) Symmetric (ii) transitive.

(a) X is a brother of Y (b) X likes Y. [I.I.T. 1972]

44. Given a relation $R = \{(1, 2)\ (2, 3)\}$ on the set of natural numbers, add a minimum number of ordered pairs so that the enlarged relation is symmetric, transitive and reflexive. [I.I.T. 1978]

45. Check the following relation R and P for reflexing symmetriy and transitivity.

(i) $a\ R\ b$ iff b is divisible by a where a and b for reflexivity symmetry and transitivity

(ii) $\alpha\ R\ \beta$ iff is perpendicular to β where α and β are straight lines in a plane [I.I.T. 1975]

46. Let L be the set of all straight lines of the Euclidean plane. Verify whether parallelogram between two straight lines is an equivalence relation on L. [I.I.T. 1980]

47. Let n be a fixed positive integer. Define a relation R on I (the set of all integers) as follows: $a\ R\ b$ iff $n/a-b$ that is iff $a-b$ is divisible by n. Show that R is an equivalence relation on I. [I.I.T. 1973; Roorkee 1978]

48. Let R be a relation defined on the set of natural numbers N as $R = \{(x, y) : x \in N, y \in N, x + y = 41\}$.

Find the domain and range of this relation R. Also verify whether R is (i) reflexive (ii) symmetric (iii) transitive. [Roorkee 1983]

Hint: From the equation $2x + y = 41$.

We obtain y be setting $x = 1, 2$ ...., 20 as 39, 37, 35, 9, 7, 5, 3, 1.

49. (i) Examine whether the following relation are reflexive, symmetric or transitive. R is defined on the set of real numbers.

(i) $a\ R\ b$ iff $|a-b| > 0$

(ii) $a\ R\ b$ iff $1 + ab > 0$

(iii) $a\ R\ b$ iff $|a| \le b$.

50. (i) N is the set of natural numbers. The relation is defined on $N \times N$ as follows $(a, b)\ R\ (c, d) \Leftrightarrow a + d = b + c$. Prove that R is an equivalence relation. [Roorkee 1982]

(ii) N is the set of positive integers and R be a relation defined on $N \times N$ as follows $(a, b) \sim (c, d)$ iff $ad = bc$. Check the relation for being an equivalence relation.

(iii) Let $S = \{1, 2, 3, 4, 5\}$ and $A = S \times S$. Define the relation R on A as follows "$(a, b) R (c, d)$ if and only if $ad = cb$".

Show that R is an equivalence relation. Compute the collection of all equivalence classes. [Roorkee 1989]

Hint: (i) R is reflexive since $\forall (a, b) \in N, (a, b) R (a, b), a + b = b + a$

R is symmetric since $(a, b) R (c, d)$

$\Rightarrow a + d = b + c \Rightarrow d + a = c + b$

$\Rightarrow c + b = d + a \Rightarrow (c + d) R (a, b)$

R is transitive for $(a, b) R (c, d)$ and $(c, d) R (e, f)$

$\Rightarrow a + d = b + c$ and $c + f = d + e$

$\therefore a + d + c + f = b + c + d + e \Rightarrow a + f = b + e$

$\Rightarrow (a, b) R (e, f)$

Hence R is an equivalence relation

(ii) $(a, b) R (c, d)$ Þ $(c, d) R (a, b) \forall a, b, c \in N$

Since $ad = bc \Rightarrow bc = ad \Rightarrow cb = da$

i.e. $(a, b) R (c, d) \Rightarrow (c, d) R (a, b)$

$\therefore$ R is symmetric.

$(a, b) R (a, b) \forall a, b \in N$

$\therefore$ R is reflexive.

$(a, b) R (c, d), (c, d) R (e, f) \Rightarrow (a, b)$ R (ef)

i.e. R is transitive $\forall a, b, c, d, e, f \in N$

Since $(a, b) R (e, d)$ iff $ad = bc$ ...(a)

$(c, d) R (e, f)$ iff $cf = de$ ...(b)

$(a, b) R (e, f)$ iff $af = be$ ...(c)

From (a) and (b)

$(a, b) R (c, d)$ and $(c, d) R (e, f)$ iff a $= cf = dcde$

i.e. iff $af = be$

$\therefore$ From (c)

$(a, b) R (c, d), (c, d) R (e, f) \Rightarrow (a, b) R (e, f)$

(iii) Do yourself. R is an equivalence relation.

Collection of equivalence classes

(1) $\{(1, 1), (2, 2), (3, 3), (4, 4), (5, 5)\}$

(2) $\{(1, 2), (2, 4),$

(3) {(2, 1), (4, 2)}

(4) {(1, 3)}

(5) {(1, 4)} .... (19) {(5, 4)}

51. (i) Prove that a relation R on a set A is transitive if $RoR \subseteq R$

(ii) Prove that the inverse of a transitive relation is also transitive.

52. (i) Show that the congruence relation R on a set x of all triangles is an equivalence relation.

(ii) If R and R^1 be two equivalence relations defined on a set A, prove that (a) $R \cap R^1$ is an equivalence relation on A and (b) $R \cup R^1$ is not an equivalence relation on A.

Hint 52: (ii) We have $R \subseteq A \times A$ and $R^1 \subseteq A \times A$ ...(1)

Thus $R \cap R^1 \subseteq A \times A \Rightarrow R \cap R^1$ is a relation on the set A.

Now $(a, b) \in R \cap R^1 \Rightarrow (a, b) \in R$ and $(a, b) \in R^1$

$\Rightarrow (b, a) \in R$ and $(b, a) \in R^1 \because R \cap R^1$ are symmetric

$\Rightarrow (b, a)\ R \cap R^1$

$\therefore R \cap R^1$ is symmetric. We see further that

$(a, a) \in R, (a, a) \in R^1\ \forall\ a \in A\ \therefore (a, a) \in R \cap R^1$

$\therefore R \cap R^1$ is reflexive $\therefore$ Again $(a, b) \in R \cap R^1, (b, c) \in R \cap R^1$

$\Rightarrow (a, b)$ and $(b, c) \in R$, (a, b) and $(b, c) \in R^1 \Rightarrow (a, c) \in R$, $(a, c) \in R^1$

(since R and R^1 transitive) $\therefore R \cap R^1$ is transitive.

We can show $R \cup R^1$ is symmetric as well as reflexive but is not transitive.

ANSWERS TO PROBLEMS AND EXERCISES 2B (I)

1. $R = \{(2, 6), (2, 10), (3, 3), (3, 6), (5, 10)\}$

2. $R = \{(3, 2), (4, 2)\}$.

3. $R = \{(3, 3), (4, 4)\}$.

4. $\{(2, 3), (2, 7), (3, 2), (3, 7), (4, 3), (4, 7), (7, 2), (7, 3), (7, 4)\}$

5. R is a relation, Yes, Yes, Yes, No.

6. (i) Yes (ii) Yes (iii) No (iv) No (v) Yes.

7. The horizontal line through c contains all the points of R in which c appears as the second element. They are (c, c) and (e, c). Thus c in related to c and e hence the desired set is $\{c, e\}$.

8. The vertical line through e contains all the points of R is which e appears as the first element. They are (e, a) (e, b) and (e, c), i.e, e is related to a, b and c. Hence $\{a, b, c\}$ is the desired set.

9. The solution set of the relation is its graph

   (1) $x^2 + y^2 < 4$ is the area shown by dotted lines inside the circle. The boundary of the circle. The boundary of the circles excluded here.

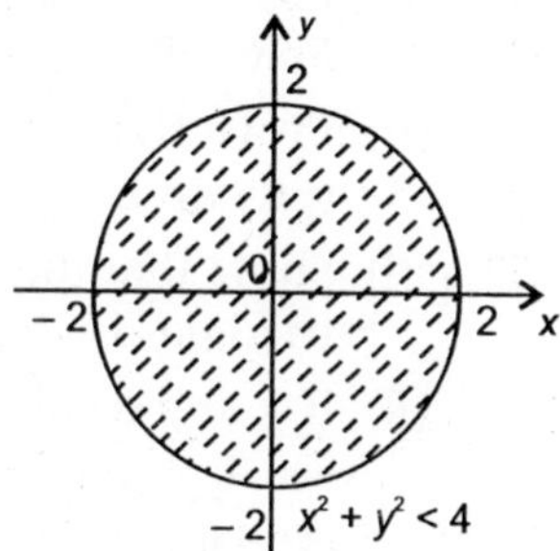

   (2) $x^2 + y^2 \geq 4$ is the area shown by the dotted lines outside the circle. The boundary of the circle is included here.

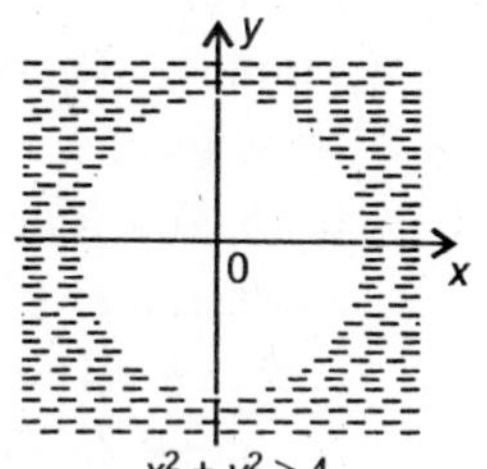

   (3)

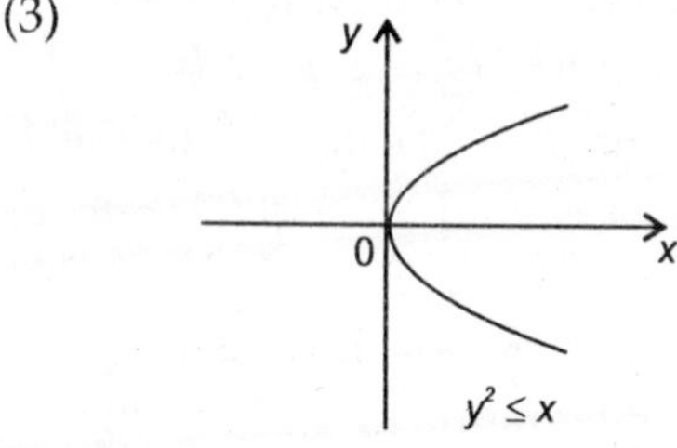

   (4) $y + x^2$ i.e. $x^2 - y \geq 0$ is shown by the dotted area. The boundary of the parabola is included here.

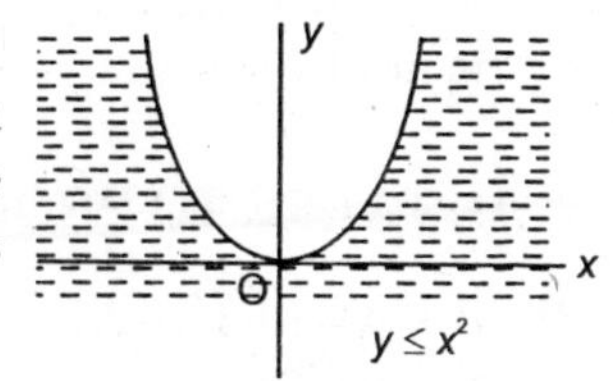

   (5) $y \geq x^3$ i.e. $x^3 - y \leq 0$ is shown by dotted area. The boundary is included here.

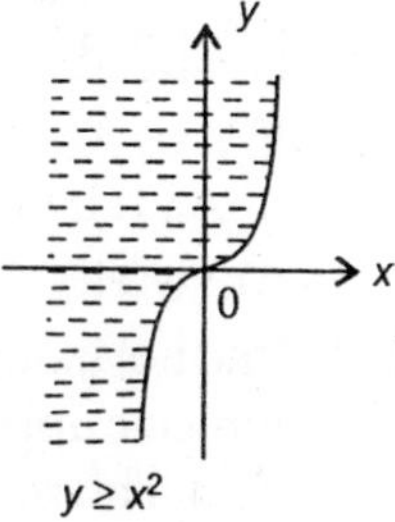

(6) $\frac{x^2}{16} - \frac{y^2}{4} \geq 1$ is shown by the area of dotted lines. The boundary of the hyperbola is included here.

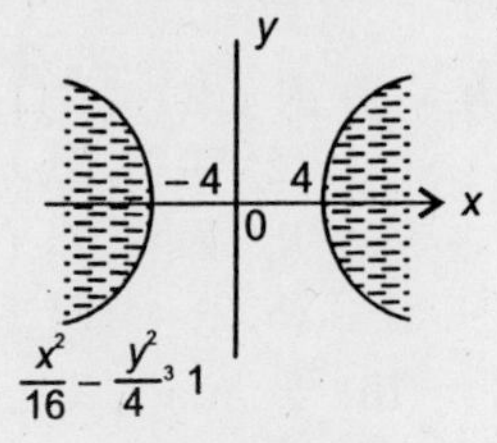

(7) The boundry is included here.

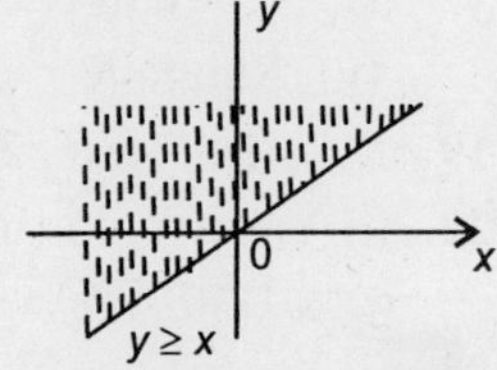

(8) The boundary in $x \geq |y|$ is included.

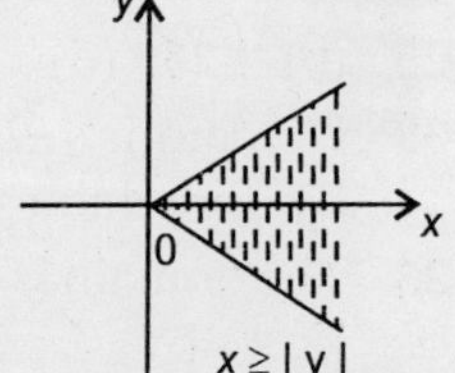

(9) $\frac{x^2}{16} - \frac{y^2}{9} < 1$ is shown by dotted lines. The bounday of the hyperbola is excluded here.

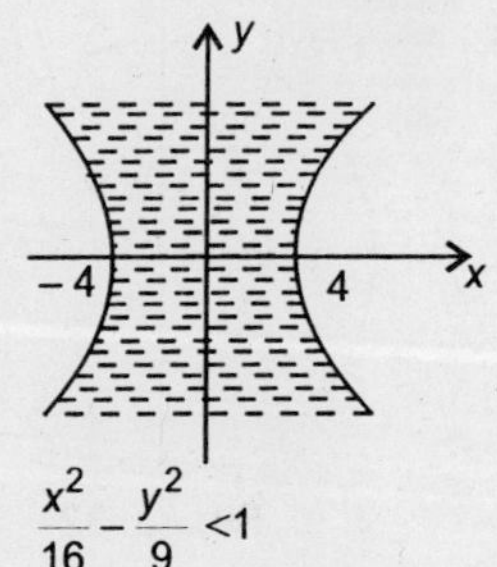

10. (1) T (2) T (3) T (4) T

11. $(-\infty, 0) \cup (0, +\infty)$.

12. 2^{12}

13. $R^{-1} = \{(y, x), (x, z), (z, z), (y, z)\}$

14. $R = \{(1, 3), (1, 5), (2, 3), (2, 5), (3, 5), (4, 5)\}$

$R^{-1} = \{(3, 1), (5, 1), (3, 2), (5, 2), (5, 3), (5, 4)\}$

16. The domain of R is the range of R^{-1} and the range of R is the domain of R^{-1} since the ordered pairs in R and R^{-1} one of reversed order.

17. $R^{-1} = \{(4, 2), (3, 4), (2, 6), (1, 8)\}$

18. (i) $R = \{(1, 1), (1, 2), (1, 3), (1, 4), (1, 5), (2, 2), (2, 3), (2, 4), (2, 5), (3, 3), (3, 4), (3, 5), (4, 4), (4, 5), (5, 5)\}$

(ii) $R^{-1} = \{(1, 1), (2, 1), (3, 1), (4, 1), (5, 1), (2, 2), (3, 2), (4, 2), (5, 2), (3, 3), (4, 3), (5, 3), (4, 4), (5, 4), (5, 5)\}$

(iii) Domain $R = \{1, 2, 3, 4, 5\}$

(iv) Domain $R^{-1} = \{1, 2, 3, 4, 5\}$

(v) Range $R^{-1} = \{1, 2, 3, 4, 5\}$

19. $R^{-1} = \{(8, 1), (6, 2), (4, 3), (2, 4)\}$

22. (i) Yes (ii) No (iii) Yes (iv) No (v) Yes (vi) Yes (vii) Yes if $a = b$ (vii) Yes.

23. (i) Yes (ii) Yes (iii) Yes.

24. (i) Anti-symmetric (ii) symmetric.

25. (b) **26.** (d) **27.** (b) **28.** (c) **29.** (b) **30.** (a)

32. Domain is $[-2\sqrt{3},\ 2\sqrt{3}]$; Range is [0, 4]. The area shown by dotted lines represents $R_1 \cap R_2$.

33. The domain is the entire axis of real numbers. The range is $[2, +\infty]$.

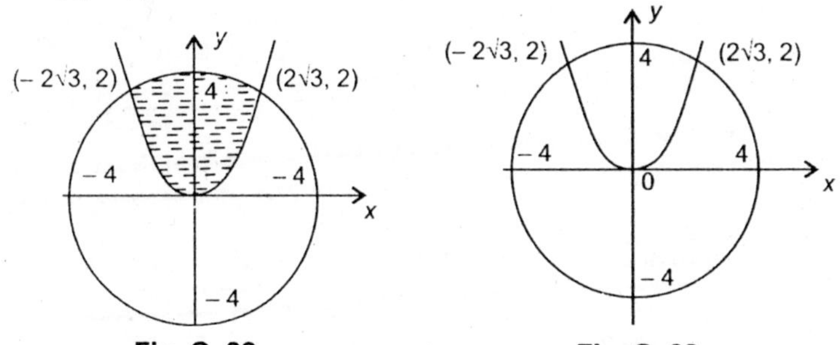

Fig. Q. 32 **Fig. Q. 33**

37. Reflexive, transitive but not symmetric.

40. (i) Consider the relation "is a facing of" or $R = \{(1, 1), (2, 2), (3, 3), (4, 4), (1, 2), (2, 3)\}$.

(ii) Consider the relation " is a multiplicative inverse of" or define R over the set A by $a\,R\,b$ iff $a + b$ is odd where $a, b \in N$.

(iii) Consider the relation "equal to".

42. No. 43 (a) The relation is not symmetric but is transitive. (b) Neither symmetric not transitive.

44. $R_1 = \{(1, 1), (2, 2), (3, 3), (4, 4), (1, 2), (2, 1)\}$.

45. (i) R is reflexive and transitive but not symmetric.

(ii) P is neither reflexive not transitive but is symmetric.

46. Yes, parallelogram between two straight lines is an equivalence relation on L.

48. Domain $R = \{1, 2, 3, ..., 18, 19, 20\}$

Range $R = \{39, 37, 35, 9, 7, 5, 3, 1\}$.

R is neither reflexive nor symmetric. R is also not transitive.

49. (i) R is symmetric but not reflexive and transitive

(ii) Reflexive, symmetric but not transitive

(iii) Neither reflexive nor symmetric but transitive.

Chapter 2 (C)
Algebra of Sets, Partition of a Set, Equivalence Class and Residue Class

2.19 ALGABRA OF SETS

In this portion we include the following laws and their consequences:

Idempotent laws: $A \cup A = A$ and $A \cap A = A$

Associative laws: $(A \cup B) \cup C = A \cup (B \cup C)$ and $(A \cap B) \cap C = A \cap (B \cap C)$

Commutative laws: $A \cup B = B \cup A$ and $A \cap B = B \cap A$

Distributive laws: $A \cup (B \cup C) = (A \cup B) \cap (A \cap C)$ and

$A \cap (B \cup C) = (A \cap B) \cup (A \cap C)$

Identity laws: $A \cup \phi = A$; $U \cap A = A$; $A \cup U = U$ and $A \cap \phi = \phi$

Complement laws: $A \cup A^1 = U$; $A \cap A^1 = \phi$; $(A^1)^1 = A$; $U^1 = \phi$ and $\phi^1 = U$

Demorgan's laws: $(A \cup B)^1 = A^1 \cap B^1$ and $(A \cap B)^1 = A^1 \cup B^1$

2.20 PRINCIPLE OF DUALITY

(i) *Principle of duality:* If the operations $\cap$ and $\cup$ and the sets U and ϕ are interchanged in a statement concerning sets, then the statement so obtained is known as the dual of the original statement. Thus $(U \cup B) \cap (A \cup \phi) = A$ has the dual $(\phi \cap B) \cup (A \cap U) = A$. The principle of duality is applied to the algebra of sets.

(ii) *Index set:* If to each element i belonging to a set Δ there is a set A_i. then the set Δ is known as the index set. The index set is generally denoted by Δ or T.

If $\Delta = \{a, b, c, d, e\}$ and $A_a = \{a, l\}$; $A_b = \{b, d, f, l\}$; $A_c = \{c, f, k\}$; $A_d = \{d, j\}$ and $A_e = \{e, f, l\}$; then Δ be the index set and the set $\{A_a, A_b, \ldots\ldots, A_e\}$ are indexed sets.

Each $i \in \Delta$ makes an index to the set A_i. Let A be the collection of sub-sets of a set S such that to each $i \in \Delta$ there is a member $A_i \in A$, then A is known as an indexed family of sets.

Then $A = \{A_i : i \in \Delta\}$ or $\{A_i\} \quad i \in \Delta$.

An index set may be infinite or finite.

An indexed family of sets $\{A_i\} \quad i \in \Delta$ is a function $f : \Delta \to \{A_i\} \quad i \in \Delta$, where Δ is the domain of f and a family of sets $\{A_i\}$ $i \in \Delta$ is the range of f.

Example 1: Define $A_n = \{x : 0 \leq x \leq \frac{1}{2n}$ where $n \in N\}$. We have $A_1 = \left[0, \frac{1}{2}\right], A_2 = \left[0, \frac{1}{4}\right], A_3 = \left[0, \frac{1}{6}\right]$ .... Here the index set is $N = \{1, 2, 3 \ldots\ldots\}$.

(iii) *Union and intersection of indexed family of sets:* Let Λ be an index set and $A = \{A_i : i \in \Delta\}$ be an indexed collection of subset of a set S then

$$\bigcup_{i=1}^{n} A_i \equiv A_1 \cup A_2 \cup A_3 \ldots\ldots \cup A_n$$

and
$$\bigcap_{i=1}^{n} A_i \equiv A_1 \cap A_2 \cap A_3 \ldots\ldots \cap A_n.$$

We generalise these concepts as follows: If $J \subseteq \Lambda$ then

$$\bigcup_{i \in J} A_i = \{x : \text{there is an } i \in J \text{ such that } x \in A_i\}$$

and
$$\bigcap_{i \in J} A_i = \{x : x \in \forall_1 \; i \in J\}.$$

Example 1: Let $A_a = \{a, l\}$; $A_b = \{b, d, f, l\}$; $A_c = \{c, f, k\}$; $A_d = \{d, j\}$ and $A_e = \{e, f, l\}$ and $J = \{b, c, e\}$ then $\bigcup_{i \in J} A_i = A_b \cup A_c \cup A_e = \{b, c, d, e, f, k, l\} = \{b, c, d, e, f, k, l\}$ and $\bigcap_{i \in J} A_i = A_b \cap A_c \cup A_e = \{f\}$.

(iv) *Partitions of sets:* Let A be a non-empty set and B_1, B_2, B_3, B_4 be the subsets of A, where $B = \{B_1, B_2, B_3, B_4\}$ then B is called a partition of the set A if (i) $A = B_1 \cup B_2 \cup B_2 \cup B_4$ i.e A is the union of the set in the family of sets B and (ii) for any B_i and B_j either $B_i = B_j$ or $B_i \cap B_j = \phi$ i.e. the intersection of two subsets of B is empty i.e. B_i and B_j are disjoint. In addition, each B_i is known as an equivalence class of A.

Example 1: Find the partition of the set T where

$$T = \{1, 2, 3, 4, 5, 6\}$$
$$A = \{1, 3\}, B = \{2, 4\}, C = \{5, 6\}$$

Solution: We see that $T = A \cup B \cup C$

$\therefore$ $\{A, B, C\}$ is the partition of the set T.

(v) *Theorem on equivalence relations:* The equivalence relation R is a set A decomposes or partitions the set A into disjoint on mutually exelusive classes known as equivalence classes, such that any two members of different classes are non-equivalent where as those of the same class are equivalent.

Proof: Let $A = \{a, a_1, a_2, a_3 \ldots\ldots, b, b_1, b_2, b_3, \ldots\ldots, c, c_1, c_2, c_3\}$.

Let the class $\{a, a_1, a_2, a_3 \ldots\}$ be denoted by $\bar{a}$, where the elements equivalent to a form a non-empty class.

If b does not belong to a, then a element equivalent to b will also not belong to $\bar{a}$. Thus all the elements equivalent to b form the class $\{b, b_1, b_2, b_3 \ldots\}$ which is denoted by $\bar{b}$ and so on.

Thus the classes $\bar{a}$, $\bar{b}$, $\bar{c}$ ... are disjoint.

Assume now that for $i \neq j$, $a_i, a_j \, R \, a$ then $a_i \, R \, a$ and $a_j \, R \, a$. Due to symmetry $a_j \, R \, a \Leftrightarrow a \, R \, a_j$.

$\therefore$ By transitivity $a_i \, R \, a_j$ i.e. the members of the class are equivalent.

If $a_i \, R \, a$ and $b_i \, R \, b$ then a_i is not equivalent to b_i. Thus memebrs of different classes are not equivalent.

The converse of this theorem i.e. "The partition of a set A into mutually exclusive or disjoint subsets defines an equivalence relation in A" also holes good.

Example 1: Find all the partitions of the set $T = \{1, 2, 3\}$.

Solution: The partitions are $[(1,2,3)], [(1), [(2,3)], [(2), (1,3)], [(3), (1, 2)], [(1), (2), (3)]$.

(vi) *Equivalence classes.* Let R be an equivalence relation on a non-empty set A. If $a \in A$ then the element $x \in A$ which satisfy $a\ R\ x$ from a subset A_a of A which is known as an equivalence class of A with respect to R determined by a.

The equivalance class or equivalence set is denoted by $[a]$ or $A_a = [x\colon x \in A \text{ and } a\ R\ x]$

Example 1: Show that the relation "$a\ R\ b$" iff $a - b$ is a mulitple of 5 defined on the set I of integers is an equivalence relation. Find equivalence classes and the quotient set.

Solution: Since $(a - b)$ is a multiple of 5 therefore $(a - b)$ is also a multiple of 5.

$\therefore a\ R\ b \Rightarrow b\ R\ a\ \forall\ a, b \in I$.

$a\ R\ a\ \forall\ a \in I$ since $a - a = 0$ is a multiple of 5. Thus R is symmetric as well as reflexive.

Now $a - c = (a - b) + (b - c)$ is a multiple of 5 if $(a - b)$ and $(b - c)$ are multiples of 5.

Thus $a\ R\ b, b\ R\ c \Rightarrow a\ R\ c\ \forall\ a, b, c \in I$

$\therefore R$ is transitive.

$\therefore R$ is an equivalence relation.

In order to collect equivalence classes we proceed as follows:

Since a belongs to I, the equivalence class of a i.e. $[a]$ is the set of integers of the form $a + 5n = x$ where $n = 0, \pm 1, \pm 2$ .... and $0 \leq a < 5$.

If $a =$ 0 and $n = 0, \pm 1, \pm 2$ .... then the class

$[0] = \{-15, -10, -5, 0, 5, 10, 15 \ldots\} = E_0$ (say for convenince)

If $a =$ 1 and $n = 0, \pm 1, \pm 2$ .... then the class

$[1] = \{\ldots -14, -9, -4, 1, 6, 11, 16 \ldots\} = E_1$

If $a =$ 2 and $n = 0, \pm 1, \pm 2$ .... then the class

$[2] = \{-11, -8, -3, 2, 7, 12, 19, \ldots\} = E_2$

In a similar way

$[3] = \{\ldots -7, -2, 3, 8, 13 \ldots\} = E_3$

$[4] = \{\ldots -11, -6, -1, 4, 9, 14, 19 \ldots\} = E_4$

The set of equivalence classes is known as the quotient set and is denoted by

$$\frac{I}{R} = \{E_0, E_1, E_2, E_3, E_4\}$$

Note: The collection of equivalence disjoint classes defined by an equivalence relation R on a set A is known as the quotient set of A relative to the given relation R. This is denoted by $\bar{A}$ or $\frac{A}{R}$.

(viii) *Properties of equivalence classes:* If R be an equivalence relation in a non-empty set A and a, b, c be any elements of × and the equivalence class be A_a then

(1) If $a \in A$ then $a = A_a$

(2) If $b \in [a]$ then $[b] = [a]$

(3) If $b, c \in A_a$ then $b\ R\ c$

(4) If $b \in A_a$ and $b\ R\ c$ then $C \in A_a$

(5) Two equivalent classes are either identical or disjoint

(6) Equivalence classes cannot be empty.

Proof: (1) R is an equivalence relation $\Rightarrow$ R is reflexive i.e., $a\ R\ a \Rightarrow a \in A_a$ from def.

(2) $b \in [a] \Rightarrow b\ R\ a \Rightarrow a\ R\ b\ \therefore\ R$ is symmetric.

If x be any element of $[b]$ then

$$x \in [b] \Rightarrow x\ R\ b$$

R is transitive $\therefore\ x\ R\ b, b\ R\ a \Rightarrow x\ R\ a$

$$\therefore \quad x \in [b] \Rightarrow x \in [a] \Rightarrow [b] \subseteq [a] \qquad \dots (1)$$

Again if y be any element of $[a]$ then

$$y \in [a] \Rightarrow y\ R\ a$$

R is transitive $\therefore\ y\ R\ a, a\ R\ b \Rightarrow y\ R\ b$

$$\therefore \quad y \in [a] \Rightarrow y \in [b]$$

$$\therefore \quad [a] \subseteq [b] \qquad \dots(2)$$

$\therefore$ from (1) and (2) $[a] = [b]$

(3) $b \in A_a \Rightarrow b\ R\ a$ and $c \in A_a \Rightarrow c\ R\ a \Rightarrow a\ R\ c$ ($\because$ R is symmetric)

$\therefore\ b, c \in A_a \Rightarrow b\ R\ a$ and $c\ R\ a \Rightarrow b\ R\ a$ and $a\ R\ c$ ($\because$ R is symmetric)

$\Rightarrow b\ R\ a$ and $a\ R\ c \Rightarrow b\ R\ c$. Since R is transitive.

(4) If $b \in A_a$ and $b\,R\,c$ then $c \in A_a$. In order to prove this we have

$b \in A_a \Rightarrow b\,R\,a \Rightarrow a\,R\,b$ ($\because$ R is symmetric)

$\therefore \quad b \in A_a \Rightarrow b\,R\,a \Rightarrow a\,R\,b$ and $b\,R\,c$

$\Rightarrow a\,R\,c$, since R is transitive

$\Rightarrow c \in A_a$.

(5) Let $A_a \cap A_b \neq \phi$, where A_a and A_b are equivalence classes of a and b respectively in A then there is at least an element $c \in A$ such that $c \in A_a \cap A_b$ i.e. $c \in A_a$ and $c \in A_b$

Where $a, b \in A$.

If there be another element $d \in A_a$ then $d \in A_a$ and $c \in A_a$ $\Rightarrow d\,R\,c$ by (1)

Now $\therefore$ $d\,R\,c$ and $c \in A_a$

$\because \qquad d \in A_b$

$\therefore \qquad A_a \subseteq A_b$ ... (3)

Similarly if $d \in A_b$ then $c \subseteq A_b$ then

$d \in A_b$ and $c \in A_b \Rightarrow d\,R\,c$ by (1)

Again $d\,R\,c$ and $c \in A_a$ and therefore $d \in A_a$ by (2)

Hence $d \in A_b \Rightarrow d \subseteq A_a$

i.e. $\qquad A_b \subseteq A_a$ ...(4)

From (3) and (4) $A_a = A_b$ if $A_a \cap A_b \neq \phi$

If $A_a \cap A_b = \phi$ and $A_a = A_b$ then $A_a = \phi$ and $A_b = \phi$ but A_a and A_b being equivalence classes cannot be empty hence $A_a \cap A_b = \phi$ or $A_a = A_b$.

(6) R is reflexive $\therefore$ $a\,R\,a$ and hence $a \in A\,a\ \forall\ a \in A$

$\therefore$ A_a is not empty.

Thus, we see that every element of A is in some equivalence class.

2.21 CONGRUENCE OF INTEGERS

An integer a is said to be congruent to other integer b module m if $m/a - b$ i.e. m is a division of $a - b$ where a is a fixed positive integer.

We write it symbolically $a \equiv b$ (modem) and read it as "a is congruent to be modulo m".

if λ is some integer then $a - b = \lambda\,m$.

Example 1: $22 \equiv 10 \pmod 3$ since $22 - 10 = 12$ and $3/12$.

Another definiton of congruence

$a \equiv b \pmod m$ iff a and b have the same remainder when divided by m, where $a, b \in I$ and m is a positive integer.

(i) **Theorems 1.** Prove that in the set of integers, the relation "congruent modulo m" is an equivalence relation.

Proof: $a \equiv b \pmod m \Rightarrow b \equiv a \pmod m$

$$[\because a - b = \lambda m \Rightarrow (b - a) = (-\lambda)\, m \Rightarrow b \equiv a \pmod m]$$

Thus the relation is symmetric.

Also $a \equiv a \pmod m$ $[\because a - a = 0.\, m]$

Hence the relation is reflexive.

We further see that

$$a \equiv b \pmod m,\ b \equiv C \pmod{\text{m}} \Rightarrow a \equiv c \pmod m$$

$$[\because a - b = \lambda_1 m;\ b - c = \lambda_2 m \ \therefore\ a - c = (a - b) + (b - c) = (\lambda_1 + \lambda_2)\, m \Rightarrow a \equiv c \pmod m]$$

Thus the relation is transitive also.

The relation is therefore equivalence relation.

Thorem 2. If $a \equiv b \pmod m$, prove that $\forall\ x \in I$

$$a + x \equiv (b + x) \pmod m$$

and $$ax \equiv bx \pmod m$$

Proof: We have $a - b = \lambda m$

and $(a + x) - (b + x) = \lambda m$ and therefore

$$(a + x) \equiv (b + x) \pmod m.$$

Also $$(a - b) = \lambda m \Rightarrow ax - bx = \lambda xm$$

Where $x \in I$.

Thus $ax \equiv bx \pmod m$

Theorem 3. (i) If $a \equiv b \pmod m$ and $c \equiv d \pmod m$

Prove that $a - c \equiv (b - d) \pmod m$

$$a + c \equiv (b + d) \pmod m$$

and $$ac \equiv bd \pmod m$$

The proof is left from readers.

(ii) If $ca = cb \pmod m$, $(c, m) = d$ and $m = m_1 d$ then $a \equiv b \pmod{m_1}$ and conversely.

(iii) If $ca = cb \pmod m$ and $(c, m) = 1$, then $a \equiv b \pmod m$.

(iv) $a \equiv b \pmod{m}$ iff a and b have the same remainder when divided by m. Every integer a is congurent (mod m) to its remainder when a is divided by m.

Note: $(c, m) = d$ means $d = \lambda c + \mu m$, where λ and μ are integers. $(c, m) = d \Rightarrow d$ is the greater common division of c and m. Theorems 3 (i) (ii) and (iii) are given without proofs. Some theorems without proofs are given below:

(1) If x_1 is a solution of congruence are $\equiv b \pmod{m}$ then any integer $x_2 \equiv x_1 \pmod{m}$ is also a solution.

(2) The congruence are $\equiv b \pmod{m}$ has a solution iff $(a, m) = d$ divides b.

(3) If $d = (a, m)$ divides b, then the congruence $ax \equiv b \pmod{m}$ has exactly d incongruent solution (mod m).

2.22 RESIDUE CLASSES

The congruence relation $\equiv \pmod{m}$ in the set of integers is an equivalence relation. If decomposes or partitions the set I into disjoint classes such that all the integers which are congruent modulo m are collected in the same class. These classes are called residue classes modulo m. Any integer a is congurent (mod m) to its remainder when divided by m gives m possible remainders 0, 1, 2 .... m –1 and hence the number of disjoint classes be m. Thus the number of residue class is m.

Residue classes are denoted as follows:

$\bar{0}$ or [0] = the class in which all integers $\equiv 0 \pmod{m}$

$\bar{1}$ or [1] = the class in which all integers $\equiv 1 \pmod{m}$

$\bar{2}$ or [2] = the class in which all integers $\equiv 2 \pmod{m}$

$\bar{3}$ or [3] = the class in which all integers $\equiv 3 \pmod{m}$

The set of residue class modulo m is generally denoted by Im or I/m. Following are the examples of residue classes:

1. The residue classes modulo 3 are as follows:

   $\bar{0}$ = [0] = {..., –9, –6, –3, 0, 3, 6, 9, ...} i.e. all integers $\equiv 0 \pmod{3}$

   $\bar{1}$ = [1] = {..., –8, –5, –2, 1, 4, 7, 10, ...} i.e. all integers $\equiv 1 \pmod{3}$

$\bar{2}$ = [2] = {..., –7, –4, –1, 2, 5, 8, 11, ...} i.e. all integers ≡ 2 (mod 3)

There are only three residue classes. The set of residue classes known as quotient set is denoted by $I/(3) = \{\bar{0}, \bar{1}, \bar{2}\}$.

2. The residue classes modulo 4 are as follows:

$\bar{0}$ = [0] = {..., –12, –8, –4, 0, 4, 8, 12, ...} i.e. all integers ≡ 0 (mod 4)

$\bar{1}$ = [1] = {..., –11, –7, –3, 1, 5, 9, 13, ...} i.e. all integers ≡ 1 (mod 4)

$\bar{2}$ = [2] = {..., –10, –6, –2, 2, 6, 10, 14, ...} i.e. all integers ≡ 2 (mod 4)

$\bar{3}$ = [3] = {..., –9, –5, –1, 3, 7, 11, 15, ...} i.e. all integers ≡ 3 (mod 3)

There are only form residue classes. The set of residue classes known as quotient set is denoted by $I/(4) = \{\bar{0}, \bar{1}, \bar{2}, \bar{3}\}$.

2.23 SOME OF THE RESIDUE CLASSES

(i) *Sum of the residue classes (mod m):* The sum $[r_1] + [r_2]$ of $[r_1]$ and $[r_2]$, two residue classes (mod m) is defined as the class in which the sum of any integer of $[r_1]$ and any integer of $[r_2]$ is included where $1 \le r_1 \le (m-1)$ and $1 \le r_2 \le (m-1)$.

We now prove $[r_1] + [r_2] = [r_1 + r_2]$

Let $a_1 \in r_1$ and $a_2 \in r_2$, then $a_1 = r_1 + \lambda_1 m$ and $a_2 = r_2 + \lambda_2 m$

$\therefore \quad (a_1 + a_2) = (r_1 + r_2) + (\lambda_1 + \lambda_2) m$

or $\quad (a_1 + a_2) \equiv (r_1 + r_2) \pmod{m}$

$\therefore \quad a_1 + a_2 \in [r_1 + r_2]$

$\therefore \quad [r_1] + [r_2] = [r_1 + r_2]$

Example 1: Let $\{\bar{0}, \bar{1}, \bar{2}, \bar{3}, \bar{4}, \bar{5}, \bar{6},\} = I/(7)$ be the set of residue classes (mod 7), then [1] + [2] = [3] and [2] + [3] = [5] (mod 7).

If $r_1 + r_2 \ge m$ then we reduce it as (mod m).

Thus [5] + [6] = [4] ∴ 5 + 6 = 11 ≡ 4 (mod 7).

(ii) Let there be two residue classes $[r_1]$ and $[r_2]$ (mod m), then we define the product of $[r_1]$ and $[r_2]$ as the class which contains the product of any integer of $[r_1]$ and any integer of $[r_2]$. We now prove $[r_1][r_2] = [r_1r_2]$

Let $a_1 \in R_1$ and $a_2 \in R_2$

$\therefore \quad a_1 = r_1 + \lambda_1 m$ and $a_2 = r_2 + \lambda_2 m$

$$\Rightarrow \quad a_1a_2 = r_1r_2 + m(\lambda_1 r_2 + \lambda_1 r_1 + \lambda_1\lambda_2 m)$$

$$= r_1r_2 + m\lambda_2$$

$$\Rightarrow \quad a_1a_2 = r_1r_2 \pmod m$$

$$\therefore \quad a_1a_2 \in [r_1r_2]$$

$$\therefore \quad [r_1][r_2] = [r_1r_2]$$

If $\quad I/(7) = \{\bar{0}, \bar{1}, \bar{2}, \bar{3}, \bar{4}, \bar{5}, \bar{6},\}$

then [2] (mod 7). [4] (mod 7) = [1] (mod 7)

$\because \quad 2.4 = 8 \equiv 1 \pmod 7$

[2] (mod 7). [3] (mod 7) = 6 (mod 7)

Example 1: Write the correct alternative, the solution $8x \equiv 6 \pmod{14}$ are

(a) [8], [6] (b) [8], [14]

(c) [6], [13] (d) [8], [14], [16] [MLNRE 1985]

Solution: $x = [0] = \{....-6-8, 6, 20, 34 ....\}$ satisfies the equation $8x \equiv 6 \pmod{14}$ since $8x - 6 = 48 - 6 = 42$ which is divisible by 14.

Similarly for $x = 13$ the equation $8x \equiv 6 \pmod{14}$ is also satisfied.

$\therefore \quad x = [13] \equiv \{... -15, -1, 13, 27, 41 ....\}$ is also a slolution.

$x = [20] \equiv \{... -8, 6, 20, 34, 48 ....\}$ is also a slolution.

$\therefore$ Alternative (*c*) is correct.

PROBLEMS AND EXERCISES 2 (C) (I)

Write the dual of the followings:

1. $(B \cap C) \cup A = (B \cup A) \cap (C \cup A)$
2. $A \cup (B \cap C) = (A \cup B) \cap (A \cup C)$
3. $A - (B \cup C)$
4. $\phi' = U$
5. $A \cap A' = \phi$
6. Define $B_n = \{x : x \text{ is a multiple of } n, n \in N\}$
7. If $A_n = \left[0, \dfrac{1}{2n}\right]$ where $n \in N$, find $\bigcup_{i \in N} A_i$ and $\bigcap_{i \in N} A_i$

8. If $N = \{1, 2, 3 \ldots\}, A = \{2, 4, 6 \ldots\}, B = \{1, 3, 5 \ldots\}$. Is $\{A, B\}$ the partition of the set N?

9. Find all the partitions of $T = \{1, 2, 3, 4\}$.

10. If $T_n = \{x : x$ is a multiple of p where $p \in N\}$, find $T_3 \cap T_5$, $T_4 \cap T_6$, $T_2 \cap T_7$ and $\bigcup_{i \in P} T_i$, where P is the set of prime numbers.

11. If $A_n = [n, n + 1]$ where $n \in I$ the integers, find,

(i) $A_1 \cup A_2$ (ii) $A_3 \cap A_4$ (iii) $\bigcup_{i=8}^{17} A_i$ (iv) $\bigcup_{i=I} A_i$

12. If $B_n = \left(0, \frac{1}{2n}\right)$ where $n \in N$, find $B_3 \cup B_7$ and $B_3 \cap B_{14}$

13. Let the indexed family $\{A_i\}_{i \in I \times I}$ of subsets $R \times R$ defined by $A(p, q) = \{(x, y): p \leq x \leq p + 1, q \leq y \leq q + 1\}$.

$x, y \in R$ and R is the set of real number, sketch the followings

(i) $A(1, 2) \cup A(1, 3)$ (ii) $\bigcup_{i=1}^{3} A(z, i)$

(**Hint:** Take the advantage of the answersheet)

14. Let the indexed family $\{A_i\}_{i \in I \times I}$ of subsets $R \times R$ be defined by

$A(p, q) = \{(x, y) : x \in R, p \leq x \leq p + 1, y \in R, q \leq y \leq q + 1\}$

where R is the set of real numbers, sketch the followings on a diagram of $R \times R$ is the coordinate plane. (1) $A(1, 2)$

(2) $T = \bigcup_{k=0}^{2}\left(\bigcup_{q=-2}^{1} A_{(j,k)}\right)$

Express T in the set builder form.

(**Hint:** See the answersheet)

15. Express (i) all integers $\equiv 4 \pmod 5$

(ii) all integers $\equiv 6 \pmod 7$

16. Prove that $(a + b)^n \equiv (a^n + b^n) \pmod n$.

17. Write down the residue class which are (i) congruent modulo y (ii) congruent modulo 5. Write down the quotient sets in both the cases.

18. Does the congruence $207x \equiv 6 \pmod{18}$ posses a solution?

(**Hint:** See the answersheet.)

ANSWERS TO PROBLEMS AND EXERCISES 2C (I)

1. $(B \cup C) \cap A = (B \cap A) \cup (C \cap A)$
2. $A \cap (B \cup C) = (A \cap B) \cup (A \cap C)$
3. $(A - B) \cap (A - C)$.
4. $U' = \phi$
5. $A \cup A' = U$
6. $B_1 = \{1, 2, 3, 4 .....\}$; $B_2 = \{2, 4, 6, 8 .....\}$;
   $B_3 = \{3, 6, 9, 12 .....\}$. The index set is $N = B$.
7. $\left[0, \frac{1}{2}\right]$, $\{0\}$.
8. Yes
9. $\{\{1, 2, 3, 4\}\}, \{\{1\}, \{2, 3, 4\}\}, \{\{2\}, \{1, 3, 4\}\},$
   $\{\{3\}, \{1, 2, 4\}\}, \{\{4\}, \{1, 2,3\}\}, \{\{1, 2\}, \{3, 4\}\},$
   $\{\{1, 3\}, \{2, 4\}\}, \{\{1, 4\}, \{2, 3\}\}, \{\{1\}, \{2\}, \{3, 4\}\},$
   $\{\{1\}, \{3\}, \{2, 4\}\}, \{\{1\}, \{4\}, \{2, 3\}\}, \{\{2\}, \{3\}, \{1, 4\}\},$
   $\{\{2\}, \{4\}, \{1, 3\}\}, \{\{3\}, \{4\}, \{1, 2\}\}, \{\{1\}, \{2\}, \{3\}, \{4\}\}$.
10. $T_3 \cap T_5 = \{15, 30, 45, ...\} = T_{15}$
    $T_4 \cap T_6 = \{12, 24, 36, ...\} = T_{12}$
    $T_2 \cap T_7 = \{14, 28, 42, ...\} = T_{14}$
11. (i) $A_1 \cup A_2 = [1, 3]$
    (ii) $A_3 \cup A_4 = [4]$
    (iii) $\bigcup_{i=8}^{17} A_i = [8, 18]$
    (iv) $\bigcup_{i \in I} A_i = [1, 2] \cup [2, 3] \cup [3, 4] .....$
12. $B_3 \cup B_7 = \left(0, \frac{1}{6}\right) = B_3$

    $B_3 \cap B_{19} = \left(0, \frac{1}{38}\right) = B_{19}$
13. **Solution:** From the definition of $A_{(p,q)}$, we have $A_{(1, 2)} = \{(x, y) : x \in [1, 2], y \in [2, 3]\}$ i.e. the set of points whose first coordinates lies between 1 and 2 and the second coordinate between 2 and 3.

Similarly $A_{(1,3)} = \{(x, y) : x \in [1, 2], y \in [3, 4]\}$.

$A_{(1,2)} \cup A_{(1,3)}$ is sketched in Fig. I by shaded portion.

$\bigcup_{i=1}^{3} A_{(2,i)} = A_{(2,1)} \cup A_{22} \cup A_{2,3}$. For $A_{(2,1)}$ $x \in [2, 3]$, $y \in [1, 2]$.

For $A_{(2,2)} x \in [2, 3], y \in [2, 3]$ and for $A_{(2,3)} x \in [2, 3], y \in [3, 4]$.

$\bigcup_{i=1}^{3} A_{(2,i)}$ is sketched as in Fig. II by the shaded portion.

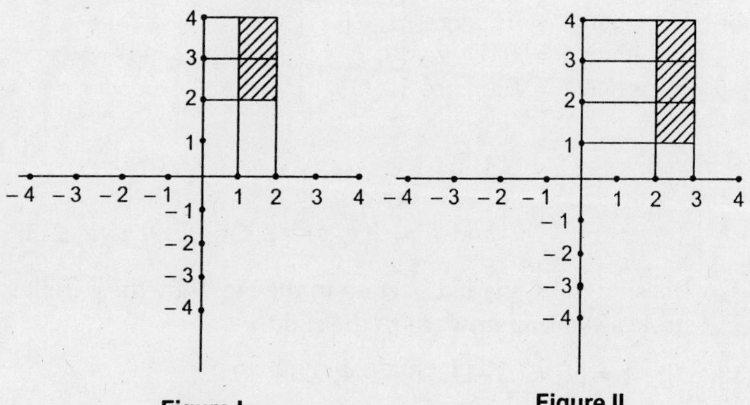

Figure I Figure II

14. Solution: From the equality $A_{(p,q)} = \{(x, y) : x \in R, p \leq x \leq p + 1, y \in R, q \leq y \leq q + 1\}$ we find that $A_{(1,2)} = \{(x, y): x \in [1, 2], y \in [2, 3]$ i.e. the set of points whose first coordinate lies between 1, 2 and the second coordinate between 2 and 3. $A(1, 2)$ is shown in Fig. I by the shaded portion.

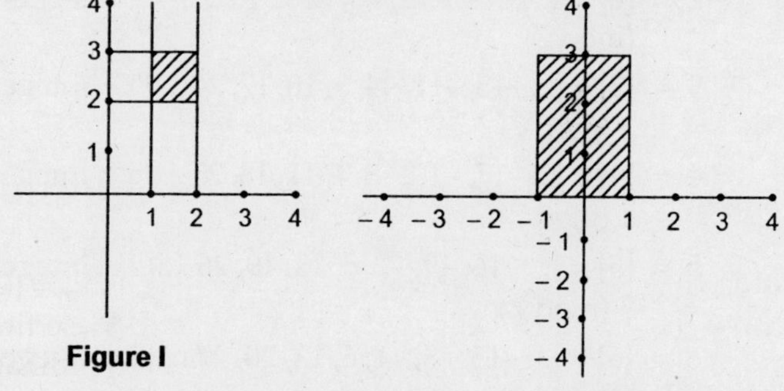

Figure I Figure II

$$T = \bigcup_{k=o}^{2}\left(\bigcup_{j=-2}^{1} A(j, k)\right)$$

$$= \bigcup_{k=c}^{2}(A(-2, k) \cup A(-1, k) \cup A(0, k) \cup A(1, k))$$

$$= A(-2, 0) \cup A(-1, 0) \cup A(0, 0) \cup A(1, 0) \cup A(-2, 1) \cup A(-1, 1) \cup A(0, 1) \cup A(1, 1) \cup A(-2, 2) \cup A(-1, 2) \cup A(0, 2) \cup A(1, 2).$$

$$\left\{\begin{array}{llll} \text{when } p & = -2 & x \in & [-2, \ -1] \\ \text{when } p & = 1 & x \in & [1, 2] \\ \text{when } q & = 0 & y \in & [0, 1] \\ \text{when } q & = 2 & y \in & [2, 3] \end{array}\right\}$$

$$\begin{cases} \text{Thus } -2 \le x \le 2 \\ \qquad\quad 0 \le y \le 3 \\ \text{and } T = \{(x, y): -2 \le x \le 2, \ 0 \le y \le 3\} \end{cases}$$

T is shown by shaded portion in the Fig. II by the parellel strokes slanting upward to the right.

15. (i) $\bar{4} = [4] = \{\ldots -11, -6, -1, 4, 9, 14, 19 \ldots.\}$

(ii) $\bar{6} = [6] = \{\ldots -15, -8, -1, 6, 13, 20, 27 \ldots.\}$

17. (i) $\bar{0} = [0] = \{\ldots -21, -14, -7, 0, 7, 14, 21 \ldots.\}$ i.e. integers ≡ (mod 7)

$\bar{1} = [1] = \{\ldots -20, -13, -6, 1, 8, 15 \ldots.\}$ i.e. integers ≡ 1 (mod 7)

$\bar{2} = [2] = \{\ldots -19, -12, -5, 2, 9, 16 \ldots.\}$ i.e. integers ≡ 2 (mod 7)

$\bar{3} = [3] = \{\ldots -18, -11, -4, 3, 10, 17, 24 \ldots.\}$ i.e. integers ≡ 3 (mod 7)

$\bar{4} = [4] = \{\ldots -17, -10, -3, 4, 11, 18, 25 \ldots.\}$ i.e. integers ≡ 4 (mod 7)

$\bar{5} = [5] = \{\ldots -16, -9, -2, 5, 12, 19, 26 \ldots.\}$ i.e. integers ≡ 5 (mod 7)

$\bar{6} = [6] = \{\ldots -15, -8, -1, 6, 13, 20, 27 \ldots.\}$ i.e. integers ≡ 6 (mod 7)

(ii) $\overline{0}$ = [0] = {... –15, –10, –5, 0, 5, 10, 15 ....} i.e. integers ≡ 0 (mod 5)

$\overline{1}$ = [1] = {... –14, –9, –4, 1, 6, 11, 16 ....} i.e. integers ≡ 1 (mod 5)

$\overline{2}$ = [2] = {... –13, –8, –3, 2, 7, 12, 17 ....} i.e. integers ≡ 2 (mod 5)

$\overline{3}$ = [3] = {... –12, –7, –2, 3, 8, 13, 18 ....} i.e. integers ≡ 3 (mod 5)

$\overline{4}$ = [4] = {... –11, –6, –1, 4, 9, 14, 19 ....} i.e. integers ≡ 4 (mod 5)

$I / (7) = \{\overline{0}, \overline{1}, \overline{2}, \overline{3}, \overline{4}, \overline{5}, \overline{6}\}$

$I / (5) = \{\overline{0}, \overline{1}, \overline{2}, \overline{3}, \overline{4}\}$

18. **Ans.** No.

Hint: $207x \equiv 6 \pmod{18} \Rightarrow 9.\,23x \equiv 6 \pmod{18}$

The greatest common divisor of 207 and 18 is 9 which does not divide 6 hence $207x$ and 6 are not congruent module 18.

Thus the given congruence does not possess a solution.

EXERCISE 2 C (II) SOME MORE IMPORTANT PROBLEMS WITH MODEL SOLUTIONS

Note: Please use the notation C instead of ⊆ for the subset of a set for this exercise only.

1. If $A \subset C$ prove that $A \times B \subset C \times B$. [I.I.T. 1972]
2. Find the smallest set Y such that $Y \cup \{1, 2\} = \{1, 2, 3, 5, 9\}$. [I.I.T. 1977]
3. If $A = \{2, 3, 4, 8, 10\}$, $B = \{3, 4, 5, 10, 12\}$ and $C = \{4, 5, 6, 12, 14\}$. Find $(A \cup B) \cap (A \cup C)$ and $(A \cap B) \cup (A \cap C)$. [Roorkee 1979]
4. Solve $3x^2 - 12x = 0$ where $x \in S = \{a + ib : b \neq 0, a, b \in R\}$.
   [**Hint:** See the solution of Q. No 13 Exercise 1 (ka)] [I.I.T. 1970]
5. If A and B are two set show that

$$A \cup B = (A - B) \cup (B - A) \cup (A \cap B)$$

Hence or otherwise prove

$$n(A \cup B) = n(A) + n(B) - n(A \cap B)$$

Where $n(A)$ denotes the number of elements in A.

[Roorkee 1978]

6. Let $A = \{\theta : 2\cos^2\theta + \sin\theta \leq 2\}$

   $B = \{\theta : \pi/2 \leq \theta \leq 3\pi/2\}$. Find $A \cap B$. [I.I.T. 1987]

7. A has 3 elements, and B has 6 elements. What can be the minimum number of elements in the set $A \cup B$?

8. Let U be the set of all people and M = {Males}, S = {College students}, T = {Teenagers i.e. youth belonging to the age groups from thirteen to nineteen years}, W = {People having heights more then five feet}. Express each of the following in the notation of set theory. (i) college students having heights more than five feet. (ii) People who are not teenagers and have their heights less than five feet. (iii) All people who are neither males nor teenages nor college students. [Roorkee 1977]

9. If $x = \{2, 3, 5, 7, 9\}$ be the universal set where $A = \{3, 7\}$ and $B = \{2, 5, 7, 9\}$ then prove that $(A \cup B)^1 = A^1 \cup B^1$.

   [MLNRE 1988]

10. Given $A = \{1, 2, 3\}$, $B = \{3, 4\}$, $C = \{4, 5, 6\}$, find $A \cup (B \cup C)$ and $(A \times B) \cap (B \times C)$. [I.I.T 1974]

11. Verify the following identities:

    (i) $A \cup (B \cap C) = (A \cup B) \cap (A \cup C)$

    (ii) $A \cap (B \cup C) = (A \cap B) \cup (A \cap C)$

    where A, B, C are three sets defined by

    $A = \{1, 2, 4, 5\}$, $B = \{2, 3, 5, 6\}$, $C = \{4, 5, 6, 7\}$ [Roorkee1975]

12. Given $A = \{2, 3\}$, $B = \{4, 5\}$, $C = \{5, 6\}$, find $A \times (B \cup C)$, $A \times (B \cap C)$, $(A \times B) \cup (B \times C)$. [I.I.T 1973]

13. Let $A = \{1, 2\}$ and $B = \{1, 3\}$. Prove that $(A \times B) \cup (B \times A) = \{(1, 3), (2, 3), (3, 1), (3, 2), (1, 1), (1, 2), (2, 1)\}$[Roorkee 1975]

14. The set A consists of all points within and on the unit circle $x^2 + y^2 = 1$, where as the set B consists of all points on and inside the rectanguler boundary $x = 0$, $x = 2$, $y = -3$, $y = 3$. Determine $A \cup B$ and $A \cap B$. Illustrate your answer by diagrams. [Roorkee 1973]

15. Suppose $A_1, A_2 \ldots A_{30}$ are thirty sets each with five elements and B_1, B_2 ... N_n are n sets each with three elements. Let

$$\bigcup_{i=1}^{30} A_i = \bigcup_{j=1}^{n} B_j = S$$

Assume that each element of S belongs to exactly ten of the Ai's and exactly to nine to the B_j's. Find n.

[I.I.T. 1981; MLNRE 1988]

16. An investigator interviewed 100 students to determine their preferences for the three drinks: milk (M), coffee (C) and tea (T). He reported the following: 10 students had all the twice drinks M, C, T; 20 had M and C only; 30 had C and T; 25 had M and T; 12 Had M only; 5 had C only, 8 had T only. Using a Venn diagram, find how many did not take any of the three drinks? [I.I.T 1978]

17. Prove $A - (B \cap C) = (A - B) \cup (A - C)$.

18. The report of one survey of 100 students stated that the numbers studying the various languages were: Sanskrit, Hindi and Tamil, 5; Hindi and Sanskrit, 10; Tamil and Sanskrit, 8; Hindi and Tamil, 20; Sanskrit, 30; Hindi 23; Tamil 50. The surveyor who prepared the report was fired. Why? [Roorkee 1983]

19. In a town of 10, 000 families it was found that 40% families buy newspaper A, 20% families buy newspaper B and 10% families buy newsaper C. 5% families buy A and B, 3% buy B and C and 4% buy A and C. If 2% families buy all the three newspapers, find the number of families which buy (i) A only (ii) B only (iii) none of A, B and C. [Roorkee 1991]

20. A survey of 500 television watchers produced the following information: 285 watch football, 195 watch hockey, 115 watch basketball, 45 watch football and basketball, 70 watch football and hockey, 50 watch hockey and basketball, 50 do not watch any of the three games. How many watch all the three games?

How many watch exactly one of the three games?

[Roorkee 1989]

21. State De-Morgan's laws. A graph of 123 workers went to a canteen for cold drinks, icecream and tea, 42 workers took icecream, 36 tea and 30 cold drinks. 15 workers purchased icecream and tea, 10 ice cream and cold drinks, and 4 cold drinks and tea but not ice cream, 11 took ice cream and tea but not cold drinks. Determine how many workers did not purchase any thing? [MLNRE 1989]

22. In a pollution study of 1500 Indian rivers the following data were reported. 520 were polluted by sulphur compounds, 335 polluted by phosphates, 425 were polluted by crude oil, 100 were followed by both crude oil and sulphur compounds, 180 were polluted by both sulphur compounds and phosphates, 150 were polluted by both phosphates and crude oil and 28 were polluted by sulphur compounds, phosphates and cude oil. How many of the rivers were polluted by at least one of the three impurities? How many of the rivers were polluted by exactly one of the three impurities? [Roorkee 1987]

23. A class has 175 students. The following table shows the number of strudents studying one or more of the following subjects in this class:

Subject	*No. of students*
Mathematics	100
Physics	70
Chemistry	46
Mathematics and Physics	30
Mathematics and Chemistry	28
Physics and Chemistry	23
Mathematics, Physics and Chemistry	18

How many students are enrolled in Mathematics alone, Physics alone and Chemistry alone?

Are there students who have not offered any of these three subjects? [Roorkee 1984]

24. Let R be a relation defined on the set of natural numbers N as $R = \{(x, y) : x \in N, y \in N, 2x + y = 41\}$.

Find the domain and range of this relation R. Also verify whether R is (i) reflexive (ii) symmetric (iii) transitive.

[Roorkee 1983]

25. If $X = \{1, 2, 3, 4, 5\}$ and $Y = \{1, 3, 5, 7, 9\}$.
Find $X \cap Y$ and $(X - Y) \cup (Y - X)$. Determine which of the following sets are (i) mappings (ii) relations.
(a) $F = \{(x, y) : y = x + 2, x \in X, y \in Y\}$
(b) $F = \{(1, 1), (2, 1), (3, 3), (4, 3), (5, 5)\}$
(c) $F = \{(1, 1), (1, 3), (3, 5), (3, 7), (5, 7)\}$
(d) $F = \{(1, 3), (2, 5), (4, 7), (5, 9), (3, 1)\}$ [Roorkee 1981]

26. What is the fundamental difference between function and relation?
Is $g = \{(1, 1), (2, 3), (3, 5), (4, 7)\}$ a function? If this is described by the formula
$g(x) = \alpha x + \beta$ then what values should be assigned to α and β. [Roorkee 1982]

27. Given $A = \{x : \pi/6 \le x \le \pi/3\}$ and $f(x) = \cos x - x\,(1+x)$; find $f(A)$. [I.I.T. 1980]

28. Let f be a one-one function with domain $\{x, y, z\}$ and range $\{1, 2\ 3\}$. If is given that exactly one of the following statements is true and the remaining two are false. $f(x) = 1$, $f(y) \ne 1, f(z) \ne 2$. Determine $f^{-1}(1)$.

29. Let A and B be two sets with a finite numebr of elements. Assume that there is injective mapping from A to B and that there is an injective mapping from B to A. Prove that there is bijective mapping form A to B. [I.I.T. 1981]

30. Let $A = \{x : -1 \le x \le 1\} = B$. For each of the following functions from A to B, find whether it is surjective, injective or bijective:
(i) $f(x) = x/2$ (ii) $g(x) = |x|$
(iii) $h(x) = x\,|x|$ (iv) $k(x) = x^2$
(v) $l(x) = \sin \pi x$

31. Let $A = \{x : 0 \le x \le 2\}$ and $B = \{1\}$. Give an example of a function from A to B. Can you define a function from B to A which is surjective. Give reasons for your answer.
[I.I.T. 1975]

32. Is the function $f : N \to N$ (N is the set of the natural numbers) defined by $f(n) = 2x + 3$ for all $n \in N$ surjective?
[I.I.T. 1974]

33. Are the followins sets of ordered pairs functions? If so, examine whether the mapping is surjective or injective?

(i) $\{(x, y) : x$ is a person, y is the mother of $x\}$

(ii) $\{(a, b) : a$ is a person, b is an ancestor of $a\}$.

[I.I.T. 1974]

34. Consider the following relations on the set of real numbers.

$$R = \{(x, y) : x, y \text{ are real } x^2 + y^2 \leq 25\}$$

$$R' = \left\{(x, y) : x, y \text{ are real } y \geq \frac{4x^2}{9}\right\}$$

Find $R \cap R'$. Is the relation $R \cap R'$ a function? [I.I.T. 1979]

35. Find the domain and range of $f(x) = \dfrac{x^2}{1+x^2}$ (x real). Is the function one to one. [I.I.T. 1978]

36. Let $A = R - \{3\}$, $B = R - \{1\}$. Let $f: A \to B$ be defined by $f(x) = \dfrac{x-2}{x-3}$. Is f bejective? Give reasons. [I.I.T. 1971]

37. (a) Let $f: R \to R$ be defined by $f(x) = \cos(5x + 2)$. Is f invertible? Justify your answer. [I.I.T. 1977]

(b) A mapping is defined as $f: R \to R$, $f(x) = \cos x$. Show that it is neither one-one nor surjective. [MLNRE 1989]

38. If R is a set of real numbers and $f: R \to R$ is given by the relation $f(x) = \sin x$, $x \in R$ and mapping $g: R \to R$ by the relation $g(x) = x^2$, $x \in R$ then prove that $fog \neq gof$.

[MLNRE 1985]

39. Choose the correct alternative.

(i) Let $f: R \to R$ be defined by $f(x) = 3x - 4$ then f^{-1} is

(a) $\frac{1}{3}(x+4)$ (b) $\frac{1}{3}x - 4$

(c) $3x + 4$ (d) not defined.

[MLNRE 1993]

(ii) Let A and B have 3 and 6 elements respectively. What can be the minimum numbers of elements in $A \cup B$?

(a) 3 (b) 6

(c) 9 (d) 18. [MLNRE 1987]

(iii) Two finite sets have m and n elements. The total number of subsets of the first set is 56 more than the total number of subsets of the second set. The values of m and n are

(a) 7, 6 (b) 6, 3

(c) 5, 1 (d) 8, 7. [MLNRE 1991]

(iv) The composite mapping fog of the maps $f : R \to R$, $f(x) = \sin x$; $g : R \to R$, $g(x) = x^2$ is

(a) $\sin x + x^2$ (b) $(\sin x)^2$

(c) $\sin x^2$ (d) $\dfrac{\sin x}{x^2}$. [MLNRE 1987]

(v) The function $f : N \to N$ (N is the set of natural numebrs) defined by $f(n) = 2x + 3$ is

(a) Surjective (b) Non surjective

(c) Injective (d) None of these.

[MLNRE 1987]

(vi) If $f : R \to R$ defined by $f(x) = x^2 + 1$ then the value of f^{-1} (17) and f^{-1} (3) respectively are

(a) ϕ, {4, –4} (b) {3, – 3}, ϕ

(c) ϕ {3, –3} (d) {4, –4}, ϕ. [MLNRE 1986]

40. Which of the four statements given below is different from the other?

(a) f: $A \to B$

(b) f: $x \to f(x)$

(c) f is a mapping of A into B

(d) f is a function of A into B. [MLNRE 1986]

41. Assume R and S are (non-empty) relations is a set A. Which of the relation given below is false.

(a) If R and S are transitive then $R \cup S$ is transitive

(b) If R and S are transitive then $R \cap S$ is transitive

(c) If R and S are transitive then $R \cup S$ is symmetric

(d) If R and S are transitive then $R \cap S$ is reflexive

[MLNRE 1986]

42. Write the correct alternative

(i) The relation less than in the set of natural number is

(a) only symmetric (b) only transitive

(c) only reflexive (d) equivalence realtion.

[MLNRE 1993]

(ii) Give the sets $A = \{1, 2, 3\}$, $B = \{3, 4\}$, $C = \{4, 5, 6\}$ then $A \cup (B \cap C)$ is

(a) $\{3\}$ (b) $\{1, 2, 3, 4\}$

(c) $\{1, 2, 5, 6\}$ (d) $\{1, 2, 3, 4, 5, 6\}$

[MLNRE 1988]

(iii) If X and Y are two sets then $X \cap (X \cup Y)$ equals

(a) X (b) Y

(c) ϕ (d) None of these. [I.I.T 1979]

(iv) Consider the set of all determinants of order 3 with entries 0 or 1 only.

Let B be the subset of A consisting of all determinants with value 1. Let C be the subset of the set of all determinants with value –1. Then

(a) C is empty

(b) B has as many elements as C

(c) $A = B \cup C$

(d) B has twice as many elements as C.

(v) Let A be a set containing 10 distinct elements, then the total number of distinct function from A to A is

(a) 101 (b) 10^{10}

(c) 2^{10} (d) $2^{10} - 1$. [MLNRE 1992]

(vi) Let $A = \{x, y, z\}$, $B = \{u, v, w\}$ the function $f: A \to B$ is defined by $f(x) = u$, $f(y) = v$, $f(z) = v$ is

(a) Surjective (b) Bijective

(c) Injective (d) None of these.

[MLNRE 1988]

(vii) If sets A and B are defined as

$A = \{(x, y) : y = e^x, x \in [R]\}$

$B = \{(x, y) : y = x, x \in [R]\}$ then

(a) $B \subset A$ (b) $A \subset B$

(c) $A \cap B = \phi$ (d) $A \cup B = A$. [MLNRE 1994]

43. Write True or False in the following problems:

(i) These exists a set of all sets.

(a) True (b) False

(ii) P, Q, R are subsets of a set A. Then

$R \times (P^c \cup Q^c) = (R \times P) \cap (R \times Q)$

(a) True (b) False [I.I.T. 1980]

(iii) For any two subsets X and Y of a set A, define $X\,O\,Y = (X^c \cap Y) \cup (X \cap Y^c)$.

Then for any three subset X, Y, and Z of a set A we have $(XOY)OZ = XO(YOZ)$

(a) True (b) False [I.I.T. 1981]

(iv) For real numbers x and y we write $x * y$ if $x - y + \sqrt{2}$ is an irrational number. Then the relation * is an equivalence relation.

(a) True (b) False [I.I.T. 1981]

44. Draw the graphs of solution set of the following inequalities.

$x^2 + y^2 - 2x \geq 0, 3x - y - 12 \leq 0, y - x \leq 0, y \geq 0$ [I.I.T. 1978]

45. Define "real valued function". Describe the algebra of real valued function.

46. We are taught "A partition of a set A is its decomposition into nonempty subsets or cells which are disjoint, whose union is A and $a \in A$ belongs to a unique subset or cell."

Are the following partitions of A where A is $\{a, b, c, d, e, f, g, h, i\}$?

(i) $[\{a, c, e\}, \{b, f\}, \{d, h, i\}]$

(ii) $[\{a, c, e\}, \{b, d, f, h\}, \{e, g, i\}]$

(iii) $[\{a, c, e\}, \{b, d, f, h\}, \{g, i\}]$

ANSWERS TO "SOME MORE IMPORTANT PROBLEMS" EXERCISE 2C(II)

(Hints and Solutions)

1. **Solution:** Let $(x, y) \in A \times B$

   Then $x \in A$ and $y \in B \Rightarrow x \in c$ and $y \in B$ [$\because A \subset C$]

   $\Rightarrow (x, y) \in C \times B$

   Thus $A \times B \subset C \times B$ Proved.

2. **Ans.** $Y = \{3, 5, 9\}$

   Hint: $Y \cup \{1, 2\} = \{1, 2, 3, 5, 9\}$

   $\therefore Y = \{3, 5, 9\}$.

3. **Ans.** $\{2, 3, 4, 5, 8, 10, 12\}$. $\{3, 4, 10\}$.

   Solution: We have $A \cup B = \{2, 3, 4, 5, 8, 10, 12\}$

   $A \cup C = \{2, 3, 4, 5, 6, 8, 10, 12, 14\}$

   $A \cap B = \{3, 4, 10\}$; $A \cap C = \{4\}$

   $\therefore \quad (A \cup B) \cap (A \cup C) = \{2, 3, 4, 5, 8, 10, 12\}$

   $(A \cap B) \cup (A \cap C) = \{3, 4, 10\}$.

4. Please see the solution of Q. No. 13 Exercise 1(ka).

5. **Solution:** We take the help of Venn diagram to prove $A \cup B = (A - B) \cup (B - A) \cup (A \cap B)$.

   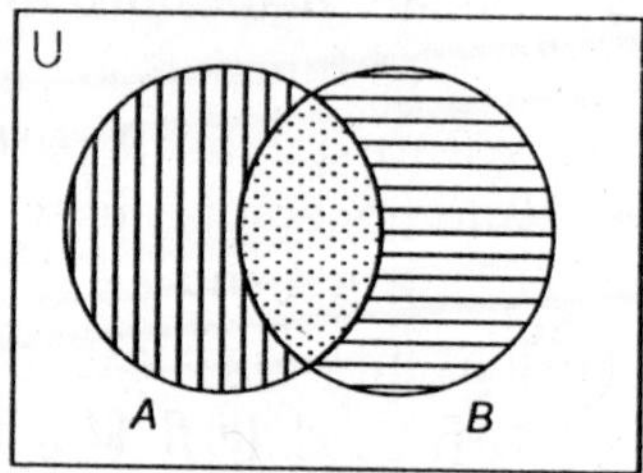

   Figure Q. 5

   The portion shaded by vertical lines shows $A - B$ and the portion shaded by horizontal lines shows $B - A$. The portion shaded by dots in $A \cap B$.

   Thus $A \cup B = (A - B) \cup (B - A) \cup (A \cap B)$.

   We have $x \in A - B \Leftrightarrow x \in A$ and $x \notin B \Leftrightarrow x \in A$ and $x \in B'$

   $x \in A \cap B'$ $\therefore A - B = A \cap B'$

   $$\therefore (A - B) \cup (A \cap B) = (A \cap B') \cup (A \cap B)$$
   $$= A \cap (B' \cap B) = A \cap U = A$$

   Thus $(A - B) \cup (A \cap B) = A$ ...(1)

   Again $(A - B) \cap (A \cap B) = (A \cap B') \cap (A \cap B) = A \cap (B' \cup B)$

   $= A \cap \phi = \phi$

Thus $(A - B) \cap (A \cap B) = \phi$ ...(2)

In a similar way we can write

$$(B - A) \cup (A \cap B) = B \quad ...(3)$$

and $(B - A) \cap (A \cap B) = \phi$ ...(4)

From (1) and (3)

$$A \cup B = [(A - B) \cup (A \cap B)] \cup [(B - A) \cup (A \cap B)]$$
$$= (A - B) \cup (A \cap B) \cup (B - A) \cup (A \cap B)$$
$$= (A - B) \cup (B - A) \cup A \cap B \quad ...(5)$$
$$(\because A \cap B \cup A \cap B = A \cap B)$$

Now the sets $A - B$, $B - A$ and $A \cap B$ are pairwise disjoint and hence

$n(A \cup B) = n(A - B) + n(B - A) + n(A \cap B)$ ...(6)

Also from the equation $A = (A - B) \cup (A \cap B)$

We can write $n(A) = n(A - B) + n(A \cap B)$

i.e. $n(A - B) = n(A) - n(A \cap B)$ ...(7)

From $B = (B - A) \cup (A \cap B)$

$n(B - A) = n(B) - n(A \cap B)$ ...(8)

$\therefore$ (6) with the help (7) and (8) gives

$n(A \cup B) = n(A) - n(A \cap B) + n(B) - n(A \cap B) + n(A \cap B)$

6. Ans. $\left\{\theta : \frac{\pi}{2} \le \theta \le \frac{5\pi}{6} \text{ or } \pi \le \theta \le \frac{3\pi}{2}\right\}$.

Solution: We have

$$2\cos^2\theta + \sin\theta \le 2 \Rightarrow 2(1 - \sin^2\theta) + \sin\theta \le 2$$
$$\Rightarrow 2 - 2\sin^2\theta + \sin\theta \le 2 \Rightarrow \sin\theta - 2\sin^2\theta \le 0$$
$$\Rightarrow 2\sin^2\theta + \sin\theta \ge 0 \Rightarrow \sin\theta\,(2\sin\theta - 1) \ge 0 \quad ...(1)$$

As $\sin\theta \le 0$ makes both the factors negative and their product is positive i.e. > 0. Thus $\sin\theta \le 0$ is one of the solutions, of inequality No. (1).

Now $\sin\theta \le 0 \Rightarrow \sin\theta \le \sin 0$ or $\sin\pi$

i.e. $0 \le \theta \le \pi$ but the permisisilde interval is given by

$$B = \left\{\theta : \frac{\pi}{2} \le \theta \le \frac{3\pi}{2}\right\}$$

hence the solution $\sin\theta \le 0$ becomes $\pi \le \theta \le \frac{3\pi}{2}$

The second solution of the inequality (1) is

$\sin\theta \ge \frac{1}{2}$ as it makes both the factors positive whose product is positive i.e. > 0.

Now $\sin\theta \ge \frac{1}{2} \Rightarrow \sin\theta \ge \sin\frac{\pi}{6}$ or $\sin\frac{5\pi}{6}$

$\Rightarrow \frac{\pi}{6} \le \theta \le \frac{5\pi}{6}$ but the interval is $\left[\frac{\pi}{2}, \frac{3\pi}{2}\right]$

$\therefore \sin\theta \ge \frac{1}{2}$ gives $\frac{\pi}{2} \le \theta \le \frac{5\pi}{6}$

$\therefore A \cap B = \left\{\theta : \frac{\pi}{2} \le \theta \le \frac{5\pi}{6} \text{ or } \pi \le \theta \le \frac{3\pi}{2}\right\}$

7. **Ans.** The minimum number of elements in $A \cup B$ is 6.
   Hint: Do yourself.
8. **Ans.** (i) $S \cap W$ (ii) $U - T$ i.e. T^1
   (iii) $U - (M \cup T \cup S)$ i.e. $(M \cup T \cup S)^1$
9. **Solution:** We have $A \cup B = \{2, 3, 5, 7, 9\}$
   $\therefore \quad (A \cup B)^1 = X - (A \cup B) = \{2, 3, 5, 7, 9\} - \{2, 3, 5, 7, 9\} = \phi$
   $B^1 = X - B = \{3\};$
   $A^1 = X - A = \{2, 5, 9\}$
   $\therefore \quad A^1 \cap B^1 = \phi$
   $\therefore \quad (A \cup B)^1 = A \cap B^1$
10. **Ans.** $(A \times B) \cap (B \times C) = \{1, 3, 4\}$
    $A \cup (B \cup C) = \{1, 2, 3, 4, 5, 6\}$
    Hint: Do yourself.
11. **Hint:** Verify yourself.
12. **Ans.** $A \times (B \cup C) = \{(2, 4), (2, 5), (2, 6), (3, 4), (3, 5), (3, 6)\}$
    $A \times (B \cap C) = \{(2, 5), (3, 5)\}.$
    $(A \times B) \cup (B \times C) = \{(2, 4), (2, 5), (3, 4), (3, 5), (4, 5), (4, 6), (5, 5), (5, 6)\}.$

    Hint: Do yourself.

13. Do yourself.

14. **Ans.** $A \cup B = \{(x, y) : x^2 + y^2 \leq 1 \text{ and } x \leq 0$ or $(0 \leq x \leq 2 \text{ and } -3 \leq y \leq 3)\}$

$A \cap B = \{(x, y) : x^2 + y^2 \leq 1 \text{ and } x \geq 0\}$.

Solution: The set $A = \{(x, y) : x^2 + y^2 \leq 1\}$.

This set consists of all points within and on the circle $x^2 + y^2 = 1$ and is shaded by horizontal lines.

The set $B = \{(x, y) : 0 \leq x \leq 2$ and $-3 \leq y \leq 3\}$

Consists of those points which line on and inside the rectangular boundary *MNPQ* and is shaded by vertical lines.

$A \cup B = LRSMNPQL$ and is $\{(x, y) : x^2 + y^2 \leq 1$ and $x \leq 0$ or $(0 \leq x \leq 2$ and $-3 \leq y \leq 3)\}$

$A \cup B = LOSTL$ and is $\{(x, y) : x^2 + y^2 \leq 1$ and $x \geq 0\}$.

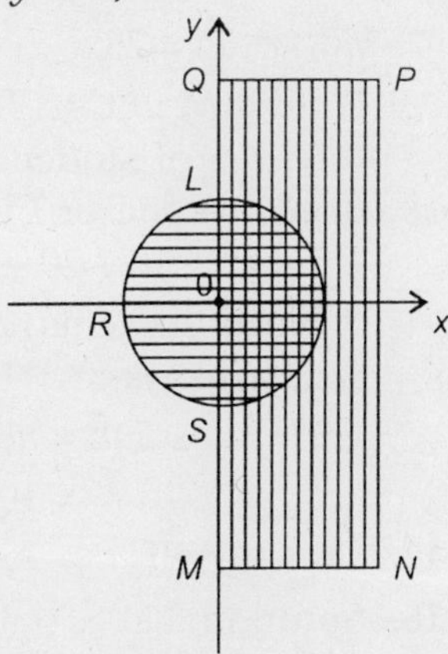

Figure Q. 14

15. **Ans.** 45.

Solution: $\bigcup_{i=1}^{30} A_i = A_1 \cup A_2 \cup A_3 \ldots \cup A_{30}$. Each A_i has five elements. $\therefore n(A_1) + n(A_2) + \ldots + n(A_{30}) = 5 \times 30 = 150$

$\bigcup_{j=1}^{n} B_j = B_1 \cup B_2 \cup B_3 \ldots \cup B_n$. Each B_j has 3 elements

$\therefore \quad n(B_1) + n(B_2) + \ldots\ldots + n(B_n) = 3 \times n = 3n.$

Let x be the no. of elements in S. Since each element of S belongs to exactly ten of the A_i's

$\therefore \quad 10x = 150$

$\Rightarrow \quad x = 15$

Each element of S belongs to exactly 9 of the B_j's

$\therefore \quad 9x = 3n$

$9 \times 15 = 3n \Rightarrow n = 45$

16. Ans. 20.

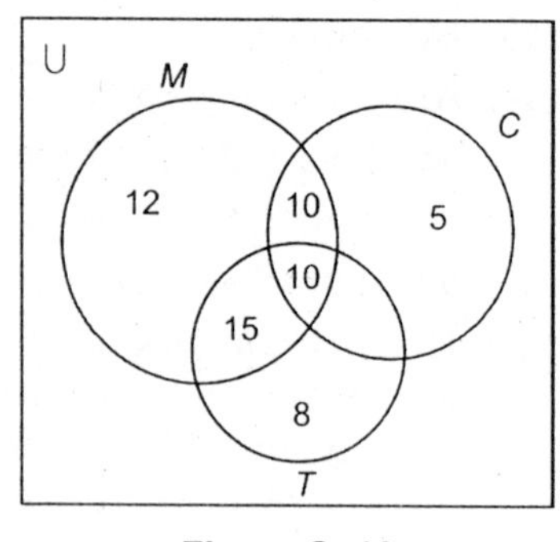

Figure Q. 16

Solution: We have

$n(M \cap C \cap T) = 10; n(M) = 12$

$n(M \cap C) = 20; n(C) = 5$

$n(C \cap T) = 30; n(T) = 8$

$n(M \cap T) = 25;$

Now $n(M \cup C \cup T)$ i.e. the total no. of students taking drinks M or C or T is $12 + 10 + 5 + 15 + 10 + 20 + 8 = 80$.

$\therefore$ No. of students not taking any drinks is

$$n(M \cup C \cup T)^1 = n(U) - n(M \cup C \cup T)$$
$$= 100 - 80 = 20.$$

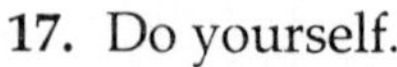

17. Do yourself.

18. Solution: Let S, H and T be the set of students who study Sanskrit, Hindi and Tamil respectively.

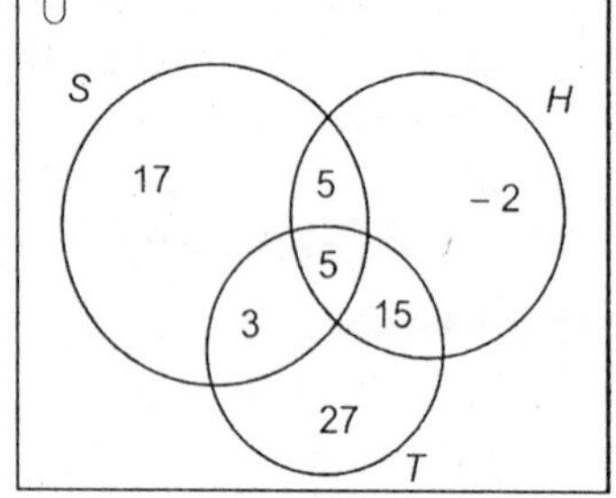

We are given

$n(S \cap H \cap T) = 5; n(S) = 30$

$n(T \cap S) = 8; n(H) = 23$

$n(H \cap T) = 20; n(T) = 50$

$n(S \cup H \cup T) = 100$ (given)

With the help of Venn diagram we have $n(S \cup H \cup T) = 17 + 5 + 5 + 3 + 15 + 27 - 2 = 72 - 2 = 70$. This does not tally with 100.

Aliter: $n(S \cup H \cup T) = n(S) + n(H \cup T) - n\{S \cap (H \cup T)\}$

$= n(S) + n(H) + n(T) - n\{(H \cap T)\} - n[(S \cap H) \cup (S \cap T)]$

$= n(S) + n(H) + n(T) - n\{(H \cap T)\} - [n[(S \cap H) + n(S \cap T) - n(S \cap H \cap T)]$

$= 30 + 23 + 50 - 20 - 10 - 8 + 5 = 70$

The surveyor was fired due to the inconsistency of the data. There should be survey of 70 students only.

19. Ans. 3300, 1400, 500, 4000.

Solution: $n(A) = 40\%$ of $10{,}000 = 4000$

$n(B) = 20\%$ of $10{,}000 = 2000$

$n(C) = 10\%$ of $10{,}000 = 1000$

$n(A \cap B) = 5\%$ of $10{,}000 = 500$

$n(B \cap C) = 3\%$ of $10{,}000 = 300$

$n(C \cap A) = 4\%$ of $10{,}000 = 400$

$n(A \cap B \cap C) = 2\%$ of $10{,}000 = 200$

$n(U) = 10{,}000$

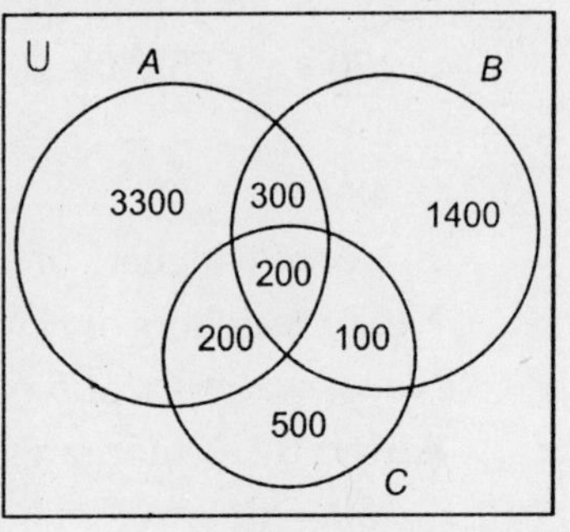

Figure Q. 19

Taking the advantage of Venn diagram we have

No. of families buying A only is $4000 - 700 = 3300$

No. of families buying B only is $2000 - 600 = 1400$

No. of families buying C only is $1000 - 500 = 500$

No. of families buying none of A, B, C is $10{,}000 - [3300 + 1400 + 500] - [300 + 200 + 200 + 100]$

$= 10{,}000 - [5200] - [800] = 10{,}000 - 6000 = 4000.$

20. Ans. 190 watch football only; 95 watch hockey only; 40 watch basketball and 20 watch all the three games.

Solution: Let F, H and B be the set of watchers watching football, hockey and basketball respectively. Let $n(F \cap H \cap B)$ be x. We have

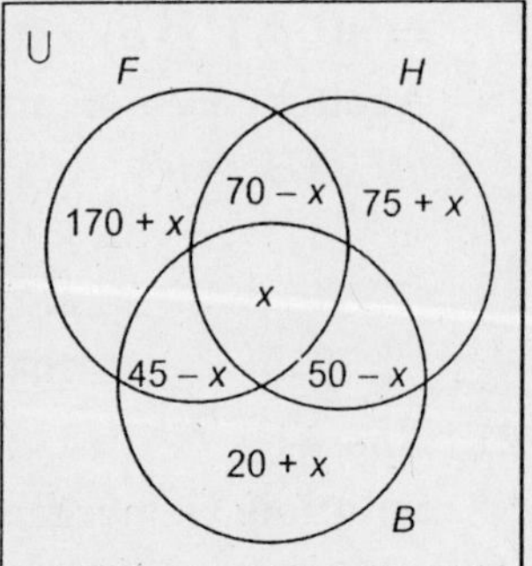

$n(F) = 285$; $n(H) = 195$; $n(B) = 115$

$n(F \cap B) = 45$; $n(F \cap H) = 70$

$n(H \cap B) = 50$;

No. of watchers of F only $= 285 - (70 - x + x + 45 - x)$

$= 285 - 115 + x = 170 + x$

No. of watchers of H only $= 195 - (70 - x + x + 50 - x)$

$= 195 - 120 + x = 75 + x$

No. of watchers of B only $= 115 - (45 - x + x + 50 - x)$

$= 115 - 95 + x = 20 + x$

Fifty are such that they do not watch any game.

$\therefore 170 + x + 75 + x + 20 + x + 70 - x + x + 45 - x + 50 - x + 50 = 500$

$\Rightarrow 480 + x = 500 \therefore x = 20$

$\therefore$ No. of watchers of F only $= 170 + 20 = 190$

No. of watchers of H only $= 75 + 20 = 95$

No. of watchers of B only $= 20 + 20 = 40$

Aliter: By Demorgan's law

$$50 = n(F' \cap H' \cap B') = n(F \cup H \cup B)'$$
$$= 500 - n(F \cup H \cup B)$$
$$\Rightarrow 50 = 500 - \{n(F) + n(H \cup B) - n[F \cap (H \cup B)]\}$$
$$= 500 - \{n(F) + n(H) + n(B) - n(H \cap B) - n[(F \cap H) \cup (F \cap B)]\}$$
$$= 500 - \{n(F) + n(H) + n(B) - n(H \cap B) - n[(F \cap H) - n(F \cap B)] + n[(F \cap H) \cap (F \cap B)]\}$$
$$= 500 - \{285 + 195 + 115 - 50 - 70 - 45 + n(F \cap H \cap B)\}$$
$$= 500 - \{575 - 165 + n(F \cap H \cap B)\}$$
$$= 50 - 500 + 430 = - n(F \cap H \cap B)$$

$\Rightarrow n(F \cap H \cap B) = 20$

Again by Demorgan's law

$$n(F \cap H' \cap B') = n\{F \cap (H \cup B)'\}$$
$$= n(F) - n\{(F \cap H) \cup (F \cap B)\}$$
$$= n(F) - \{n(F \cap H) + n(F \cap B) - n(F \cap H \cap B)\}$$
$$= 285 - 70 - 45 + 20 = 190.$$

21. Ans. 44

Solution: Demorgan's law status

(1) $A - (B \cup C) = (A - B) \cap (A - C)$

(2) $A - (B \cap C) = (A - B) \cup (A - C)$

(3) $(A \cup B)' = A' \cap B'$

(4) $(A \cap B)' = A' \cup B'$

(5) $n(A' \cap B' \cap C') = n(A \cup B \cup C)'$

$$= n(U) - n(A \cup B \cup C)$$

$n(U) = 123;\ n(I) = 42;\ n(T) = 36,\ n(C) = 30$

$n(I \cap T) = 15;\ n(I \cap C) = 10;\ n(C \cap T \cap I') = 4$

$n(I \cap T \cap C') = 11$

We have to find $n(I' \cap T' \cap C')$.

Now 4 $= n(C \cap T \cap I') = n(A \cap I')$ where $A = C \cap T$

$= n(A) - n(A \cap I) = n(C \cap T) - n(C \cap T \cap I)$

Thus $4 = n(C \cap T \cap I') = n(C \cap T) - n(C \cap T \cap I)$ ...(1)

Also $11 = n(C \cap T \cap I') = n(I \cap T) - n(I \cap T \cap C)$

$\therefore 11 = 15 - n(I \cap T \cap C)$

$\therefore n(I \cap T \cap C) = 4$

From (1) $4 = n(C \cap T) - 4$

$\therefore n(C \cap T) = 8$

$\therefore n(I' \cap T' \cap C')$

$= n(I \cup T \cup C)'$

$= n(U) - n(I \cup T \cup C)$

$= n(U) - \{n(I) + n(T) + n(C) - n(I \cap T) - n(T \cap C) - n(C \cap I)$
$+ n(I \cap T \cap C)\}$

$= 123 - \{42 + 36 + 30 - 15 - 8 - 10 + 4\} = 44$

Note: $n(C \cap T \cap I')$ stands for the element which belong to C and T but not I.

22. Ans. 268, 33, 878, 203

Solution: Let S, P and C be the set of Indian reviews polluted by sulphur compounds, phosphates and crude oil. We are given

$n(U) = 1500, n(S) = 520, n(P) = 335$

$n(C) = 425; n(C \cap S) = 100; n(S \cap P) = 180$

$n(P \cap C) = 150$ and $n(S \cap P \cap C) = 28$.

We have to determine $n(S \cup P \cup C)$ and $n(S \cap P' \cap C')$.

We $n(S \cap P' \cap C') = n[S \cap (P \cap C)']$

$= n(S) - [(S \cap P) \cup (S \cap C)]$

$= n(S) - \{n(S \cap P) + (S \cap C) - n(S \cap P \cap C)\}$

$= 520 - \{180 + 100 - 28\}$

$= 520 - \{252\} = 268.$

$n(S \cup P \cup S)$

$= n(S) + n(P) + n(C) - n(P \cap C) - \{n(S \cap P) + n(S \cap C) - n(S \cap P \cap C)\}$

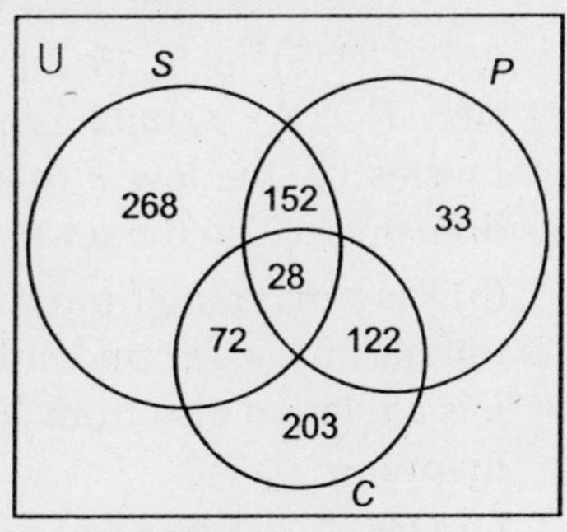

Figure Q. 22

$= 520 + 335 + 425 - 150 - \{180 + 100 - 28\}$

$= 1280 - 150 - \{252\}$

$= 1280 - 402 - 878.$

By Venn diagram, the rivers polluted by only C is $425 - [28 + 72 + 22]$

$= 425 - 222 = 203$

The rivers polluted by only P is $335 - [152 + 122 + 28]$

$= 335 - 302 = 33.$

23. Ans. 60, 35, 13, 22

Hint: Given $n(U) = 175$, $n(M) = 100$; $n(P) = 70$;

$n(C) = 46$; $n(M \cap P) = 30$; $n(M \cap C) = 28$;

$n(P \cap C) = 23$ and $n(M \cap P \cap C) = 18$

Now do yourself.

24. Ans. $\{1, 2, 3, \ldots, 19, 20\}$; $\{39, 37, \ldots, 3, 1\}$.

Solution: We have $R = \{(x, y) : x \in N, y \in N \text{ and } 2x + y = 41\}$

This relation R can be written as

$R = \{(1, 39)(2, 37)\ldots\ldots(19, 3)(20, 1)\}$

$\therefore$ Domain of R is $\{1, 2, 3 \ldots\ldots 19, 20\}$

Range of R is $\{39, 37 \ldots\ldots 3, 1\}$

sin $(x, x) \notin R \;\forall\; x \in N$ $\therefore$ R is not reflexive. We see $(2, 2) \notin R$.

$\therefore$ R is not symmetric.

25. Ans. $X \cap Y = \{1, 3, 5\}$; $(X - Y) \cup (Y - X) = \{2, 4, 7, 9\}$.

Solution: (a) $F = \{(1, 3), (2, 4), (3, 5), (4, 6), (5, 7)\}$ $4 \in X$ and $6 \notin Y$

$\therefore$ $(4, 6) \notin F$. Similarly $(2, 4) \notin F$.

$\therefore$ $F = \{(1, 3), (3, 5), (5, 7)\}$. Thus F is a relation from X to Y since $F \subset (X \times Y)$ but it is not a mapping as 2 and 4 have no images i.e. the law F does not transform 2 and 4 of the domain set X in the set Y.

(b) F is a mapping from X to Y as every element of X has a unique image in Y under the correspondence F. In addition F is a relation also from X to Y. Hence F is many one into mapping.

(c) Here $1 \in X$ has two images 1 and 3 in Y so f is not a mapping. $F \subset X \times Y$. $\therefore$ F is a relation.

(d) Here F is a bijective (one-one and onto) mapping and it is also relation.

26. Ans. $\alpha = 2$ and $\beta = -1$

Solution: Fundamental difference between function and relation: A function f from A to B is a subset of $A \times B$. In this subset $a \in A$ is seen in one and only one ordered pair belonging to f. Every subset of $A \times B$ is a relation. Both have domain and range. In relation more than one ordered pair may have the same first component where as in function this is not possible. A function is a special type of relation where the image of every element of the domain is unique.

$g = \{(1, 1), (2, 3), (3, 5), (4, 7)\}$ is a function as every element of the set $\{1, 2, 3, 4\}$ has unique image.

$g(x) = \alpha x + \beta \Rightarrow 1 = \alpha + \beta$ and $3 = 2\alpha + \beta$.

These two give $\alpha = 2$ and $\beta = -1$

Note: The difference between a function and a relation can also be understood with the help of a diagram in the coordinate plan, described in the previous article.

27. Ans. $f(A) = \left\{u : \frac{1}{2} - \frac{\pi}{3}\left(1 + \frac{\pi}{3}\right) \le f(u) \le \frac{\sqrt{3}}{2} - \frac{\pi}{6}\left(1 + \frac{\pi}{6}\right)\right\}$

Solution: x lies in $\left[\frac{\pi}{6}, \frac{\pi}{3}\right]$ where $A = \left\{x : \frac{\pi}{6} \le x \le \frac{\pi}{3}\right\}$

$$f(x) = \cos x - x(1 - x)$$

$$\therefore f(A) = \cos A - A(1 - A)$$

$$\because \frac{\pi}{6} \le x \le \frac{\pi}{3}$$

$$\therefore \cos\frac{\pi}{6} \ge x \ge \cos\frac{\pi}{3} \Rightarrow \frac{\sqrt{3}}{2} \ge x \ge \frac{1}{2}$$

$$\Rightarrow \frac{1}{2} \le x \le \frac{\sqrt{3}}{2} \qquad ...(1)$$

$$\text{Again } \frac{\pi}{6} \le x \le \frac{\pi}{3} \qquad ...(2)$$

$$\therefore 1 + \frac{\pi}{6} \le 1 + x \le 1 + \frac{\pi}{3} \qquad ...(3)$$

∴ Multiplying (2) by (3), we get

$$\frac{\pi}{6}\left(1+\frac{\pi}{6}\right)\le x(1+x)\le\frac{\pi}{3}\left(1+\frac{\pi}{3}\right)$$

$$\Rightarrow -\frac{\pi}{6}\left(1+\frac{\pi}{6}\right)\ge -x(1+x)\ge -\frac{\pi}{3}\left(1+\frac{\pi}{3}\right)$$

$$\Rightarrow -\frac{\pi}{3}\left(1+\frac{\pi}{3}\right)\le -x(1+x)\le -\frac{\pi}{6}\left(1+\frac{\pi}{6}\right) \qquad ...(4)$$

Adding (1) and (4), we get

$$\frac{1}{2}-\frac{\pi}{3}\left(1+\frac{\pi}{3}\right)\le \cos x - x(1+x)\le\frac{\sqrt{3}}{2}-\frac{\pi}{6}\left(1+\frac{\pi}{6}\right)$$

i.e. $\frac{1}{2}-\frac{\pi}{3}\left(1+\frac{\pi}{3}\right)\le f(x)\le\frac{\sqrt{3}}{2}-\frac{\pi}{6}\left(1+\frac{\pi}{6}\right)$

Thus $f(A) = \left\{4:\frac{1}{2}-\frac{\pi}{3}\left(1+\frac{\pi}{3}\right)\le f(u)\le\frac{\sqrt{3}}{2}-\frac{\pi}{6}\left(1+\frac{\pi}{6}\right)\right\}$

28. We have the following three possibilities

(i) $f(x) = 1$ is true and $f(y) \ne 1, f(z) \ne 2$ are false.

(ii) $f(y) \ne 1$ is true and $f(y) = 1, f(z) \ne 2$ are false.

(iii) $f(z) \ne 2$ is true and $f(x) = 1, f(y) \ne 1$ are false.

In (i) the true statements are

$f(x) = 1, f(y) = 1$ and $f(z) = 2$,

where x, y have the same image 1 and that is why f in not a one-one mapping and hence this possibility is excluded.

In (ii) the true statements are

$f(x) \ne 1, f(y) \ne 1$ and $f(z) = 2$

or $f(x) = 2$ or 3 $f(y) = 2$ or 3 and $f(z) = 2$

In this case, two of the elements x, y, z have the same image ∴ f is not one-one mapping hence this possibility is also excluded.

In (iii) the true statements are

$f(x) = 2$ or $3, f(y) = 1$ and $f(z) = 1, 3$

If f is one-one mapping then $f(z) = 3$

$\because f(y) = 1 \quad \because f(x) = 2$

$\therefore f^{-1}(1) = \{y\}$

This possibility is taken into consideration.

29. Solution: By injective mapping we mean one-one mapping or an injective or monomorphism in which no two different elements in A have the same image is B where $f: A \to B$.

$\therefore$ The no. of elements in $A \leq$ the no. of elements in B.

Again $g: B \to A$ is an injective mapping.

$\therefore$ no. of elements in $B \leq$ the no. of elements in A.

Thus the no. of elements in A = no. of elements in B.

Thus if $A = \{a_1, a_2, a_3, ..., a_n\}$ and $B = \{b_1, b_2, b_3....b_n\}$

Then $\phi = \{(a_1\ b_1)\ (a_2\ b_2)\ ...\ (a_n\ b_n)\}$ is a bijective mapping from A to B.

30. Ans. (i) f is injective (ii) g is neither surjective nor injective (iii) h is bijective (iv) k is bijective (v) l is bijective.

Solution: (i) We have $\forall\ x, y \in A \qquad x \neq y \Rightarrow \frac{1}{2}x \neq \frac{1}{2}y$

i.e. $f(x) \neq f(y)$ i.e. f is one-one i.e. injective. The set B has an element l which is not the image of any elements belonging to A and hence f is not an onto i.e. surjective function.

Here $f(A) = \left\{x : -\frac{1}{2} \leq x \leq \frac{1}{2}\right\}$ is a proper subset of B.

(ii) $g(1) = 1$ and $g(-1) = 1$

$\therefore$ g is many one mapping. $g(A) = \{x: 0 \leq x \leq 1\}$. This is a proper subset of B.

$\therefore$ g is into mapping.

$\therefore$ g is neither surjective nor injective function.

(iii) $h(x) = x\,|\,x\,|$ $\therefore$ $h(x) = x^2$ when $x \geq 0$ and $h(x) = -x^2$ where x < 0, thus h is a objective function i.e. into and onto both.

(iv) $k(x) = x^2$. This is a many one and into mapping since $k(1) = 1$ and $k(-1) = 1$.

(v) $lx = \sin \pi x$ here $l(-1) = \sin(-\pi) = 0$ and $l(1) = \sin \pi = 0$

Thus l is many one onto function. The values of $\sin \pi x$ lies in $[-1, 1]$ as x vanies from -1 to 1.

31. Ans. No.

Hint: The set B has only one element. The set has infinite no. of elements. It is not possible to define an onto function i.e. surjective function from B to A. All the elements of B. If this is possible, then the definition of onto function will be vorilatel.

32. Ans. No.

Solution: $f(N) = \{5, 7, 9 ....\}$ a proper subset of N. Therefore f is not surjective.

33. Ans. (i) Yes, surjective (ii) No.

Solution: (i) The given ordered pairs is a surjective function not injective as each person has one and only mother. Every mother has a child in A. (ii) The given ordered pairs is not a function as a person has many ancestors. The image of an element of the domain is not unique here.

34. Ans. Domain is $\{x : x \text{ is real and } -3 \leq x \leq 3\}$.

Range is $\{y : y \text{ is real and } 0 \leq y \leq 5\}$.

Solution: The set R consists all points or inside the circle $x^2 + y^2 = 25$ shown by horizontal lines.

The set R' consists of all points on or above the parabola $y^2 = \frac{4}{9}x^2$ shown by vertical lines.

$\therefore$ $R \cap R'$ consists of points which are common to both the region. This common portion is shown in the figure by horizontal and vertical lines both.

The region is $O\,A\,B\,C\,O$.

We can write

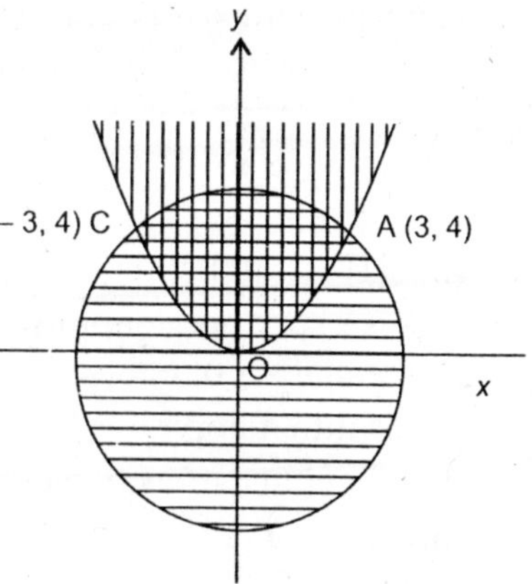

Figure Q. 34

$$R \cap R' = \{(x, y) : x, y \text{ are real}, \left\{x^2 + y^2 \leq 25 \text{ and } y^2 \geq \frac{4}{9}x\right\}$$

Solving $x^2 + y^2 = 25$ and $y^2 = \frac{4}{9}x$. We get the coordinates of the points A and C as (3, 4) and (–3, 4) respectively. The point B is (0, 5).

The domain of $R \cap R'$ is $\{x : x \text{ is real and } -3 \le x \le 3\}$ and the range of $R \cap R'$ is $\{y : y \text{ is real and } 0 \le y \le 5\}$. $R \cap R'$ is not a function since 0 is related to more than one member.

35. Ans. Domain is the set of real numbers, the range is $\{y : y \text{ is real } 0 \le y \le 1\}$

The function is not one-one.

Solution: $f(x) = \dfrac{x^2}{1+x^2}$; Put $x = 3$

$$\therefore f(x) = \frac{3^2}{1+3^2} = \frac{9}{10}$$

Again $x = -3$ gives $f(x) = \dfrac{(-3)^2}{1+(-9)^2} = \dfrac{9}{10}$

Here different elements 3 and – 3 of the domain of f have the same image 9/10 is the codomain. Hence f is not one-one. For every real $x, l + x^2 \ne 0. f(x) = \dfrac{x^2}{1+x^2}$ is a real number $\forall\, x$.

$\therefore$ The domain of f is the set of real numbers.

For the range we have $f(x) = \dfrac{x^2}{1+x^2} = y$

$$\therefore x = \sqrt{\frac{y}{1-y}}$$

Since x is real $\quad \therefore \dfrac{y}{1-y} \ge 0 \; (y \ne 1)$

Which is possible when $0 \le y < 1$

$\therefore f$ has the range $\{y : y \text{ is real}, 0 \le y < 1\}$

36. Ans. f is bijective.

Solution: $x_1\, x_2 \le A, f(x_1) = f(x_2)$

$$\Rightarrow \frac{x_1 - 2}{x_1 - 3} = \frac{x_2 - 2}{x_2 - 3}$$

$\Rightarrow (x_1 - 2)(x_2 - 3) = (x_2 - 2)(x_1 - 3)$
$\Rightarrow x_1x_2 - 3x_1 - 2x_2 + 6 = x_1x_2 - 3x_2 - 2x_1 + 6$
$\Rightarrow - 3x_1 + 2x_1 = - 3x_2 + 2x_2$
$\Rightarrow x_1 = x_2$ therefore f is injective.
Let $y \in B$

Solving $f(x) = y = \frac{x-2}{x-3}$, we get $x = \frac{2-3y}{1-y}$, since $y \neq 1$ x is real. The value $x = 3$ gives the absurd result as $3y - 3 = 3y - 2$.

$\therefore x = \frac{2-3y}{1-y} \in A$ and $f(x) = y$ and thus f is surjective. Thus f is bijective.

37. (a) **Ans.** No.

Solution: cos $(5x + 2)$ has the same values for may value of x hence f is many one. The value of cos $(5x + 2)$ is in the interval $[-1, 1]$. The interval $[-1, 1]$ is a proper subset of the co-domain R. Therefore f is not surjective.

In order to prove that f is in variable it is necessary that it should be bijective.

(b) Do yourself.

38. **Solution:** $(fog)(x) = f(g(x)) = f(x^2) = \sin x^2$
and $(gof)(x) = g(f(x)) = g(\sin x) = \sin^2 x$
$\because \sin x^2 \neq \sin^2 x \ \forall \ x \in R$
$\therefore gof \neq fog$

39. (i) **Ans.** (a)

Hint: $y = f(x) = 3x - 4 \Rightarrow x = f^{-1}(y)$

$$= \frac{1}{3}(y + 4) \Rightarrow f^{-1}(y) = \frac{1}{3}(x + 4)$$

$\therefore$ (a) is correct.

(ii) **Ans.** (b)

Hint: $A \cup B$ contains minimum number of elements if $A \subset B$ so that $n(A \cup B) = n(B) = 6$

$\therefore$ (b) is correct

(iii) **Ans.** (b)

Hint: We have $2^m - 2^n = 56$

By trial we get $m = 6$ and $n = 3$ and therefore (b) is correct.

(iv) **Ans.** (c)

Hint: $fog(x) = f(g(x)) = f(x^2) = \sin x^2$

$\therefore$ (*c*) is correct.

(v) **Ans.** (b) and (c)

Hint: $n, m \in N$ and $n \neq m \Rightarrow 2n + 3 \neq 2m + 3$

$\Rightarrow f(n) \neq f(m)$ $\therefore$ *f* is injective

Since 1 is not the image of any element of the domain and hence *f* is not surjective.

(vi) **Ans.** (d)

Hint: $f(\pm 4) = 17 \therefore f^{-1}(17) = \pm 4; f(\pm\sqrt{2})23$

$\therefore f(3) = \pm\sqrt{2}$.

40. **Ans.** (a) All statements are the same.

41. **Ans.** (a) is false

42. (i) **Ans.** (b)

Hint: Since $1 < 2, 2 < 3 \Rightarrow 1 < 3$

(ii) **Ans.** (b)

(iii) **Ans.** (a)

(iv) **Ans.** (b)

(v) **Ans.** (b) One element of the codomain is the image of 10 elements of the domain. Similarly other element of the domain do. Total no. of distinct function is 10^{10}.

(vi) **Ans.** (d)

Hint: Here $f(A) \neq f(B)$ and $f(y) = f(z) \not\Rightarrow y = z$.

(vii) **Ans.** (c)

Hint: Since *A* and *B* have no elements in common.

43. (i) **Ans** (b).

Solution: Let *V* be the set of all sets. Then every subset of *V* is also an element of *V*. Therefore, the power set *P*(*V*) or 2^V of *V* is a subset of *V*.

Thus $P(V)\ CV \Rightarrow n(P(V)) \leq n(V)$ ...(1)

But the cardinal number of a set *V* is always less than the cardinal no. of *P*(*V*) i.e. the no. of elements in *V* is less than the number of elements in *P*(*V*).

i.e. $n(V) < n(P(V))$ ...(2)

(1) and (2) leads to a contradiction and hence the assumption is wrong. Therefore, the alternative (b) is correct

(ii) **Ans.** (a)

Hint: We have $R \times (P^c \cup Q^c)^c$
$= R \times [(P^c)^c \cap Q^c)^c]$
$= R \times (P \cap Q) = (R \times P) \cap (R \times Q)$
Therefore, the alternative (a) is correct.
(iii) **Ans.** (a)
Solution: We have $XOY = (X^c \cap Y) \cup (X \cap Y^c)$
$= (X^c \cup X) \cap (X^c \cap Y^c) \cap (Y \cup X) \cap (Y \cup Y^c)$ ...(1)
(By distributive law)
$= U \cap (X^c \cup Y^c) \cap (Y \cup X) \cap U$. When U is an universal set.
$= (X^c \cup Y^c) \cap (Y \cup X)$ ...(A) $(\because U \cap A = A)$
$(XOY)OZ = [(X \cup Y) \cap (X^c \cup Y^c)]OZ$
$= [\{X \cup Y\} \cap (X^c \cup Y^c) \cup Z\}] \cap \{(X \cup Y) \cup (X^c \cup Y^c)\} \cup Z^c]$ by (A)
$= \{X \cup Y \cup Z\} \cap (X^c \cup Y^c \cup Z)\} \cap \{(X \cup Y)^c \cup (X^c \cup Y^c)^c \cup Z^c\}$
By Demorgan's law
$= [\{X \cup Y \cup Z\} \cap (X^c \cup Y^c \cup Z)\} \cap \{(X^c \cup Y^c) \cup (X \cup Y)\} \cup Z^c\}$ ...(2)
By Demorgan's law
Now $[(X^c \cup Y^c) \cup (X \cap Y)] \cup Z^c$
$= [(X^c \cup X)\} \cap (X^c \cup Y) \cap (Y^c \cup X) \cap (Y^c \cup Y)] \cup Z^c$
$= [U \cap (X^c \cup Y) \cap (Y^c \cup X \cap U)] \cup Z^c$
$= [(X^c \cup Y) \cap (Y^c \cup X)] \cup Z^c$
$= [(X^c \cup Y \cup Z) \cap (Y^c \cup X \cup Z^c)]$ ...(3)
Substituting from (3) is (2) we get
$(X\, o\, Y)OZ = [\{(X \cup Y \cup Z) \cap (X^c \cup Y^c \cup Z)\} \cap \{(X^c \cup Y \cup Z)$
$\cap (Y^c \cup X \cup Z^c)\}]$
We can get the same result by expanding.
$XO(YOZ)$ $\therefore$ $(XOY)OZ = XO\,(YOZ)$ $\therefore$ (a) is correct.
(iv) **Ans.** (b)
Hint: x is related to x, since $x - x + \sqrt{2} = \sqrt{2}$ (an irrational number).
Thus the relation * is reflexive.
The relation * is not symmmetric
$\therefore x - y + \sqrt{2} = \sqrt{2} - 1 + \sqrt{2} = \sqrt{2} - 1$ (an integral)

where $x = \sqrt{2}$ and $y = 1$

By $y - x + \sqrt{2} = (-\sqrt{2} + \sqrt{2}) = 1$.

Thus x is related to y but y is not related to x, and hence * is not an equivalence relation.

Therefore, the alternative (b) is corect.

44. Solution: Graph of $x^2 + y^2 - 2x \geq 0$.

We first draw the graph of $x^2 + y^2 - 2x = 0$. The equation is $(x-1)^2 - y^2 = 1$.

Which is a circle of radius 1 and centre (1, 0).

The points are on or above the circle as $x^2 + y^2 - 2x \geq 0$.

These are shown by horizontal lines.

Graph of $3x - y - 12 \leq 0$. We draw the graph of $y = 3x - 12$.

The points will be on or above the lines $y = 3x - 12$. These are shown by vertical lines.

Graph of $y - x \leq 0$.

We draw the graph of $y = x$.

All the points which satisfy $y - x \leq 0$ will lie either on or below the line $y = x$. These are shown by small circles 0.

Graph of $y \geq 0$. All the points will lie either on x axis or above it (not shown shaded in the figure).

The area is *PQRNP*.

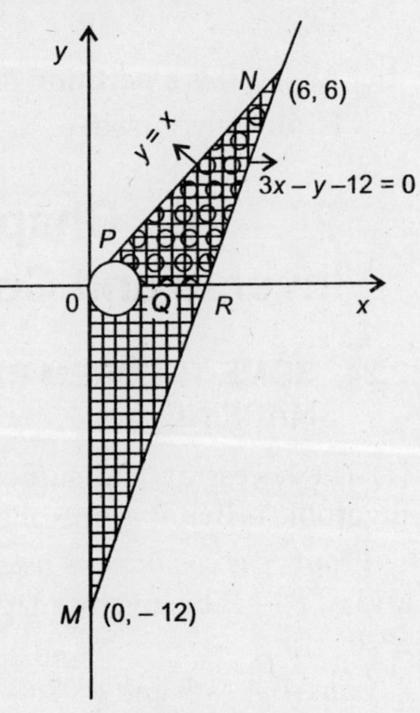

Figure Q. 44

45. Ans. A function $f : A \rightarrow R$ is called a real valued function if it maps the set A into the set of reals R.

Polynomials, trigonometic function, exponential and logarithmic functions are the examples of real valued functions.

Algebra of real valued function: Let R^A be the family of real valued function. D is its domin. Then may algebraic operations viz addition, multiplication etc. are defined is R^A.

Let $f: D \to R$ and $g: D \to R$ and $l \to R$

Then we define

$(f + l) : D \to R$ by $(f + k)(x) \equiv f(x) + l$

$(|f| + l) : D \to R$ by $(|f|)(x) \equiv |f(x)|$

$(f^n) : D \to R$ by $(f^n)(x) \equiv (f(x))^n$

$(f \pm g) : D \to R$ by $(f \pm g)(x) \equiv f(x) \pm g(x)$

$(lf) : D \to R$ by $(lf)(x) \equiv lf(x)$

$(fg) : D \to R$ by $(fg)(x) \equiv f(x)g(x)$

$$\left(\frac{f}{g}\right) : D \to R \text{ by} \left(\frac{f}{g}\right)(x) \equiv \frac{f(x)}{g(x)}$$

46. Ans. (iii) is a partition of A.

Hint: Do yourself.

Chapter 2 (D)
Inverse and Composite Mapping

2.24 SOME THEOREM RELATED TO INVERSE MAPPING

(1) The necessray and sufficient condition that a mapping be invertible is that it is one-one and onto.

Proof: *The condition is necessary:* Let the mappings $f: A \to B$ and $g : B \to A$ be inverse mappings and let $f(x_1) = f(x_2)$ for $x_1, x_2 \in A$.

Since $f: A \to B$ and $g : B \to A$ are said to be the inverse of the other if $g[f(x)] = x \ \forall \ x \in A$ and $f[g(y)] = y \ \forall \ x \in B$.

Therefore $x_1 = g[f(x_1)] = g[f(x_2)] = x_2$

Thus f is one-one i.e. if $(x_1, f(x_1))$ and $(x_2, f(x_2))$ be two ordered pairs such that $f(x_1) = f(x_2)$ then $x_1 = x_2$ and this implies f is one-one.

Let $y \in B$ then $g(y) \in A$ and $g\,[f(y)] = y$

($\because$ f and g are inverse mappings)

$\therefore$ If $x = g(y)$ then $f(x) = f[g(y)] = y$ i.e. for every $y \in B$ there is $x \in A$ $\therefore$ f is onto.

The condition is sufficient: Let f: $A \rightarrow B$ be onto and one-one mapping then for each $y \in B$ $f(x) = y$ for some $x \in A$.

In addition only one element $x \in A$ will satisfy

$$f(x) = y \text{ as } f \text{ is one-one} \quad \text{...(1)}$$

Let g: $B \rightarrow A$ be another mapping such that

$$g(y) = x \text{ for } x \in B$$

Then $\quad f[g(y)] = f(x) = y$ from (1) ...(2)

Suppose $g[f(x)] = x$, then $f(x_1) = f[g[f(x)]] = f[g(y)]$

$$= y \text{ from (2)}$$

$$= f(x) \text{ from (1)}$$

$\Rightarrow$ $f(x_1) = f(x)$. Again as f is one-one so we have

$x_1 = x = g[f(x)]$ $\therefore$ f and g are inverse mappings.

(2) If f: $A \rightarrow B$ is one-one and onto, then prove that f^{-1}: $B \rightarrow A$ is also one-one and onto.

This theorem may also be stoped as "Prove that the inverse of an invertible function is invertilate".

Or

"Prove that the inverse of a bijective is also a bijection".

Proof: Let y_1 and $y_2 \in B$ then

$$f^{-1}(y_1) = x_1 \text{ where } x_1 \in A$$

$$f^{-1}(y_2) = x_2 \text{ where } x_2 \in A$$

Thus $\quad y_1 = f(x_1)$ and $y = f(x_2)$

$$y_1 \neq y_2 \Rightarrow f(x_1) \neq f(x_2)$$

$\Rightarrow \quad x_1 \neq x_2$ as f is one-one and onto.

$\Rightarrow \quad f^{-1}(y_1) \neq f^{-1}(y_2)$

$\Rightarrow f^{-1}$ is one-one.

In order to prove f^{-1} onto mapping we assume $x \in A$, then there is $y \in B$ such that $y = f(x)$ or $x = f^{-1}(y)$ i.e. x is the f^{-1} image of $y \in B$.

$\therefore$ f^{-1} is into mapping.

(3) If f: $A \rightarrow B$ and g: $B \rightarrow A$ are inverse mappings and f: $A \rightarrow B$ and g': $B \rightarrow A$ are also inverse mappings then g and g' are equal.

Proof: $f: A \to B$ and $g': B \to A$ are inverse mappings then

$$f[g(y)] = y \ \forall \ y \in B \quad ...(1)$$

Similarly $g'[f(x)] = x \ \forall \ x \in A \quad ...(2)$

Again $g'(y) = g'[f[g(y)]]$ for (1)

$= g(y)$ for (2)

i.e. $g'(y) = g(y)$

$\Rightarrow g$ and g' are equal and the mapping inverse to f is unique.

2.25 SOME THEROM ON COMPOSITE MAPPING

(1) If $f: A \to B$ be one-one and onto this $fof^{-1} = I_B$ and $f^{-1}of = I_A$

Proof: If the function $f: A \to B$ be defined by

$$f(a) = b \text{ where } a \in A, b \in B$$

then $a = f^{-1}(b)$ i.e. a is the inverse image of b under the corrospondnce f.

Thus $f^{-1}: B \to A$ is defined by $f^{-1}(b) = a$

$\therefore \ (f^{-1}of)a = f^{-1}(f(a)) = f^{-1}(b) = a$

Thus the function $f^{-1}of$ maps the element $a \in A$ onto itself.

$\therefore \quad f^{-1}of = I_A$ the identity maps A onto itself.

$(fof^{-1})b = f(f^{-1}(b)) = f(a) = b$

$\therefore \quad fof^{-1} = I_B$

Note: This theorem may also be asked as "If the map $f: A \to B$ be one-one and onto map, then the maps fof^{-1} and $f^{-1}of$ define identity maps on B and A respectively.

(2) If $f: A \to B$ and $g: B \to C$ be two one-one onto mappings, then $gof: A \to C$ is also one-one onto and

$$(gof)^{-1} = f^{-1}og^{-1}$$

Proof: Let $x_1 \ x_2 \in A$ then $(gof)\ x_1 = (gof)x_2$

$\Rightarrow \quad g[f(x_1)] = g[f(x_2)] \Rightarrow f(x_1) = f(x_2)$

$\Rightarrow \quad x_1 = x_2$ if f is one-one $\therefore$ gof is one-one mapping.

Again as g is an onto mapping, so far every $z \in c$ there exists an element y (B) such that $g(y) = z$.

Also as f is an onto mapping so for every $y \in B$ there is an element $x \in A$ such that $f(x) = y$

$\therefore \quad z = g(y) = g[f(x)] = (gof)x$

$\therefore$ (gof) is an onto mapping.

(iii) We have $z = g(y)$ and $f(x) = y$

$f^{-1} : B \to A$ i.e. the inverse mapping of $f : A \to B$ gives $f^{-1}(y) = x$ and $g^{-1} : C \to B$ i.e. the inverse mapping of $g : B \to C$ gives $f^{-1}(z) = y$.

The composite mappings $gof : A \to e$ is given by $(gof)x = g(f(x)) = g(y) = z$

$\therefore (gof)^{-1} : C \to A$ where $(gof)^{-1}z = x$

But $\quad x = f^{-1}(y) = f^{-1}(g^{-1}(z))$

$\quad = (f^{1}og^{-1})z$

$\therefore \quad (gof)^{-1} = f^{-1}og^{-1}$

(3) If $f: A \to A$ is any mapping and I_A is the identity mapping on A then $foI_A = I_Aof = f$.

Proof: Let $x \in A$ then $(foI_A)x = f[I_A(x)] = f(x)$

$\Rightarrow \quad foI_A = f$

Again $\quad (I_Aof)x = I_A[f(x)] = f(x)$

thus $\quad I_Aof = f \quad \therefore foI_A = I_Aof$

(4) The mappings $f : A \to B$ is one-one and onto iff there exists *a* mapping $g : B \to A$ such that gof and fog are the identity mappings on A and B respectively.

The readers are advised to prove this therom themselves.

(5) If $f: A \to B$ and $g : B \to C$ are each one-one and onto mapping, then $gof: A \to C$ is also one-one onto mapping.

This theorem may also be asked as –11 if f and g are each one-one and onto mapping and f, g are composite then gof is also one-one and onto mapping.

Proof: Let x_1, x_2 be two elements of A, then $(gof)x_1 = g[f(x_1)] = (gof)x_2 = g[f(x_2)]$

$\Rightarrow f(x_1) = f(x_2) \Rightarrow x_1 = x_2$ [$\therefore$ g is one-one and f is one-one.]

$\therefore$ gof is a one-one mapping.

If z be an element of C, then $g(y) = z$ ...(1)

where $y \in B$ and g is an onto mapping.

Let $x \in A$ then $f(x) = y$ since f is an onto mapping.

$\therefore$ F is each $z \in C \ \exists\, x \in A$ such that

$$z = g(y) = g[f(x)] = (gof)x \text{ [From (1)]}$$

$\therefore$ gof is an onto mapping.

Some worked out examples:

(1) Prove that

(i) $f^{-1}[A^c] = [f^{-1}(A)]^c$

(ii) Let $f: R \to R$ defined by $f(x) = ax + b$ where $a, b, x \in R$ and $a \neq 0$. Prove that f is invertible.

(iii) What do you mean by characteristics function. Give an example.

(iv) Define equivalent set.

(i) ***Proof:*** Let x be any element of $f^{-1}[A^c]$

$\therefore \quad f(x) \in A^c$

$\Rightarrow \quad f(x) \notin A \quad \because A$ is the compliment of A^c

$\Rightarrow \quad x \notin f^{-1}(A) \Rightarrow x \in [f^{-1}(A)]^c$

$\therefore \quad f^{-1}[A^c] \subseteq [f^{-1}(A)]^c$ ...(1)

Again let y be any element of $[f^{-1}(A)]^c$

$\Rightarrow \quad f(y) \notin f^{-1}(A)$

$\Rightarrow \quad f(y) \notin A \Rightarrow f(y) \in A^c \Rightarrow y \in f^{-1}(A^c)$

$\therefore [f^{-1}(A)]^c \subseteq f^{-1}(A)^c$ ...(2)

$\therefore$ From (1) and (2) the result follows.

(ii) ***Proof:*** Let x_1, x_2 be any two elements or R, where $f(x_1) = f(x_2)$

$\therefore ax_1 + b = ax_2 + b \Rightarrow x_1 = x_2$

$\therefore a \neq 0$

$\therefore f$ is one-one.

Let $y \in R$ i.e. y be an element of R, the co-domain of f and x be its pre-image into the correspondence f.

$\therefore \quad f(x) = y$

$\Rightarrow \quad ax + b = y$

$$\Rightarrow \quad x = \frac{y-b}{a} \in R$$

$\therefore f$ is onto as every element of y of the co-domain R has its pre-image under f. Thus f is invertible.

(iii) *Characterstic function:* If A is a subset of B, the function f is defined on the set B to the set $[0, 1]$ such that $f(x) = 1$ if $x \in A$ and $f(x) = 0$ if $x \in B - A$, then f is known as the characteristic function of A.

Example: $B = \{1, 2, 3, 4 .....\}$; $A = \{2, 4, 6....\}$

$f(x) = 1$ if x is even i.e. $x \in A$ and $f(x) = 0$ if x is odd i.e. $x \in B - A$.

Hence f is a characteristic function of A.

(iv) *Equivalent sets:* If there is a function $f : A \to B$ which is one-one and onto then the two sets A and B are known as equivalent sets. Such sets have the same cardinal number.

$A \sim B$ (A wiggle B) is used to denote equivalent sets. In other words two sets are said to be equivalent if there is one to one correspondence between their elements. If two sets A and B one equivalent then we say that they have the same power.

Example: $A = \{1, 2, 3, 4, ...\}$

$B = \{2, 4, 8, 16, ... \}$

These sets are equivalent since every numebr n from A is put into correspondance with the number in from B.

EXERCISE – 2 (D) (i) SIMPLE QUESTIONS

1. Explain with examples the following relations reflexive, symmetric and transitive.
2. Following relation are expressed from N to N, where N is the set of natural numbers. Express them by rule method.
   $R_1 = \{(1, 1), (2, 4), (3, 9), (4, 16) ....\}$
   $R_2 = \{(1, 3), (2, 4), (3, 5), (4, 6) ....\}$
3. If $A = \{1, 2, 3, 4, 5\}$ and $R = \{(x, y): x > 2, y = 3\}$, write down the domain and range of R.
   [**Hint:** $R = \{(3, 3), (4, 3), (5, 3)\}$
4. If A $\{(1, 2, 3, 4\}$, define the follwoing relation in A.
   (i) reflexive, transitive but not symmetric
   (ii) symmetric but not reflexive and transitive
   (iii) reflexive, symmetric and transitive, [IIT 1970]
5. Find whether the follwing relations are reflexive, equivalence, symmetrice and transitive
   (i) $a\ R\ b$ iff a/b; $a, b \in N$ '/' means a is divisible by b.
   (ii) $a\ R\ b$ iff $a \perp b$; a, b are straight lines.
6. Examine whether the following relations are reflexive, symmetric and transitive:
   $m, n \in I$, where $m\ R\ n$ iff m is a muliple of n [IIT 1974]

7. Is it true – 'a symmetric and transitive relation is always necessarily reflexive also'. Give reasons.

[IIT 1970, Merrut B.Sc. 1974]

[**Hint:** No. Let R be the set of real numbers where $x, y \in R$ and $x\ R\ y$ iff $x, y \neq 0$

(i) $xy \neq 0 \Rightarrow yx \neq 0$ hence the relation is symmetric.

(ii) $xy \neq 0, yz \neq 0 \Rightarrow zx \neq 0$ hence the relation is transitive.
Now $xy \neq 0, yz \neq 0 \Rightarrow zx \neq 0$ $(xz \neq 0 \Rightarrow zx \neq 0)$.

Therefore $xz \neq 0, zx \neq 0 \Rightarrow x.x \neq 0$ but thin is not true since $0 \in R, 0.0 = 0$ so $0 \not R\ 0$ or $(0,0) \notin R$]

8. If $a, b \in I$ and $a\ R\ b$ iff a and b are odd numbers, show that the relation is symmetric, transitive but not reflexive.

[Merrut B.Sc. 1974]

[**Hint:** If $a = 2$, then 2, and 2 are not odd i.e. $2 \not R\ 2$ similarly if $a = 4$, then $4 \not R\ 4$]

9. In the set of real numbers the relation R is defined by

(i) $a\ R\ b \Rightarrow |\ a\ | = |\ b\ |$ [Merrut B.Sc. 1982]

(ii) $a\ R\ b \Rightarrow |\ a\ | \geq |\ b\ |$ [Merrut B.Sc. 1981]

(iii) $a\ R\ b \Rightarrow a - b \geq 0$ [Maghadh B.Sc. 1974]

Which one is an equivalence relation?

10. If $R_1 = \{(1, 2), (2, 1), (1, 1), (2, 2)\}$ and $R_2 = \{(2, 3), (3, 2), (2, 2), (3, 3)\}$ are two transitive relations on the set $S = \{1, 2, 3,\}$, show that $R_1 \cup R_2$ is not transitive.

[**Hint:** $R_1 \cup R_2 = \{(1, 2), (2, 1), (1, 1), (2, 3), (3, 2), (2, 2), (3, 3)\}$, $(1, 2) \in R_1 \cup R_2$ $(2, 3) \in R_1 \cup R_2$ but $(1, 3) \notin R_1 \cup R_2$]

11. The relations R and R' are symmetric in a set A, prove that $R \cup R'$ and $R \cap R'$ are also symmetric [Ranchi B.Sc. 1975]

[**Hint:** R and R' are relation in $A \therefore R \subseteq A \times A$ and $R' \subseteq A \times A$. Therefore $R \cup R' \subseteq A \times A$ and $R \cap R' \subseteq A \times A$ are also relation in A.

Now $(a, b), \in R \cup R' \Rightarrow (a, b) \in R$ or $(a, b) \in R' \Rightarrow (b, a) \in R$ or $(b, a) \in R' \Rightarrow (b, a) \in R \cap R'$ (in symmetric), similarly $(a, b) \in R \cap R' \Rightarrow (b, a) \in R \cap R'$]

12. In the set of positive integers $a\ R\ b$ if $a^b = b^a$, prove that the relation R is reflexive and symmetric.

13. For the relation R and its inverse R^{-1} a set A prove

(i) If R is reflexive then R^{-1} is reflexive

(ii) If R is symmetric then R^{-1} is symmetric

(iii) If R is transitive then R^{-1} is transitive.

[**Hint:** (i) $(a, a) \in R \Rightarrow (a, a) \in R^{-1}$ ($\therefore R^{-1}$ is reflexive)

(ii) Let $(a, b) \in R^{-1}$ then $(b, a) \in R$.

Now $(b, a) \in R \Rightarrow (a, b) \in R$ ($\therefore R$ is symmetric)

$\Rightarrow (b\ a) \in R^{-1}$

$\therefore (a, b) \in R^{-1} \Rightarrow (b, a) \in R^{-1}$ $\therefore$ is symmetric

(iii) Let $(a, b) \in R^{-1}, (b, c) \in R^{-1}$,

Then $(b, a) \in R, (c, b) \in R$

Thus $(c, b) \in R, (b, a) \in R \Rightarrow (c, a) \in R$ ($\therefore R$ is transitive)

$\Rightarrow (a, c) \in R^{-1}$

$\therefore (a, b) \in R^{-1}, (b, c) \in R^{-1} \Rightarrow (a, c) \in R^{-1}$ hence R^{-1} is transitive.

Note: Thus we see that if R is an equivalence relation then R^{-1} is also an equivalence relation.

14. Let $R = \{(4, 5), (1, 4), (4, 6), (7, 6), (3, 7)\}$,

find the value of (i) $R^{-1}\ o\ R^{-1}$ and (ii) $(R^{-1}\ o\ R)^{-1}$

[**Hint:** $R^{-1}\ o\ R^{-1} = (R\ o\ R)^{-1}, (R^{-1}\ o\ R)^{-1} = R^{-1}\ o\ R$]

15. N is the set of positive integers and R be a relation on $N \times N$ defined by $(a, b)\ R\ (c, d) \Rightarrow ad = be$.

Show that the relation R is an equivalence relation.

[Gorakhpur B.Sc. 1977; Roorkee 1989]

16. N is the set of natural numbers. The relation R is defined on $N \times N$ as $(a, b)\ R\ (c, d) \Rightarrow a + d = b + c$, prove that R is an equivalence relation.

[U.P. 1984, Roorkee 1982, Gorakhpur B.Sc. 1977]

17. A relation R on the set of complex numbers (except o) in defined by $z_1\ R\ z_2 \Rightarrow \dfrac{z_1 - z_2}{z_1 + z_2}$ is a real number. Show that R is an equivalence.

[IIT 1982]

[**Hint:** In the given set we do not consider o, since $\dfrac{o - o}{o + o} = \dfrac{o}{o}$ is not real.]

(i) If $\frac{z_1 - z_2}{z_1 + z_2} = 0$ is a real number, then the relation is reflexive.

(ii) If $\frac{z_1 - z_2}{z_1 + z_2}$ is real, then $\frac{z_1 - z_2}{z_2 + z_1}$ is also real and therefore $z_1 \, R \, z_2 \Rightarrow z_2 \, R \, z_1$ and thus R is symmetric.

(iii) Let $z_1 = x_1 + i\, y,;\, z_2 = x_2 + i\, y_2;\, z_3 = x_3 + i\, y_3$ and $z_1 \, R \, z_2$ and $z_2 \, R \, z_3$ be true, then $z_1 \, R \, z_2 \Rightarrow \frac{z_1 - z_2}{z_1 + z_2}$ is real.

$$\Rightarrow \frac{(x_1 - x_2) + i(y_1 - y_2)}{(x_1 + x_2) + i(y_1 + y_2)} \text{ is real}$$

$$\Rightarrow \frac{[(x_1 - x_2) + i(y_1 - y_2)]\ [(x_1 + x_2) - i(y_1 + y_2)]}{(x_1 + x_2)^2 + i(y_1 + y_2)^2} \text{ is real}$$

$$\Rightarrow [(x_1 - x_2)\,(x_1 + x_2) + (y_1 + y_2)\,(y_1 + y_2)]$$
$$+ i\,[(y_1 - y_2)\,(x_1 + x_2) - (x_1 - x_2)\,(y_1 + y_2)] \quad \text{is real}$$
$$\Rightarrow (y_1 - y_2)\,(x_1 + x_2) - (x_1 - x_2)\,(y_1 + y_2) = 0$$
$$\Rightarrow 2x_2\, y_1 - 2y_2\, x_1 = 0 \Rightarrow y_1\, x_2 = y_2\, x_1$$

$$\Rightarrow \frac{x_1}{y_1} = \frac{x_2}{y_2} \qquad \text{(i)}$$

Similarly $z_2 \, R \, z_3 \Rightarrow \frac{x_2}{y_2} = \frac{x_3}{y_3}$ (ii)

Now from (i) and (ii)

$\frac{x_1}{y_1} = \frac{x_3}{y_3}$ and hence $z_1 \, R \, z_3$

Thus $z_1 \, R \, z_2,\, z_2 \, R \, z_3 \Rightarrow z_1 \, R \, z_3$

Therefore R is transitive.

Therefore R is an equivalence relation.

Select the correct alternative(ves) in the following Questions:

18. Let l be the set of all straight linse in a plane. R is the relation defined by $a \, R \, b \Rightarrow a \perp b,\, a,\, b \in l$. Then R is

(a) reflexive (b) symmetric (c) transitive (d) none of these.

19. In oder that a relation R defined on a non-empty set A is an equivalence relation it is sufficient if R
(a) is reflexive (b) is symmetric (c) is transitive (d) possesses all the above three properties. [CET 1990]

20. A function f: $R \to R$ is defined by $f(x) = \dfrac{\alpha x^2 + 6x - 8}{\alpha + 6x - 8x^2}$, find the interval of values of α for which f is onto. Is the function one to one for $\alpha = 3$. Justify your answer.

21. Which of the following functions are periodic
(i) $f(x) = x + \sin x$.
(ii) $f(x) = \{x\}$, where $x = [x] + \{x\}$
(iii) $f(x) = 1 \cos x^1$

(iv) $f(x) = 1 - \dfrac{\sin^2 x}{1 + \cot x} - \dfrac{\cos^2 x}{1 + \tan x}$

22. If $f(x) = \{x\}$ the fractional part of x and $g(x) = \dfrac{1}{2} \sin [x]^x$ where $[x]$ denotes the integral part of x. Find the range of $g \, o \, f$.

ANSWER TO EXERCISE 2 D (i)

(Hints and Solutions)

1. See Article 2.16. Types of relation parts (2), (3) and (5).

2. Ans. $R_1 \{ (x, y): y = x^2, x, y \in N\}$; $R_2 = \{(x, y): y = x + 2, x, y \in N\}$.

Solution: R_1 is the set of such ordered pairs in which second component y is the square of the first component x, i.e. $y = x^2$, where $x, y \in N$ $\therefore$ $R_1 = \{(x, y): y = x^2, x, y \in N\}$.

R_2 is the set of such ordered pairs in which the second component y is real to the first component plus 2.

i.e. $y = x + 2$, where $x, y \in N$

$\therefore R_2 = \{(x, y): y = x + 2, x, y \in N\}$

3. Ans. $\{3, 4, 5\}$, $\{3\}$,

Solution: $R = \{(3, 3), (4, 3), (5, 3)\}$

$\therefore$ The domain of R is $\{3, 4, 5\}$.

The range of R is $\{3\}$.

4. See the answer sheet of Q. No. 40 of Problems and Exercise 2B (i).

5. **Ans.** (i) Reflexive, transitive but not symmetric (ii) symmetric but not reflexive and transitive.

   Solution: (i) Let a be any natural number. Since each natural number divides itself i.e. a/a hence

   $a\,R\,a$ i.e. R is reflexive.

   Thus $a\,R\,a \Rightarrow R$ is reflexive.

   Again 3 divides 6 but 6 does not divide 3.

   i.e. $(3, 6) \in R$ but $(6, 3) \notin R$

   $\Rightarrow a\,R\,b \Rightarrow b \not R\, a$, where $a, b \in N$

   Thus R is not symmetric

   3 divides 6, 6 divides 12 implies 3 divides 12

   $\therefore (3, 6) \in R, (6, 12) \in R \Rightarrow (3, 12) \in R$

   $\therefore R$ is transitive

   (ii) Let a be any straight line. Since a straight line is not perpendicular to itself hence $a \not R\; a$ and therefore R is not reflexive.

   If a and b be two straight lines then $a \perp b \Rightarrow b \perp a$

   $\therefore a\,R\,b \Rightarrow b\,R\,a \therefore R$ is symmetric.

   If a, b and c be three srtaight lines then $a \perp b, b \perp c \not\Rightarrow a \perp c$

   $\therefore a\,R\,b, b\,R\,c \Rightarrow a \not R\; b$

   $\therefore R$ is not transitive.

6. **Ans.** Reflexive, transitive but not symmetric.

   Solution: $m\ R\ m$ since 1 in the multiple of 1. Thus R is reflexive.

   We have $12 = 2 \times 6$, 12 is a multiple of 6 but 6 cannot be a multiple of 12 and hence R is not symmetric.

   Let m be a multiple of n and n a multiple of p then $m = k_1 n$ and $n = k_2 p$ where $k_1\, k_2 \in I$.

   Thus $m = k_1\, k_2\, p$ i.e. m is a multiple of p.

   Therefore $m\,R\,n, n\,R\,p \Rightarrow m\,R\,p$

   $\therefore R$ in transitive.

7. **Ans. Hint:** Define a relative R by $a\,R\,b$ iff $a + b$ is even on the set of positive integers including o and $a, b \in$ I

Or

Define a relative R by $a\ R\ b$ iff a and b are both odd on the set of integers I.

Or

Take the solution from the Hint of the question given.

8. The solution is given in the book. We can take the advantage for the Hint given in Q. No. 7.

9. Ans. (i) is equivalence relation (ii) not an equivalence relation (iii) not an equivalence relation.

Solution: (i) See the Hint of the Q. No. 36 of Problems and Exercises 6.

(ii) If $a \geq b$ then $b \not\geq a$ hence the relation is not symmetric. The relation is reflexive.

$\therefore a \geq a \therefore R$ is not an equivalence relation.

(iii) $5 - 3 \geq 0$ but $3 - 5 \not\geq 0$ hence the relation is not symmetric.

$\therefore R$ is not an equivalence relation.

10. Hint: (1, 2) and (2, 3) both are in $R_1 \cup R_2$ but the ordered pair (1, 3) dose not belong to $R_1 \cup R_2$

$\therefore R_1 \cup R_2$ is not transitive.

11. Hint: $R \subseteq A \times A$ (1)

$R^1 \subseteq A \times A$ (2)

From (1) and (2) $R \cup R^1 \subseteq A \times A \Rightarrow R \cup R^1$ is a relation is A.

Now $(a, b) \in R \cup R^1$ (assume)

$\Rightarrow (a, b) \in R$ or $(a, b) \in R^1 \Rightarrow (b, a) \in R$ or $(b, a) \in R^1$

$\therefore$ (R and R' are symmetric)

$\Rightarrow (b, a) \in R \cup R'$

$\therefore (a, b) \in R \cup R' \Rightarrow (b, a) \in R \cup R^1$

$\therefore R \cup R^1$ is symmetric.

Again $R \subseteq A \times A$ and $R' \subseteq A \times A$

$\therefore R \cap R' \subseteq A \times A$

$\Rightarrow R \cap R'$ is a relation in A.

Now let $(a, b) \in R \cap R'$

$\Rightarrow (a, b) \in R \cap R' \Rightarrow (a, b) \in R$ and $(a, b) \in R'$

$\Rightarrow (b, a) \in R$ and $(b, a) \in R'$

$\Rightarrow (b, a) \in R \cap R'$

$\therefore (a, b) \in R \cap R' \Rightarrow (b, a) \in R \cap R'$

$\therefore R \cap R'$ in symmetric.

12. Hint: Here $a\ R\ b$ if $a^b = b^a\ \forall\ a, b \in N$

Let $a = b = x$, then $a^b = x^x$ and $b^a = x^x$

$\therefore a^b = b^a \Rightarrow a\ R\ b$, where $a = b = x \Rightarrow x\ R\ x$

R is reflexive.

Let $x\ R\ y$ where $x, y \in N$

$\therefore x^y = y^x$ (i)

Now $y\ R\ x$ iff $y^x = x^y$ and $x^y = y^x$ is true from (i)

$\therefore x\ R\ y \Rightarrow y\ R\ x\ \forall\ x, y \in N$

$\therefore R$ is symmetric.

13. Solution: (i) If R is reflexive then $\forall\ a \in A$

$(a, a) \in R \Rightarrow (a, a) \in R^{-1}$ (changing the components)

$\Rightarrow R^{-1}$ is reflexive.

(ii) $(a, b) \in R^{-1}$, where $a, b \in A$

Then $(b, a) \in R \Rightarrow (a, b) \in R$ [since R is symmetric]

$\Rightarrow (b, a) \in R^{-1}$ (from def.)

$\therefore$ If R is symmetric then R^{-1} is also symmetric.

(iii) Let $(a, b) \in R^{-1}$ and $(b, c) \in R^{-1}$, where $a, b, c \in A$

Then $(a, b) \in R^{-1} \Rightarrow (b, a)\ R$ (from def.) and $(b, c) \in R^{-1}$

$\Rightarrow (c, b) \in R$

$\therefore (c, b) \in R$ and $(b, a) \in R$

$\Rightarrow (c, a) \in R\ \therefore R$ is transitive

$\Rightarrow (a, c) \in R^{-1}$

$\therefore (a, b)\ R^{-1}$ and $(b, c) \in R^{-1} \Rightarrow (a, c) \in R^{-1}$

$\therefore$ If R is transitive then R^{-1} is also transitive.

14. Ans. (i) $R^{-1}\ o\ R^{-1} = \{(5, 1), (6, 1), (6, 3)\}$

(ii) $(R^{-1}\ o\ R)^{-1} = \{(1, 1), (3, 3), (4, 4), (4, 7), (7, 4), (7, 7)\}$

Solution: By graphical method:

(i) We have $R = \{(4, 5), (1, 4), (4, 6), (7, 6), (3, 7)\}$ the domain and range of which are respectively.

$\{1, 3, 4, 7\}$ and $\{4, 5, 6, 7\}$. In the figure given below $R\ o\ R$ has been displayed in which we see

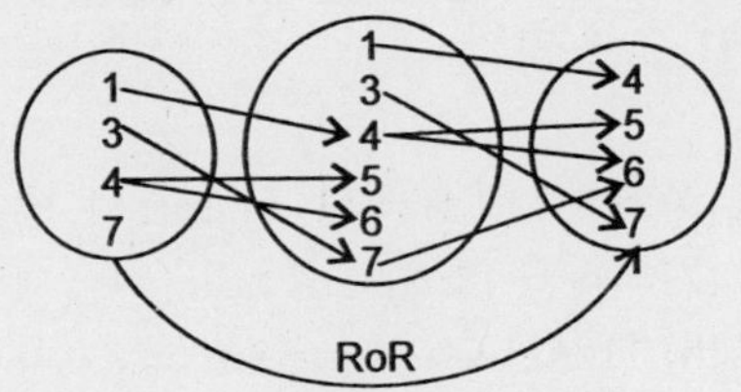

Figure Q. 14

$$1 \xrightarrow{R} 4 \xrightarrow{R} 5 \Rightarrow (1,5) \in R\, o\, R$$

$$1 \xrightarrow{R} 4 \xrightarrow{R} 6 \Rightarrow (1,6) \in R\, o\, R$$

$$3 \xrightarrow{R} 7 \xrightarrow{R} 6 \Rightarrow (3,6) \in R\, o\, R$$

No other relation besides this can be restored from A to C and hence

$$R\, o\, R = \{(1,5), (1,6), (3,6)\}$$

Therefore $R^{-1}\, o\, R^{-1} = (R\, o\, R)^{-1} = \{(5, 1), (6, 1), (6, 3)\}$

(ii) We know $(R^{-1}\, o\, R)^{-1} = R^{-1}\, o\, (R^{-1})^{-1} = R^{-1}\, o\, R$

$\therefore (R^{-1}\, o\, R)^{-1} = R^{-1}\, o\, R.$

Now $R^{-1}\, o\, R$ represents the composition of the relation R and R^{-1}, we have $R = \{(4,5), (1,4), (4,6), (7,6), (3,7)\}$

$\therefore \qquad R^{-1} = \{(5,4), (4,1), (6,4)\ (6,7), (7,3)\}$

$$1 \xrightarrow{R} 4 \xrightarrow{R^{-1}} 1 \Rightarrow (1,1) \in R^{-1}\, o\, R$$

$$3 \xrightarrow{R} 7 \xrightarrow{R^{-1}} 3 \Rightarrow (3,3) \in R^{-1} o\, R$$

$$4 \xrightarrow{R} 5 \xrightarrow{R^{-1}} 4 \Rightarrow (4,4) \in R^{-1} o\, R$$

$$4 \xrightarrow{R} 6 \xrightarrow{R^{-1}} 7 \Rightarrow (4,7) \in R^{-1}\, o\, R$$

$$7 \xrightarrow{R} 6 \longrightarrow 4 \Rightarrow (7,4) \in R^{-1}\, o\, R$$

$$7 \xrightarrow{R} 7 \xrightarrow{R^{-1}} 7 \Rightarrow (7,7) \in R^{-1}\, o\, R$$

$\therefore (R^{-1}\, oR)^{-1} = R^{-1} o\, R = \{(1,1), (3,3), (4,4), (4,7), (7,4), (7,7)\}$

Analytic method: We have $R = \{(4, 5), (1, 4), (4, 6), (7, 6), (3,7)\}$.

We have to determine $R \, o \, R$ and for this we first collect the domain of R i.e. $\{1, 3, 4, 7\}$.

Now

$(R \, o \, R)(1) = R(4) = 5$ and $6 \Rightarrow (1, 5)$ and $(1, 6) \in R \, o \, R$.

$(R \, o \, R)(3) = R(7) = 6 \Rightarrow (3, 6) \in R \, o \, R$.

$(R \, o \, R)(4) = R(5)$ This does not exist.

$(R \, o \, R)(7) = R(6)$ This does not exist.

Hence $R \, o \, R$ is $\{(1, 5), (1, 6), (6, 3)\}$.

$\therefore (R \, o \, R)^{-1} = \{(5, 1), (6, 1), (6, 3)\}$.

We have $R^{-1} = \{(5, 4), (4, 1), (6, 4), (6, 7), (7, 3)\}$.

$\therefore$ The domain of R^{-1} is $\{4, 5, 6, 7\}$

$(R^{-1} \, o \, R^{-1})(4) = R^{-1}$ This does not exist.

$(R^{-1} \, o \, R^{-1})(5) = R^{-1}(4) = 1 \Rightarrow (5, 1) \in R^{-1} \, o \, R^{-1}$

$(R^{-1} \, o \, R^{-1})(6) = R^{-1}(4) = 1 \Rightarrow (6, 1) \in R^{-1} \, o \, R^{-1}$

$= R^{-1}(7) = 3 \Rightarrow (6, 3) \in R^{-1} \, o \, R^{-1}$

$(R^{-1} \, o \, R^{-1})(7) = R^{-1}(3)$ This does not exist.

$\therefore$ The composite relation

$R^{-1} \, o \, R = \{(5, 1), (6, 1), (6, 3)\}$.

We thus see that $[R \, o \, R]^{-1} = [R^{-1} \, o \, R^{-1}]$.

We have to determine now $(R^{-1} \, o \, R)^{-1}$ and for this we try to find out $R^{-1} \, oR$ as follows:

$(R^{-1} \, o \, R)(1) = R^{-1}(4) = 1 \Rightarrow (1, 1) \in R^{-1} \, o \, R$

$(R^{-1} \, o \, R)(3) = R^{-1}(7) = 3 \Rightarrow (3, 3) \in R^{-1} \, o \, R$

$(R^{-1} \, o \, R)(4) = R^{-1}(5) = 4 \Rightarrow (4, 4) \in R^{-1} \, o \, R$

$= R^{-1}(6) = 7 \Rightarrow (4, 7) \in R^{-1} \, o \, R$

$(R^{-1} \, o \, R)(7) = R^{-1}(6) = 4 \Rightarrow (7, 4) \in R^{-1} \, o \, R$

$= 7 \Rightarrow (7, 7) \in R^{-1} \, o \, R$

Thus $R^{-1} \, o \, R = \{(1, 1), (3, 3), (4, 4), (4, 7), (7, 4), (7, 7)\}$.

$\therefore [R^{-1} \, oR]^{-1} = \{(1, 1), (3, 3), (4, 4), (7, 4), (4, 7), (7, 7)\}$

15. **Solution:** $(a, b) \, R \, (c, d) \Rightarrow (c, d) \, R \, (a, b)$, where $a, b, c \Rightarrow N$.

Since $ad = bc \Rightarrow bc = ad = cb = da$

$\therefore (a, d) \, R \, (c, d) \Rightarrow (c, d) \, R \, (a, b) \therefore R$ is symmetric.

Again $(a, b) \, R \, (a, b) \, \forall \, a, b \in N$.

Since $ab = ba : R$ is reflexive.

Further we see $(a, b)\ R\ (c, d), (c\ , d)\ R\ (e, f) \Rightarrow (a, b)\ R\ (e, f)$ i.e. R is transitive $\forall\ a, b, c, d, e, f \in N$

$\therefore \quad (a, b)\ R\ (c, d) \Rightarrow ad = be$ ...(A)

$(c, d)\ R\ (e, f) \Rightarrow ef = de$ ...(B)

$(a, b)\ R\ (e, f) \Rightarrow af = be$ ...(C)

$\therefore$ From these three relations (A), (B) and(C) we have $(a, b)\ R\ (c, d), (c, d)\ R\ (e, f) \Rightarrow ad\ ef = be\ de \Rightarrow ef = be$ which is (C)

Thus symmetry, reflexivity and transitivity are satisfied and hence R is an equivalence relation.

16. Please see that Hint of Q. No. 50 (i) of Problems and Exercises 2B (i).

17. Please see that Hint of Q. No. 39 of Problems and Exercises 2B (i).

18. **Ans.** (*b*).

19. **Ans.** (*d*).

20. **Solution:** $F : R \to R$ is an onto function $\therefore$ Range of $f = R$.

$\therefore \quad \dfrac{\alpha x^2 + 6x - 8}{\alpha + 6x - 8x^2}$ assumes all real values for real x.

Put $y = \dfrac{\alpha x^2 + 6x - 8}{\alpha + 6x - 8x^2}$

$\Rightarrow x^2 (\alpha + 8y) + 6x (1 - y) - (8 + \alpha y) \geq 0\ \forall\ y \in R$

$\therefore$ The discriminate.

$36 (1 - y)^2 + 4 (\alpha + 8y)(8 + \alpha y) \geq 0\ \forall\ y \in R$ ($\therefore x$ is real)

$\Rightarrow y^2 [8\alpha + 9] + y [\alpha^2 + 46] + [8\alpha + 9] \geq 0$

$\therefore \quad (\alpha^2 + 46)^2 - 4 (8\alpha + 9)^2 \geq 0$

$\Rightarrow (\alpha^2 + 16\alpha + 64)(\alpha^2 + 16\alpha + 28) \geq 0$

$\Rightarrow (\alpha + 8)^2 (\alpha - 14)(\alpha - 2) \geq 0\ \therefore\ 2 \leq \alpha \leq 14$

$\therefore \quad \alpha \in [2, 14]$, where $\alpha = 3, f(x) = \dfrac{3x^2 + 6x - 8}{3 + 6x - 8x^2}$

gives $f(1)$ and $f(-1) = 1\ \therefore f$ is not one-one for $\alpha = 3$.

21. **Solution:** (i) The function $f(x) = x + \sin x$ is not periodic

(ii) The function $f(x) = \{x\}$ is periodic with period 1.

(iii) $f(x) = |\cos x|$ is periodic with period π.

(iv) $f(x) = 1 - \dfrac{\sin^3 x}{\sin x + \cos x} - \dfrac{\cos^3 x}{\sin x + \cos x}$

$= 1 - 1 + \sin x \cos x$

$= \dfrac{\sin 2x}{2}$ $\therefore f(x)$ is periodic with period π.

22. Solution: $g \, o \, f(x) = g(f(x)) = g\{x\}$

$= \frac{1}{2} \sin [\{x\}] \pi = 0 \; \forall \; x \in R \; \therefore \; g \, o \, f$ is $\{0\}$.

EXERCISE – 2 D (ii) SIMPLE QUESTIONS

1. What do you mean by a mapping? Explain with examples. [Magadh B.Sc. 1977, 1976]
2. What do you mean by the domain, codomain and range of a mapping or function? [Ranchi B.Sc. 1974]
3. Explain the into and onto mappings with examples. [Meerut B.Sc. 1969, 1970, 1978]
4. Find the domain and range of the following relations:
   (i) $\{(x, y): x$ is multiples of 3 and y is multiples of 5$\}$.
   (ii) $\{(x, y): x, y \in N$ and $x + y = 0\}$.
   (iii) $\{(x, y): x = 3y, x, y \in N$ but less then 6$\}$.
5. Examine the kinds of the following mappings:
   (i) $\{(a, 1), (b, 1), (c, 1), (d, 1)\}$
   (ii) $\{(3, 2), (6, 4), (9, 2), (12, 4)\}$
   (iii) $\{(x, 1), (y, 2), (z, 3), (u, 4)\}$
6. Prove that the mapping $f: R \to R$ defined by $f(x) = x + 1$, where R is a set of real numbers, is one-one onto mapping.
7. Prove that the mapping $f: R \to R$ defined by $f(x) = e^x$, where R is a set of real numbers and $x \in R$ is one-one mapping. [Allahabad B.Sc. 1977]
8. Prove that the function on mapping $f: N \to N$ (where N is the set of the natural numbers) defined by $f(n) = 2n + 3 \; \forall \; n \in N$ is one-one and into mapping. [MLNRE 1987, I.I.T. 1974]

9. Prove that the function $f: N \to N$ defined by $f(x) = 2x, \forall x \in N$ (where N is the set of the natural numbers) is one-one and into mappimg.

10. Prove that the mapping $f: R \to R$ defined by $f(x) = \cos x$, $x \in R$ is neither one-one nor onto mapping.

[U.P. 1981, 1985, MLNRE 1989]

[**Hint:** Let $x_1, x_2 \in R$ then $f(x_1) = \cos x_1$ and $f(x_2) = \cos x_2$ and hence $f(x_1) = f(x_2) \Rightarrow \cos x_1 = \cos x_2$

$\Rightarrow x_1 = 2n\,\pi \pm x_2 \Rightarrow x_1 \neq x_2$

Therefore f is not one-one.

Again the f image of x lies in $[-1, 1]$,

i.e. $f[R] = \{f(x): -1 \leq f(x) \leq 1\}$.

Thus the other elements of co-domain except $[-1, 1]$ are not the f image of x $\therefore f[R] \subset R$.

$\therefore f$ is not onto mapping. Thus f is neither one-one nor onto.

11. Prove that the mapping $f: R \to R$ defined by $f(x) = \sin x \ \forall x \in R$ is neither one-one nor onto.

[Merrut B.Sc. 1981, U.P 1984, 1985]

12. Let $X = \left\{x : x \in R \text{ and} \frac{\pi}{2} \leq x \leq \frac{\pi}{2}\right\}$ i.e. $X = \left\{-\frac{\pi}{2}, \frac{\pi}{2}\right\}$ and $Y = \{y: y \in R \text{ and } -1 \leq y \leq 1\}$ i.e. $Y = \{-1, 1\}$, then prove that the mepping $f: X \to Y$ defined by $f(x) = \sin x \ \forall x \in X$ is one-one as well as onto.

13. Prove that $f: R \to R$ defined by $f(x) = \frac{1}{x} x \neq 0 \ x \in R$ is one-one and onto mapping. [U.P. 1980, Merrut B.Sc. 1978]

14. $f: R \to R$ and $g: R \to R$ defined by $f(x) = \sin x$, and $g(X) = x^2$, find $(f \circ g)(x)$ and $(g \circ f)(x)$ [U.P. 1987]

15. Let there be two mappings, $f: R \to R$ and $g: R \to R$ defined by $f(x) = 2x$ and $g(x) = x^2 + 2$, prove that (i) f is a one-one and onto mapping.

(ii) g is a many one into mapping.

16. Two mappings $f: R \to R$ and $g: R \to R$ are defined as $f(x) = 2x$ and $g(x) = x^2 + 2$, prove that (i) $f \circ g \neq g \circ f$

(ii) Find the values of $(f \circ g)(2)$ and $(g \circ g)(1)$.

17. Find the value of $X \cap Y$ and $(X - Y) \cup (Y - X)$ if $X = \{1, 2, 3, 4, 5\}$ and $Y = \{1, 3, 5, 7, 9\}$. Which of the followings are mappings from X to Y ?

(a) $R = \{(x, y): y = x + 2, x \in x, y \in Y\}$

(b) $R = \{(1, 1), (2, 1), (3, 3), (4, 3), (5, 5)\}$

(c) $R = \{(1, 1), (1, 3), (3, 5), (3, 7), (5, 7)\}$

(d) $R = \{(1, 3), (2, 5), (4, 7), (5, 9), (3, 1)\}$ [Roorkee 1918]

[**Hint:** $X \cap Y = \{1, 3, 5\}$, $(X - Y) \cup (Y - X) = \{2, 4\} \cup \{7, 9\}$
$= \{2, 4, 7, 9\}$

(a) $R = \{(x, y): y = x + 2, x \in x, y \in Y\}$

$X = \{1, 2, 3, 4, 5,\}$, $Y = \{1, 3, 5, 7, 9\}$

$x = 1 \in X$ and $y = x + 2 = 1 + 2 = 3 \in Y \therefore (1, 3) \in R$

$x = 2 \in x$ and $y = x + 2 = 2 + 2 = 4 \notin Y \therefore (2, 4) \notin R$

$x = 3 \in x$ and $y = x + 2 = 3 + 2 = 5 \in Y \therefore (3, 5) \in R$

$x = 4 \in x$ and $y = x + 2 = 4 + 2 = 6 \notin Y \therefore (4, 6) \notin R$

$x = 5 \in x$ and $y = x + 2 = 5 + 2 = 7 \in Y \therefore (5, 7) \in R$

Thus $R = \{(1, 3), (3, 5), (5, 7)\}$, therefore R is a relation from X to Y but this is not a mapping, since 2, 4 are the elements of the domain X where images is Y do not exist.

(b) This is a many one into mapping.

(c) This is not a mapping since $1 \in x$ has two images 1 and 3 in Y.

(d) This is a one-one onto mapping.

18. Let $A = \{x: -1 \le x \le 1\} = B$ find the nature of two following mappings. (i) $f(x) = \frac{x}{2}$ (ii) $g(x) = |x|$ (iii) $h(x) = x|x|$ (iv) $k\,x = x^2$ (v) $l(x) = \sin \pi x$. [I.I.T. 1976]

[**Hint:** (i) $x, y \in A, x \ne y \Rightarrow \frac{1}{2}x \ne \frac{1}{2}y \Rightarrow f(x) \ne f(y)$.

Therefore this is a one-one mapping.

Again $f(A) = \left\{x : -\frac{1}{2} \le x \le \frac{1}{2}\right\}$ or $f(A) \subset B$

Therefore this is an into mapping.

(ii) $g(1) = 1, g(-1) = 1$. Therefore this is many one.

Again $f(A) = \{x: 0 \le x \le 1\}$ or $f(A) \subset B$. Therefore this is an into mapping.

(iii) $h(x) = x^2$ if $x \geq 0$. This is one-one and onto.
$h(x) = -x^2$ if $x < 0$
(iv) and (v) have already been explained.]

19. Find the number of surjections from
$A = \{1, 2, 3....n\}$ $n \geq 2$ to $B = \{a, b\}$. [EAMCET 1992]
[**Hint:** The number of onto function or surjections.

Form A to B is given by $\sum_{r=1}^{n}(-1)^{n-r}\ {}^{n}c_r\, r^m$

where A and B have m and n elements such $1 \leq n \leq m$
$\therefore$ The number of surjections from A to B in the given question

$$= \sum_{r=1}^{2}(-1)^{2-r}\ {}^{2}c_r r^n = (-1)^1\ {}^{2}c_1(1)^n + (-1)^0\ {}^{2}c_2 2^n = 2^n - 2.$$

20. If $f(x) = \dfrac{x}{1+x^2}$ and $g(x) = \dfrac{e^{-x}}{1+[x]}$ where $[x] \leq x$ find domain $(f+g)$ and Range $f \cap g$.

Solution: Domain of $f = R$ and Domain of g
$= \{x: 1 + [x] \neq 0\} = \{x: x \notin [-1, 0)\}$
$\therefore$ Domain of $g = R - [-1, 0)$
$\therefore$ Domain is $(f + g) = R - [-1, 0)$

Let $y = \dfrac{x}{1+x^2}$ $\therefore$ $x = \dfrac{1 \pm \sqrt{1-4y^2}}{2y}$ $\therefore$ $y \neq 0$ and $1 - 4y^2 \geq 0$

$\therefore$ $y \in \left[-\dfrac{1}{2}, \dfrac{1}{2}\right] - \{0\}$ $\therefore$ Range $f = \left[-\dfrac{1}{2}, \dfrac{1}{2}\right] - \{0\}$

If we put $y = \dfrac{e-x}{1+[x]}$ $y > 0 \Rightarrow 1 + [x] > 0$

$\therefore$ $\dfrac{1}{e^x} > 0$ $\therefore$ $[x] > -1$. Also $y < 0 \Rightarrow [x] < -1$

$y > 0 \Rightarrow x \in [0, \infty]$ and $y < 0 \Rightarrow x \in (-\infty, -1)$

$\therefore$ Range of $g = R - \{0\}$ $\therefore$ Range $f \cap g = \left[-\dfrac{1}{2}, \dfrac{1}{2}\right] - \{0\}$.

ANSWERS TO EXERCISE 2 D (ii)

(Hints and Solutions)

1. **Hint:** Please consult Articles 2.5 and 2.7.
2. **Hint:** Please consult Article 2.5.
3. **Hint:** Please consult Article 2.8 (4).
4. **Ans.** (i) Domain = $\{0, \pm 3, \pm 6, \pm 9....\}$,

   Range = $\{0, \pm 5, \pm 10, \pm 15....\}$.

   (ii) Domain = $\{1, 2, 3, 4, 5, 6, 7, 8, 9\}$,

   Range = $\{9, 8, 7, 6, 5, 4, 3, 2, 1\}$.

   (iii) Domain = $\{3\}$, Range = $\{1\}$.

   Solution: (i) The first component of the ordered pair (x, y) is x which is multiples of 3 and hence the domain is $\{x: x$ is multiples of $3\}$ i.e. $\{0, \pm 3, \pm 6, \pm 9....\}$.

   The second component of the ordered pair (x, y) is y which is multiples of 5 as described in the question and hence the range is $\{y: y$ is multiples of $5\}$ i.e. $\{0, \pm 5, \pm 10, \pm 15....\}$.

   (ii) The values of x and y must satisfy the equation $x + y = 10$ and hence

   $x = 1\ 2\ 3\ 4\ 5\ 6\ 7\ 8\ 9$

   $y = 9\ 8\ 7\ 6\ 5\ 4\ 3\ 2\ 1$

   $\therefore$ The domain is $\{1, 2, 3, ... 8, 9\}$ and the range is $\{9, 8, 7, 6, 5, 4, 3, 2, 1\}$.

   (iii) We have $N = \{1, 2, 3, 4, 5\} < 6$.

   The values of x and y which satisfy the equation $x = 3y$ are respectively 3 and 1 and hence the domain is $\{3\}$ and the range is $\{1\}$.
5. **Ans.** (i) Constant mapping (ii) many one mapping (iii) one-one and onto mapping.

   Solution: (i) Each element of the domain $\{a, b, c, d\}$ has the same f image 1 and therefore the mapping is a constant mapping.

   (ii) The domain is $\{3, 6, 9, 12\}$ and the range is $\{2, 4\}$. 6 and 12 are related to 4 whereas 3 and 9 are related to 2. Thus the mapping is many one.

(iii) The domain is $\{x, y, z, u\}$ and the range is $\{1, 2, 3, 4,\}$. The different elements of the domain are related to different elements of the range and hence the mapping is, one-one. In addition, every element of the range are the f image of the elements of the domain.

$\therefore$ The mapping is onto.

6. **Hint.** Let x_1 and x_2 be the elements of the domain R, then

$$f(x_1) = f(x_2) \Rightarrow x_1 + 1 = x_2 + 1 \Rightarrow x_1 = x_2$$

$\therefore f$ is one-one mapping.

Let y be an arbitrary element of the range R of the mapping f. If $y = x + 1$ then $x = y - 1$ which is a real number.

Also $f(y - 1) = y - 1 + 1 = y$.

This shows that pre-image of every element of R is in the domain of R.

$\therefore f$ is onto mapping.

7. **Hint.** Let x_1 and x_2 be any two real numbers, then their images under f are $f(x_1)$ and $f(x_2)$ respectively.

$\therefore f(x_1) = f(x_2) \Rightarrow e^{x_1} = e^{x_2}$

$\Rightarrow x_1 = x_2$. $\therefore f$ is one-one mapping.

8. **Hint.** Please see the solution of Q. No. 32 and Q. No. 39 (v) of "Some More Important Problems". Exercises 2 C (ii).

9. **Solution:** Let x_1 and x_2 be any two arbitrary elements of the domain N, then $x_1\ x_2 \in N$.

$\therefore f(x_1) = f(x_2) \Rightarrow 2x_1 = 2x_2$

$\Rightarrow x_1 = x_2$

$\therefore f$ is one-one mapping.

Again $f(x) = 2x$. Putting $x = 1, 2, 3$ .... we get

$$f(1) = 2, f(2) = 4, f(3) = 6 \ldots.$$

$\therefore$ The ramge of $f = \{2, 4, 6....\} \subset N$

$\therefore f$ is into mapping.

10. **Hint.** The solution has been give in the question.

11. **Solution:** Put $x = 0$ and π.

Then $f(0) = \sin 0 = 0$ and $f(\pi) = \sin \pi = 0$.

Thus two elements 0 and π of the domain R have the same f image in the range R. $\therefore f$ is not one-one mapping.

We know $-1 \leq \sin x \leq 1$ and hence only those elements of the codomain which are contained in $[-1, 1]$ are the f image of the elements of the domain R.

$\therefore$ range $\subseteq$ codomain.

$\therefore f$ is not onto mapping.

12. Solution: Let there be two arbitrary real numbers m and n of $\left[-\frac{\pi}{2}, \frac{\pi}{2}\right]$

$\therefore m \neq n \Rightarrow \sin m \neq \sin n$

$\therefore f(m) \neq f(n)$

$\therefore f$ is one-one.

Again $-1 \leq \sin x \leq 1$ hence the real number y in between -1 and $+1$ which is the f image of x of $\left[-\frac{\pi}{2}, \frac{\pi}{2}\right]$ i.e. $\sin x = y$.

For example if $y = \frac{\sqrt{3}}{2}$ then $x = \frac{\pi}{2}$

Such that $\sin \frac{\pi}{3} = \frac{\sqrt{3}}{2}$ i.e. $\sin x = y$.

$\therefore$ The range of $f = Y$

$\therefore f$ is onto mapping.

13. Solution: Let the real numbers x_1 and x_2 are any two arbitrary elements of the domain R, where $x_1 \neq 0$ and $x_2 \neq 0$.

Then $f(x_1) = f(x_2) \Rightarrow \frac{1}{x_1} = \frac{1}{x_2}$

$\Rightarrow x_1 = x_2 \therefore f$ is one-one.

Again let $y \neq 0$ be an arbitrary element of the codomain R.

If $y = \frac{1}{x}$ then $x = \frac{1}{y}$

$$\therefore f\left(\frac{1}{y}\right) = \left(\frac{1}{\frac{1}{y}}\right) = y.$$

$\therefore$ y of the codomain R is the f image of $\frac{1}{y}$ of the domain R.

$\therefore$ The range of R = codomain R.

$\therefore$ f is onto.

14. $(f \circ g)(x) = \sin x^2$

$(g \circ f)(x) = \sin x^2$

Solution: $(f \circ g)(x) = f[g(x)] = f(x^2) = \sin x^2$

$(g \circ f)(x) = g[f(x)] = g(\sin x) = \sin^2 x$.

15. Solution: (i) The mapping $f: R \to R$ is defined by $f(x) = 2x$, $x \in R$.

For x_1 and $x_2 \in$ Domain R we have

$f(x_1) = f(x_2) \Rightarrow 2x_1 = 2x_2 \Rightarrow x_1 = x_2$

$\therefore$ f is one-one mapping.

Let R be an arbitrary element of codomain R then if

$y = 2x$.We can oblain $x = \frac{1}{2}\ y \in R$

$$\therefore f\left(\frac{y}{2}\right) = 2\left(\frac{1}{2}y\right) = y.$$

Therefore every element of the codomain R is the f image of element of the domain R.

$\therefore$ range of f = codomain R

$\therefore$ f is onto mapping.

(ii) We have $g: R \to R$ defined by $g(x) = x^2 + 2\ \forall\ x \in R$.

Let p and $-p \in$ to the domain R

then $g(p) = p^2 + 2$ and $g(-p) = p^2 + 2$

$\therefore$ g is many one mapping.

In addition, we see $x^2 + 2$ is always positive for negative and positive x and is never equal to zero.

The negative numbers including zero of the codomain are not the g image of any element of the domain R.

$\therefore$ range of g C codomain R.

$\therefore$ g is an into mapping.

16. Ans. $(f \circ g)(2) = 12$ and $(g \circ f)(1) = 11$

Solution: (i) Let $x \in R$, then

$(f \circ g)(x) = f[g(x)] = f(x^2 + 2) = 2(x^2 + 2) = 2x^2 + 4.$

$(g \circ f)(x) = g[f(x)] = g(2x) = (2x)^2 + 2 = 4x^2 + 4.$

$\therefore f \circ g \neq g \circ f$

(ii) $(f \circ g)(2) = f[g(2)] = f[(2)^2 + 2] = f(6) = 2 \times 6 = 12$

$(g \circ g)(1) = g[g^{(1)}] = g[1^2 + 2] = g^{(3)} = (3)^2 + 2 = 11.$

17. **Hint:** The solution has already been given in the question. Also consult the solution of Q. No. 25 of "Some More Important Problems". Exercise 2C (ii).

18. **Hint:** Though the solution has been given in the question but the reader is advised to consult the solution of Q. No. 30 of "Some More Important Problems". Exercise 2C (ii).

Chapter 2 (E)
A Glimpse of Mathematical Logic

2.26 MATHEMATICAL LOGIC

In order to study mathematical logic we have to be acquainted first with the term "statement".

"A statement is an assertion which may be true or false and which when spoken gives a good return for facts".

Consider the following assertions:

(1) Delhi is the capital of India.

(2) $2H_2 + O_2 = 2H_2O$.

(3) The tiger is two footed.

(4) $3 > 4$.

(5) Two is a prime number.

(6) Eight is divisible by four.

Here the assertions 1, 2, 5, 6 are true while 3 and 4 are false.

Those sentences are generally called statements whose truthfulness or falsity can be decided by us. We can frame statements with words or symbols also. Assertions like definitions, calls, questions etc. are not generally statements.

A statement is either true or false but it can not be both true and false at the same time.

If we write $x > 0$, then it is the impossible to decide whether it is true or false and therefore the sentence "x is greater than two" is not a statement. Statements are generally denoted by p, q, r ....

2.27 LOGICAL OPERATIONS

We very often obtain the new sets with the help of set operations on the given sets. In the statememts there are logical connectives. With the help of logical connectives between the given statements we obtain new statements. The logical connectives are as follows: "not", "and", "or", "if", "then", and "if and only if".

Compossite statements are composed with the help of logical operations.

(i) *Conjunction of statements:* Logical connectives "and" and "or" are known as conjunctions. We can obtain new statements with the aid of a conjunction. Let there be two statements, "America is rich". "India is a poor". We obtain a new statement with the help of "and" as "America is rich and India is poor". A statement composed of two statements p and q with the help of conjunction "and" is denoted as $p \wedge q$. We say "and" is the conjunction of p and q. The statements $p \wedge q$ is true if and only if both p and q are true. If p be the statement $5 < 6$ and q be the statement $6 < 7$ then $p \wedge q$ is shown by the inequality $5 < 6 < 7$. In this case, $p \wedge q$ are true since p is true and q is true. The logical symbol $\wedge$ can be used to define the intersection of two sets A and B viz. $A \cap B = \{x: x \in A \wedge x \in B\}$.

(ii) *Disjunction of a statement:* We can form new statement with the help of conjunction "or".

A statement composed of two statements p and q connected by "or" is denoted by $p \vee q$. Here "or" is called the disjunction of p and q.

The disjunction $p \vee q$ is true statements if and only if at least one of the given statements is true. In the definition of union of two sets A and B we can use the logical symbol $\vee$ viz, $A \cup B = \{x: x \in A \vee x \in B\}$.

Let there be two statements $6 < 8$ and $6 = 8$, denoted by p and q respectively, then $p \vee q$ is $6 \leq 8$. Since the first statement is true hence the disjunction is also true.

Following are the two statements:

He reads Geography today. He reads History today. The new statement composed of the above two statements is "He reads Geography or History today". This is true if the first statement is true and is false if the first statement is false.

(iii) *Implication of statements:* Two statements connected with "if then" form is termed as an implication and is denoted as $p \Rightarrow q$. We read it as if p, then q or p implies q. The statement p is called the premise of the implication and the statement q is called the conclusion of the implication. An implication $p \Rightarrow q$ is false if the premise is true and the conclusion is false. Example of false implication is – "If 45 is divisible by 3 and 5 then it is divisible by 16".

Example of true implication is – "If 45 is divisible by 3 and 5 then it is divisible by 15".

$p \Rightarrow q$ is a conditional implication and $p \Leftrightarrow q$ is a biconditional implication.

(iv) *Logical equivalence:* A statement formed by the given statements p and q with the help of the group of words "if and only if" is known as a logical equivalence. A logical equivalence is also a biconditional implication. We denote it as $p \Leftrightarrow q$. A logical equivalence $p \Leftrightarrow q$ is true if and only if both the statements p and q are true or if both are false.

For instance, the statements – "45 is divisible by 15" if and only if it is divisible by 3 and 5" and "45 is divisible by 6 if and only if it is divisible by 4" are true statements.

The equivalence – "The number 15 is divisible by 5 if and only if it is divisible by 4" is a false statement since one of the components is false and the other is true.

(v) *A brief and comprehensive concept of logical sum, product, equivalence and implication:* Logical sum of two statements is known as the disjunction of the sentences. This type of sentence is formed by connecting two sentences with the word "or".

By logical product of two sentences we mean the conjunction of those sentences. This type of sentence is formed by connecting the two sentences with the word "and".

By logical equivalence we mean those sentences which are formed by two sentences by connecting them with the words or a group of words "if and only if", whereas an implication is formed by connectiong two sentences by the group of words "if... then".

Consider the statements:

$p \equiv \{4 < 5\}$; $q \equiv \{4$ is prime$\}$. We form the following statements with p and q as follows:

$A = \{4 < 5$ or the number four is prime$\}$.

$B = \{4 < 5$ and the number four is prime$\}$.

$C = \{4 < 5$ if and only if the number four is prime$\}$.

$D = \{$If $4 < 5$ then the number four is prime$\}$.

The composite statements A, B, C and D are respectively a disjunction, conjunction, equivalence and implication of the sentences p and q.

(vi) *Tautologies:* A statement which is always true is known as a tautology. The statement $(p \vee q) \Rightarrow q \vee p$ is a tautology. Propositions which contain only T in the last column of their truth table are known as tautologies. A contradiction contains only F in the last column of its truth table.

(vii) *Truth value:* The truth or falsify of a statement is known as its truth value.

(viii) *Denial or negation of a statement:* A denial is also a logical operation which corresponds to the logical connective "not". Consider two false statements:

1. "3 is an even number". 2. "7 is divisible by 3". If we deny them then we write "3 is not an even number" and "7 is not divisible by 3". If p be a statement then $\overline{p}$ be its negation. The statement $\overline{p}$ states that p is false. We can say that $\overline{p}$ is true if p is false and vice versa, $\overline{p}$ is false if p is true. If $3 \in N$ is true, then $3 \notin N$ is false.

If $5 < 6$ is true, then $5 > 6$ is false.

Consider the statement: $p \equiv \{$the number four is a prime number$\}$. The denial of p is $\overline{p} \equiv \{$the number four is a composite number$\}$ or $\overline{p} \equiv \{$the number four is not a prime number$\}$. The negation or denial of p is also denoted by $\sim p$ or $-p$.

(ix) *Truth table:* The disjunction (sum) of statements p and q is denoted by $p + q$ or $p \vee q$, the conjunction (product) by $p\,q$ or $p \wedge q$, the equivalence by $p \Leftrightarrow q$ or $p \sim q$ implication by $p \Rightarrow q$ respectively. We read $p \Rightarrow q$ as q follows from p or if p then q.

The sum or disjunction of statements is true iff at least one of the statements p and q is true. The truth table for $p + q$ is (1) where T stands for true statement and F stands for false statement.

p	q	$p + q$ or $p \vee q$
T	T	T
T	F	T
F	T	T
F	F	F

(1)

p	q	pq or $p \wedge q$
T	T	T
T	F	F
F	T	F
F	F	F

(2)

The conjunction $p\,q$ statements is true iff both the statements are true. The truth table for $q \wedge q$ is (2).

The equivalence $p \Leftrightarrow q$ is false if one of the sentences is true and other is false. The equivalence is true when both p and q are true or both p and q are false. The truth table for $p \Leftrightarrow q$ is (3)

p	q	$p \Leftrightarrow q$
T	T	T
T	F	F
F	T	F
F	F	T

(3)

p	q	$p \Rightarrow q$
T	T	T
T	F	F
F	T	T
F	F	T

(4)

p	$\bar{p}$
T	F
F	T

(5)

The implication $p \Rightarrow q$ is false iff p is true and q is false. $p \Rightarrow q$ is true if

(i) p is true and q is true. (ii) p is false but q is true

(iii) p is false and q is false. The truth table for $p \Rightarrow q$ is (4).

The truth table for negation is (5).

Example 1: Prove the formula $p \Rightarrow q = \bar{p} + q$ by truth table.

Solution:

p	q	$p \Rightarrow q$	$\bar{p}$	$\bar{p} + q$
T	T	T	F	T
T	F	F	F	F
F	T	T	T	T
F	F	T	T	T

Since $\bar{p} + q$ coincides with $p \Rightarrow q$ hence $p \Rightarrow q = \bar{p} + q$.

Example 2: Prove the formula $\overline{p+q} = \bar{p}.\bar{q}$.

Solution:

p	q	$p+q$	$\overline{p+q}$	$\bar{p}$	$\bar{q}$	$\bar{p}.\bar{q}$
T	T	T	F	F	F	F
T	F	T	F	F	T	F
F	T	T	F	T	F	F
F	F	F	T	T	T	T

Since $\overline{p+q}$ concides with $\bar{p}.\bar{q}$ hence $\overline{p+q} = \bar{p}.\bar{q}$.

Example 3: Construct the truth table for (1) $p \Rightarrow p \wedge q$ (2) $p \Rightarrow p \vee q$ and prove that the latter is a tautology.

Solution:

p	q	$p \wedge q$	$p \Rightarrow (p \wedge q)$	$p \vee q$	$p \Rightarrow (p \vee q)$
T	T	T	T	T	T
T	F	F	F	T	T
F	T	F	T	T	T
F	F	F	T	F	T

We see that $p \Rightarrow (q \wedge q)$ is not a tautology but $p \Rightarrow (p \vee q)$ is a tautology.

Example 4: Determine the truth value of the composite statement – "If 5 + 3 = 8 then 6 + 6 = 10".

Solution: If p then q i.e. $p \Rightarrow q$. This is an implication of the statements p and q. Since p is true and q is false hence $p \Rightarrow q$ is false.

2.28 IDENTICALLY TRUE AND FALSE SENTENCES

Identically true sentences are always true irrespective of whether the sentences constituting them are true or false. Examples of identically true sentences are: $p + q, p \Leftrightarrow \bar{\bar{p}}, (p \Rightarrow q) \Leftrightarrow (\bar{q} = \bar{p})$.

Identically true sentences are denoted by the letter I. Identically false sentences are always false. Examples of false sentences are:

$p\,\bar{p}, (q\,p)\,\bar{p}, p\,L$. Identically false sentences are denoted by L.

Example 1: Three shots are fired at a target. "If the first shot hits the target, then the second also hits" is true, "If the third shot hits the target then the second also hits" is false. Determine which of the shots hits the target.

Solution: Let p, q and r be the propositions that the first, second and third shot hit the target respectively.

Since $p \Rightarrow q$ and $\overline{r \Rightarrow q}$ are true their product P is also true.

$\therefore P = (q \Rightarrow q)\left(\overline{r \Rightarrow q}\right)$

But from truth table $p \Rightarrow q = \bar{p} + q$

$\therefore P = (\bar{p} + q)\left(\overline{\bar{r} + q}\right)$

But $\overline{p + q} = \bar{p}\,\bar{q}$ and $\bar{\bar{p}} = p$

$\therefore P = (\bar{p} + q)\left(\bar{\bar{r}}\,\bar{q}\right) = (\bar{p} + q)\,r\,\bar{q}$

$\therefore P = \bar{p}\;r\;\bar{q} + r\,q\,\bar{q} = \bar{p}\;r\;\bar{q} + L$

i.e. $P = \bar{p}\;r\;\bar{q}$.

$\therefore$ Third shot hits the target.

2.29 (I) POLYNOMIALS AND BOOLEAN POLYNOMIALS

A polynomial is the sum of a finite number of monomials known as the terms of the polynomials and is formed as the finite sums (+), products (·) and differences (–) of the followings are the examples of polynomials in two variables:

$$f(x, y) = x \cdot x - x \cdot y - x \cdot y + y \cdot y = x^2 - 2xy + y^2.$$

$$g(x, y) = (x + y)\,(x \cdot x - x \cdot y + y \cdot y)$$

$$= (x + y)\,(x^2 - xy + y^2) = x^3 + y^3.$$

If we denote the variables by the statements p, q r .... and connect them by logical symbols $\wedge$, $\vee$, $\overline{}$, $\Rightarrow$, and $\Leftrightarrow$ then expressions formed are known as Boolean polynomials.

Some examples of Boolean polynomials are

$$f(p, q) = q \vee (\bar{p} \Rightarrow q) \text{ and } g(p, q) = (p \Leftrightarrow \bar{q}) \wedge q.$$

Example 1: The Boolean polynomial is given as $f(p, q) = \bar{p} \vee (p \Rightarrow q)$ and $p_0 \equiv 4 + 4 = 9$ and $q_0 \equiv 2 + 2 = 4$. What does $f(p_0\, q_0)$ read?

Solution: Since $f(p, q) = \overline{p} \vee (p \Rightarrow q)$

$\therefore f(p_0, q_0) = \overline{p}_0 \vee (p_0 \Rightarrow q_0)$

$\therefore f(p_0, q_0)$ = reads 4+4 ≠ 9 or if 4+4 = 9 then 2+2 = 4.

(II) EXCLUSIVE DISJUNCTION

The connective $\veebar$ is called the exclusive disjunction. We read $p \veebar q$ as—"*p* or *q* but not both" and obtain truth table for $p \veebar q$ as follows:

p	q	$p \veebar q$
T	T	F
T	F	T
F	T	T
F	F	F

(III) JOINT DENIAL

The propositional connectives ↓ is used to denote joint denial. By $p \downarrow q$ we mean "Neither *p* nor *q*" and therefore the truth table for $p \downarrow q$ is formed as follows:

p	q	$p \downarrow q$
T	T	F
T	F	F
F	T	F
F	F	T

(IV) A COMPREHENSIVE DESCRIPTION OF BOOLEAN ALGEBRA

Boolean algebra is the triplet $(B, +, \cdot)$, where B represents the set of elements a, b, c ..... and "+ (sum)" and "· (product)" represent two binary operations such that the following laws hold good.

(A) $a + b = b + a$ and $a \cdot b + b \cdot a$ i.e. commutative law for addition and multiplication holds true.

(B) $(a + b) + c = a + (b + c)$ and $(a \cdot b) \cdot c = a \cdot (b \cdot c)$ i.e. associative law for addition and multiplication holds true.

(C) $a + (b \cdot c) = (a + b) \cdot (a + c)$ and $a \cdot (b + c) = a \cdot b + a \cdot c$ i.e. distributive law holds true.

(D) $a + 0 = a$ and $a \cdot U = a$ i.e. an additive identify 0 and multiplicative identify U exist.

(E) $a + a' = U$ and $a \cdot a' = 0$ i.e. for $a \in B \exists a' \in B$ such that (E) holds good where a' is the compliment of a.

(F) $a + b$ and $a \cdot b$ exist and they belong to B i.e. closure law holds true.

Boolean algebra is also defined under the operation of the set i.e. union, intersection and compliment. The triplet $(\mathcal{A}, \cap, \cup)$ defines Boolean algebra where $\mathcal{A}$ is a family of sets closed under the operations of union, intersection and compliment. Here the universal set is the unit element and the empty set ϕ is the zero element. This algebra is also an algebra of elementary logical properties of statements (propositions).

Boolean algebra when defined on the set of proposition formed by the variables gives another triplet $(B, \wedge, \vee)$, where B is the set of propositions and the statements $p, q\ r$ .... are the variables which generate the former.

2.30 SWITCHING CIRCUIT DIAGRAM

A switching circuit diagram is that diagram which contains only "on, off" switches.

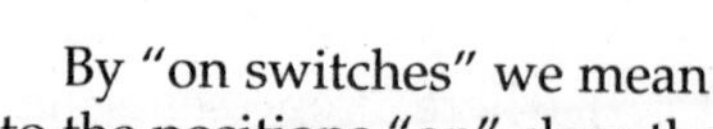

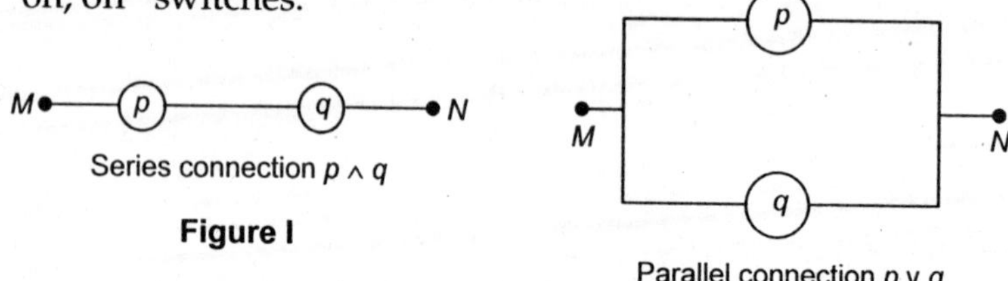

Series connection $p \wedge q$

Figure I

Parallel connection $p \vee q$

Figure II

By "on switches" we mean those switches which when put to the positions "on" close the circuit and the current flows in it. On the other hand, "off switches" are those switches which when put to the position "off" open or break the circuit and the current ceases to flow in it.

Two switches p and q can be connected by wires in series (Fig. I) or parallel (Fig. II) which correspond to conjunction or disjunction respectively of the statements p and q. Every switch is associated with a statement. Switches are denoted by the same letters or their statements. This is the relation established between the switching circuit and the algebra of propositions.

If two switches are such that one of them is cut in, while the other is cut out and vice versa then they correspond to the statement p and $\overline{p}$. When the switch is off the statement is considered to be false and when the switch is on the statement is considered to be true.

Some worked out examples:

Example 1: Replace the given diagram of (Fig. III) by a simple diagram and find out the condition under which the current flows in it.

Solution: The diagram given in Fig. III corresponds to the statements $(p \wedge q) \vee (p \wedge r)$.

But we have $p \wedge (q \vee r) = (p \wedge q) \vee (p \wedge r)$

$\therefore$ Hence the statement $(p \wedge q) \vee (p \wedge r)$ is equivalent to the statement $p \wedge (q \wedge r)$ and hence the diagram of Fig. III can be replaced by simple diagram given is Fig. IV.

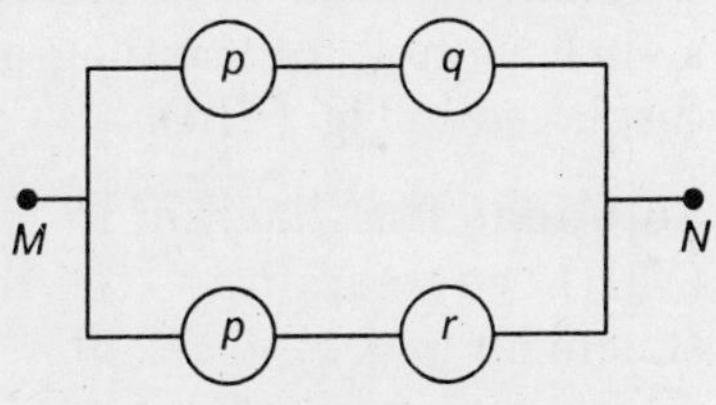

Figure III

Now $p \wedge (q \vee r)$ is true if at least one of $(p \wedge q)$ or $(p \vee q)$ is true.

$\therefore$ The current will flow if both the switches p and q are on.

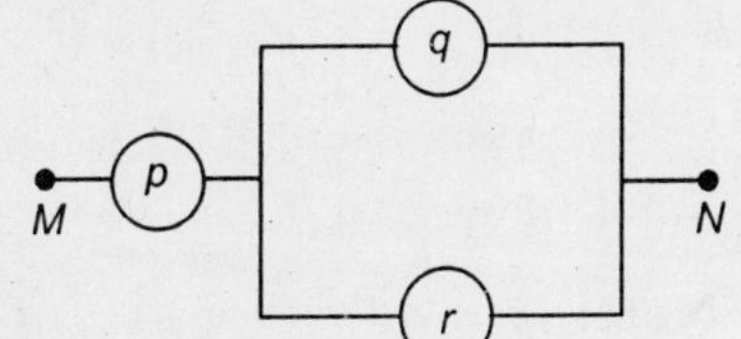

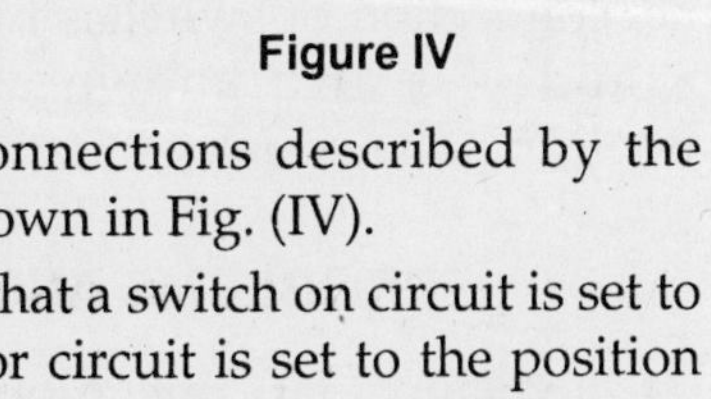

Figure IV

Note: Boolean switching circuit diagram which consists of repeated series and parallel connections described by the connectives $\wedge$ and $\vee$ has been shown in Fig. (IV).

If 1 and 0 denote respectively that a switch on circuit is set to the position "on" and a switch or circuit is set to the position "off", then we denote a series circuit $p \wedge q$ and a parallel circuit $p \vee q$ by the truth tables described below in Fig. (V) and Fig. (VI):

p	q	$p \wedge q$
1	1	1
1	0	0
0	1	0
0	0	0

Series circuit

Figure V

p	q	$p \vee q$
1	1	1
1	0	1
0	1	1
0	0	0

Parallel circuit

Figure VI

The relation between p and $\bar{p}$ is as follows given in Fig. (VII)

p	$\bar{p}$
1	0
0	1

Figure VII

Example 2: Substitute a simple diagram which consists of three switches only, for the diagram displayed in Fig. (VIII).

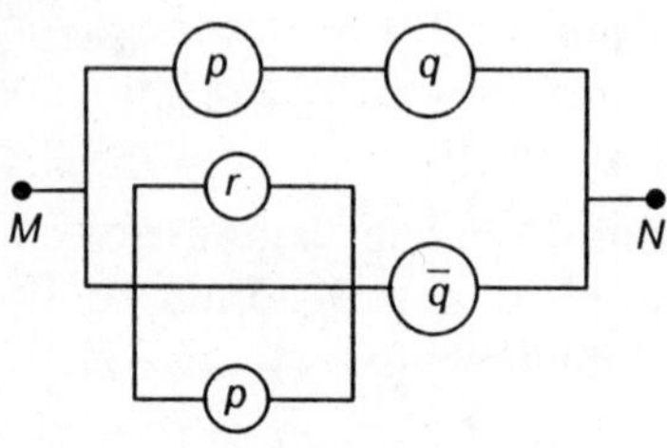

Figure VIII

Solution: The diagram in Fig. (VIII) corresponds to the statement $(p \wedge q) \vee (r \wedge p) \wedge \bar{q}$ which is equivalent to

$$(p \wedge q) \vee (r \wedge \bar{q}) \vee (p \wedge \bar{q})$$

$$= (p \wedge q) \vee (p \wedge \bar{q}) \vee (r \wedge \bar{q})$$

$$= p \wedge (q \wedge \bar{q}) \vee (r \vee \bar{q}) = p \vee (r \wedge \bar{q})$$

$\therefore q \vee \bar{q} = L$ which is shown in Fig. (IX).

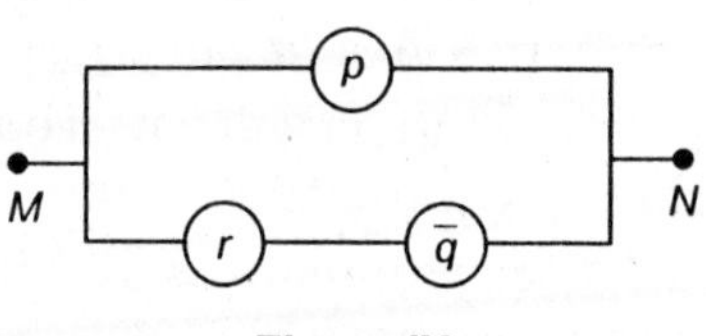

Figure IX

Note: $(p \wedge q) \vee (r \vee q) \wedge \bar{q}$ i.e. connection of switches by $\wedge$ and $\vee$ is also known as Boolean polynomial.

PROBLEMS AND EXERCISES 2 E (I)

1. Explain binary operations.
   (**Hint:** See the answer sheet.)
2. Which of the following sentences are statements: (i) x is greater than 5. (ii) Ram is rich and Mohan is poor. (iii) Four is greater than five. (iv) Hydrogen when combines with oxygen gives water. (v) The moon revolves round the sun.
3. We have two statements

   p: It is hot

   q: It is raining

What do the following statements consist in:

(i) $\overline{p}$ (ii) $p \vee q$ (iii) $p \wedge q$ (iv) $p \Rightarrow q$ (v) $p \Leftrightarrow \overline{q}$.

4. We have the following composite statements.

Determine the truth value of each.

(i) If 2 + 3 = 6 then 2 + 2 = 4

(ii) If is not true that 2 + 2 = 7 if and only if 3 + 3 = 8

(iii) Patna is in U.P. or Lucknow is in Bihar

(iv) It is not true 2 + 5 = 7 or 3 + 5 = 8

(v) It is false that if Patna is in U.P. then Lucknow is in Bihar.

5. Prove that the followings are tautologies.

(i) $p \vee \overline{p}$

(ii) $(p \wedge q) \Rightarrow (p \wedge q)$

(iii) $(p \vee q) \Leftrightarrow (q \vee p)$

(iv) $p \wedge q \Rightarrow q$

6. Prove the following algebric propositions by truth table.

(i) $p + q = q + p$

(ii) $p\,q = q\,p$

(iii) $p \vee (q \vee r) = (p \vee q) \vee r$

(iv) $p \wedge (q \wedge r) = (p \wedge q) \wedge r$

(v) $p\,(q + r) = pq + qr.$

(vi) $(p + q)\,(p + r) = p + qr$

(vii) $\overline{p+q} = \overline{p}.\overline{q}$

(viii) $\overline{p.q} = \overline{p} + \overline{q}$

(ix) $\overline{\overline{p}} = p$

(x) $p \veebar q = (p \vee q) \wedge \left(\overline{p \wedge q}\right)$

(xi) $p + p = p$

(xii) $pp = p$

(xiii) $p + \overline{p} = I$

(xiv) $p \veebar p = (p \downarrow q)\,(p \downarrow q)$

(xv) $p\,\overline{p} = L$

(xvi) $p + I = I$

(xvii) $p\,I = p$

(xviii) $p + L = p$

(xix) $pL = L$

(xx) $p \wedge \bar{p}$ is a contradiction.

7. Write down the Boolean polynomial for the following switching circuit diagrams.

(i)

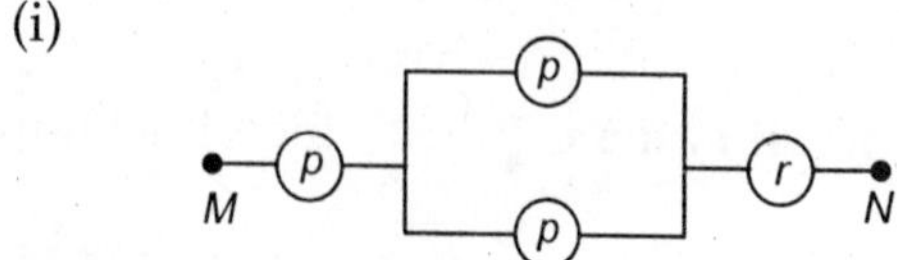

(ii)

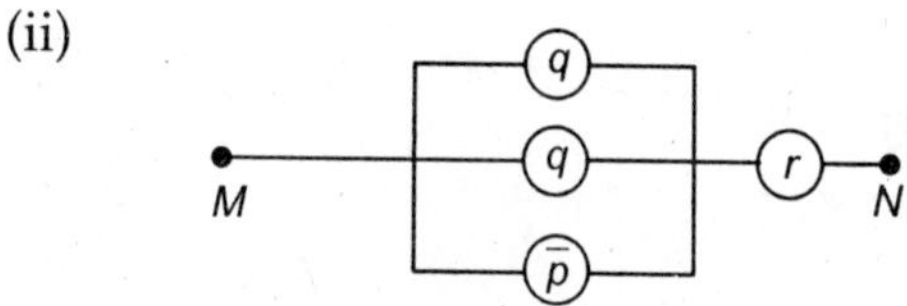

8. Construct the switching circuit diagram for the following Boolean polynomials.

(i) $(p \wedge q) \vee (r \wedge \bar{q})$ (ii) $(p \wedge q) \vee r \vee (\bar{p} \wedge \bar{q})$

9. Simplify the Boolean polynomial

$(p \wedge q) \vee (p \wedge \bar{q}) \vee (\bar{p} \wedge \bar{q})$

10. Ram, Shyam and Mohan are charged in a bank robbery. The robbers escaped in a car that was waiting for them. At the inquest Ram stated that robbers escaped in a blue Maruti, Shyam stated that it had been black Chevrolet and Mohan said that it hed been Ambassador and by no means blue. In order to make the court confused each of them only indicated correctly either the make of the car or only its colour. What clour was the car and of what make?

11. (i) For any two sets A and B prove that $(A \cup B) \cap B' = A$ if and only if $A \cap B = \phi$

(ii) Prove that $A \cap (B - C) = (A \cap B) - (A \cap C)$

(iii) Prove that $A \cap (B \cap C) = (A \cap B) \cap (A \cap C)$ (Please see the answer sheets.)

ANSWERS TO PROBLEMS AND EXERCISES 2 E (i)

1. **Hint:** A binary operation. "o" on a set A is a mapping of the Cartesian product $A \times A$ into A.

   Let A be any set and "o" be an operation, $a \ o \ b \in A \ \forall \ a$, $b \in A$ i.e. $o : A \times A \to A$ be a mapping then 'o' be a binary operation on A.

   A binary operation obeys the following laws

   (i) Cumulative law
   i.e. $a \ o \ b = b \ o \ a \ \forall \ a, b \in A$.

   (ii) Associative law
   i.e. $(a \ o \ b) \ o \ c = a \ o \ (b \ o \ c) \ \forall \ a, b, c \in A$.

   (iii) Identity element
   i.e. $e \ o \ a = a = a \ o \ e \ \forall \ a \in A$ where $e \in A$ is called an indentity element.

   (iv) Inverse element
   i.e. $a \ o \ b = e = b \ o \ a \ \forall \ a, b, \in A$ where b is the inverse of a and a is the inverse of b.

2. **Ans.** (ii) (iii) (iv) (v)

3. (i) It is not hot
   (ii) It is hot or it is raining
   (iii) It is hot and it is raining
   (iv) If it is hot then it is raining
   (v) It is hot if and only if it is not raining.

4. (i) p is false and q is true hence $p \Rightarrow q$ is true.
   (ii) Each of p and q one false and hence $p \Leftrightarrow q$ is true. The statement is the negation of $p \Leftrightarrow q$ and hence it is false. (Here p: $2 + 2 = 7$; q: $3 + 3 = 8$)
   (iii) Each of p and q are false hence $p \vee q$ is false.
   (iv) The given statement is the negation of the true statements $p \vee q$ hence it is false.
   (v) The given statement is the negation of the true statement $p \Rightarrow q$ and hence it is false.

7. (i) $p \wedge (p \vee q) \wedge r$ (ii) $(p \vee q \vee \bar{p}) \wedge r$

8. (i)

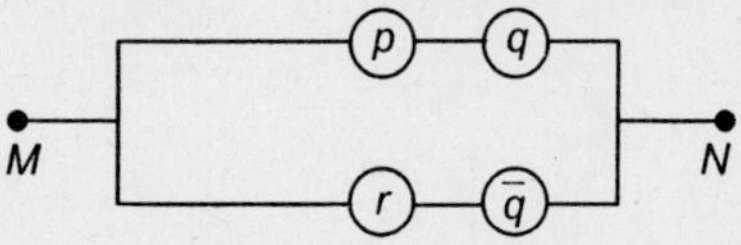

M N
p q
r $\bar{q}$

(ii)

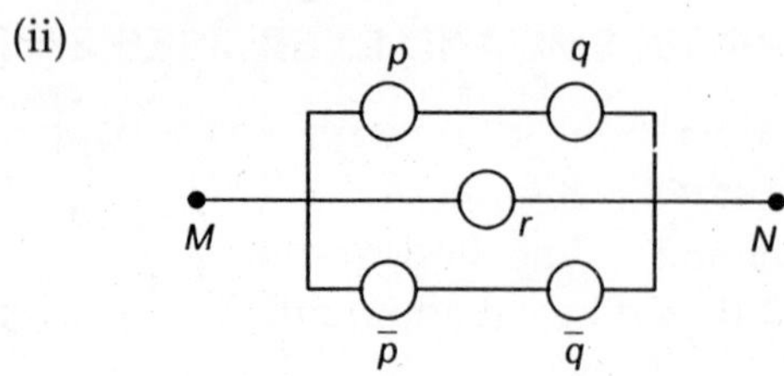

9. **Ans.** $p \vee \bar{q}$.
10. **Ans.** The robbers escaped in a black maruti car.
11. (i) **Hint:** We know $(B \cup C) \cap A = (B \cap A) \cup (C \cap A)$
Substitute B', A and B for A, B and C we get
$(A \cup B) \cap B' = (A \cap B') \cup (B \cap B') = (A \cap B') \cup = \phi\ A \cap B'$
Now we have to prove $A \cap B' = A \Leftrightarrow A \cap B = \phi$
For this assume $A \cap B' = A \Rightarrow A\ C\ B' \Rightarrow A$ and B are disjoint sets $\Rightarrow A \cap B = \phi$.
Again suppose $A \cap B = \phi \Rightarrow A\ C\ B'$ $\therefore$ A and B are disjoints
$\Rightarrow A \cap B' = A$
$\therefore$ For $A \cup \phi = A$ we get
$(A \cup B) \cap B' = A$
(ii) Let $x \in A \cap (B - C) \Rightarrow x \in A$ and $x \in B - C$
$\Rightarrow x \in A$ and $x \in B$ but $x \notin C$
$\Rightarrow (x \in A$ and $x \in B)$ but $(A \in A, x \notin C)$
$\Rightarrow x \in A \cap B$ but $x \notin A \cap C$
$\Rightarrow x \in (A \cap B) - (A \cap C)$ ...(1)
Again if $x \in (A \cap B) - (A \cap C) \Rightarrow x \in (A \cap B)$ but $x \notin A \cap C$
$\Rightarrow x \in (A \cap B)$ but $x \notin$ to A and C both
$\Rightarrow x \in A \cap B$ but $(x \in A, x \notin C)$
$\Rightarrow (x \in A$ and $x \in B)$ but $(x \in A, x \notin C)$
$\Rightarrow x \in A$ and $(x \in B$ but $x \notin C)$
$\Rightarrow x \in A \cap (B - C)$ ...(2)
For (1) and (2) the result follows.
(iii) $x \in A \cap (B \cap C) \Rightarrow x \in A$ and $x \in (B \cap C)$
$\Rightarrow (x \in A$ and $x \in B)$ and $(x \in A$ and $x \in C)$
$\Rightarrow x \in (A \cap B)$ and $x \in (A \cap C)$
$\Rightarrow x \in (A \cap B) \cap (A \cap C)$

$\therefore A \cap (B \cap C) \in (A \cap B) \cap (A \cap C)$ ...(1)

Assuming $y \in (A \cap) \cap (A \cap C)$ we can prove

$y \in A \cap (B \cap C)$ ...(2)

For (1) and (2) the result follows.

CHAPTER

Number System

3.1 INTRODUCTION

The great mathematician Guass (1777– 1855) had rightly said – "Mathematics is the queen of science and arithmetic is the queen of mathematics". The arithmetic is the mathematics of digits. As a matter of fact arithmetic is based on digits. Algebra, analysis and other branches of mathematics are also based on the properties of numbers. Numbers like one, two, three, four ... are represented by International symbols 1, 2, 3, 4 ...

From primitive time numbers have been used in a natural way for counting objects and for the solutions of practical problems hence they are known as natural numbers. They came into being from primitive time.

Definition: Natural numbers also known as positive integers or whole numbers is the set of numbers 1, 2, 3, ... which are used for counting objects and is denoted as $N = \{1, 2, 3 ...\}$. Every element of N is a natural number. The set N is an infinite set and hence the number of natural numbers is infinite. The set $N = \{1, 2, 3 ...\}$ is known as a natural scale.

Arranging the natural numbers in the increasing order we obtain unity as the first member, two as second member and three as the third member and so on of the set N. "$m > n$; $m < n$; and $m = n \ \forall \ m, n \in N$" reveals the fact respectively that "m is greater than n, m is less than n, and m and n are the same natural numbers".

If $p = m + n$ then m and n are called summands and p is the sum of the natural numbers m and n. If $q = m \ n$ the m is a multiplicand, n is a multiplier, q is a product; m and n are also called factors $\forall \ m, n \ q \in N$.

3.2 PROPERTIES OF NATURAL NUMBERS

(1) **Successor or consequent:** For every natural number there exists one natural number n^+ called the successor of n i.e. $n^+ = n + 1$.

The smallest of the natural numbers i.e. one is not a successor of any natural number i.e. $n^+ \neq 1$. The greatest on the last number does not exist in the natural numbers. The mapping $S: N \to N$ where $S(n) = n^+ \ \forall \ n \in N$ and $S(N) = \{2, 3, 4, 5...\}$, $1 \neq S(N)$ is known as successor mapping which is one-one into.

(2) **The operations addition and multiplication on natural numbers obey the following laws:**

(i) *Closure law:* If p, q be natural numbers then $p + q \in N \ \forall \ p, q \in N$ and $p \ q \in N \ \forall \ p, q \in N$. These laws are known as closure laws of addition and multiplication respectively.

Note: Addition on N is defined by

(A) $p + 1 = p^+ \ \forall \ p \in N$

(B) $p + q^+ = (p + q)^+$ where p and q are natural numbers.

(ii) *Cumulative law:* If p and q are natural numbers, then $p + q = q + p$ and $p \times q = q \times p$.

Note: Multiplication on N is defined by

(A) $p \cdot 1 = 1 \cdot p = p \ \forall \ p \in N$

Here 1 is called the natural element for multiplication.

(B) $p \cdot q^+ = p \ q + p$ where p and $q \in N$.

(iii) *Associative law:* If p, q, r be three natural numbers, then $(p + q) + r = p + (q + r)$ and $(p \times q) \times r = q \times (q \times r) \ \forall \ p, q, r \in N$.

Multiplicative identity: For each natural number there is a natural number 1 known as multiplicative identity such that

$$p \cdot 1 = 1 \cdot p = p.$$

(v) *Cancellation law:* $\forall\ p, q, r \in N$

If $p + q = r + q$ then $p = r$

and if $p \times q = r \times q$ then $p = r$

These laws are respectively known as cancellation law for addition and multiplication.

(vi) *Distributive law:* $\forall\ p\ , q\ r \in N$ we have

$$p \times (q + r) = p \times q + p \times r.$$

(vii) Natural numbers are not closed for the operations "difference" and "division".

(viii) *Even, odd, prime and composite natural numbers:* A prime number is that natural number which only two divisors unity and the number itself.

Thus the set of prime numbers of first ten natural number is {2, 3, 5, 7}.

The numbers 2, 4, 6 ... are divisible by 2 and hence they are even natural numbers.

The numbers 1, 3, 5, 7 ... are not divisible by 2 and hence they are odd natural numbers. Natural numbers greater than unity and having atleast one division different from unity and itself are composite numbers.

(ix) If m is taken K times to be multiplied then $m^K = m, m, m, \ldots$ upto K factors.

∴ We have the following properties for the natural number m, n, K

(A) $m^{K+n} = m^K\ m^n$

(B) $m^{Kn} = (m^K)^n$

(C) $(m\ n)^K = m^K\ n^K$

If $n - m = t$, where $n > m$ and $m, n\ t \in N$, then t is the difference of n and m.

n is the minuend and m is the subtraherd.

3.3 PEANO'S AXIOMS

Guiseppe Peano (1858–1932) gave the following statements in 1899. According to him N is an abstract set and elements belonging to it are known as natural numbers. The axiom is a statement which need no proof. It is generally accepted as true.

Peano's Postulates or Axioms:

Postulate 1 or P_1: $1 \in N$, where N is the set of natural numbers i.e. 1 is a natural number and N is non-empty.

Postulate 2 or P_2: For each $n \in N$ there is unique n^+ which is the successor of n i.e $\forall\ n \in N\ \exists$ unique $n^+ \in N$.

Postulate 3 or P_3: $\forall\ n \in N\ n^+ \neq 1$ i.e. 1 is not the successor of any natural number.

Postulate 4 or P_4: $m^+ = n^+ \Rightarrow m = n, m, n \in N$ i.e. if the successors of two natural numbers are equal, then those natural numbers are equal.

Postulate 5 or P_5: If $M \subseteq N$ such that (i) $1 \in N$ (ii) $\forall\ m \in M \Rightarrow m^+ \in m$ then $M = N$.

Note: Postulate 5 is called the postrate of induction. Principle of mathematical induction is based on P_5.

3.4 DIRECT CONSEQUENCES OF PEANO'S POSTULATES

Theorem 1: For any two natural numbers $m, n \in N$ we have

(i) $m = n \Rightarrow m^+ = n^+$

(ii) $m \neq n \Rightarrow m^+ \neq n^+$.

Proof: (i) $m \in N \Rightarrow m^+ \in N$

$n \in N \Rightarrow n^+ \in N$

$\therefore\ m = n \Rightarrow m^+ = n^+$

(ii) If possible assume

$m \neq n \Rightarrow m^+ = n^+$

$\therefore\ m \neq n \Rightarrow m^+ = n^+ \Rightarrow m = n$

which is not possible hence $m \neq n \Rightarrow m^+ = n^+$ is not true

$\therefore\ m \neq n \Rightarrow m^+ \neq n^+$

Theorem 2: "1 is the only natural number which is "non-successor" or "Every natural number except 1 is the successor of some natural number".

Proof: Let $S: N \rightarrow A$ be a successor mapping. The domain of S is N and the range of S is A. Clearly the elements of A are the successors of all the natural numbers $\in N$.

But according to P_3 one is not the successor of any natural number $\therefore 1 \in A$.

Now we substitute $A \cup \{1\}$ for the set B

i.e. $B = A \cup \{1\}$ then $1 \in B$

Let m be any arbitrary element belonging to B then $m \in A$

$\therefore \quad B = A \cup \{1\}$

$\therefore \quad m \in B \Rightarrow m \in A$

$\Rightarrow m$ is the successor of some natural number.

Assume now $m = n^+$

$\therefore \quad n^+ \in B$ since $m \in B$

$\Rightarrow (n^+)^+ = m^+ \in B$ ($\therefore$ The successor of every natural number is in the set B)

$\therefore \quad m \in B \Rightarrow m^+ \in B$

$\therefore \quad B = N \Rightarrow B = (N - \{1\}) \cup \{1\}$ ...(1)

But $B = A \cup \{1\}$ ...(2)

$\therefore$ from (1) and (2) $A = N - \{1\}$

$\therefore$ Every number except 1 is in A.

Thus every natural number except 1 is the successor of some natural number.

Theorem 3 (i) *First Principle of Mathematical Induction:*

A statement $P(n)$ is true for all $n \in N$, where N is the set of natural number if

(i) $P(1)$ is true and (ii) $P(r)$ is true $\Rightarrow P(r^+)$ is true.

Proof: We first verity the truth of the statement for $n = 1$, then we assume that the statement is true for $n = r$ and in the last we prove the statement for $n = r + 1$ on the assumption that the statement is true for $n = r$.

Let A be the set of those natural numbers r for which $P(r)$ is true.

$\therefore P(1)$ is true, as $1 \in A$

Also $A \in N \Rightarrow P(r)$ is true by definition

$\Rightarrow P(r^+)$ is true by hypothesis

$\Rightarrow r^+$ i.e. $r + 1 \in A$

$\therefore A = N$ i.e. $P(n)$ is true for all $n \in N$.

Note: Induction method gives the proof of specified assertions. It does not serve as a derivation of such assertions. For example we can not obtain the formula for general term of an A.P. by induction method. If we have found the formula by trial and error or by any other method, then the proof of this formula can be carried out by the method of induction.

(ii) If a natural number m is a divisor of natural numbers p and q then it is also a divisor of $p + q$.

Proof: Since m is a divisor of p $\therefore$ $p_1 = K_1\, m$, similarly $K_2\, m = q$

$\therefore p + q = m\,(K_1 + K_2) \Rightarrow p + q$ is divisible by m.

(iii) If a natural number m is a divisor of natural number p and q then it is also a divisor of $p - q$ if $p > q$.

Proof: The proof follows in a similar fashion as given in (ii).

(iv) *Extended series of natural numbers:* When zero is included in the set of natural numbers then the series formed by them is known as the extended series of natural numbers.

Theorem 4 (i) No natural number is equal to its successor i.e. $n \neq n^+, n \in N$.

Proof: Assume $P(n)$: $n \neq n^+$

(i) For $n = 1$ $P(1)$: $1 \neq 1^+$

$\therefore$ $P(1)$ is true.

(ii) For $n = r$. Assume $P(r)$: $r \neq r^+$ is true.

then $r \neq r^+ \Rightarrow r^+ \neq (r^+)^+$

$\therefore$ $P(r^+)$: $r^+ \neq (r^+)^+$ is also true.

Thus the statement $P(n)$: $n \neq n^+$ is true for all natural numbers.

(ii) Decimal number of system: We introduce ten symbols 1, 2, 3, 4, 5, 6, 7, 8, 9 in this system known as digits. Symbol 0 denotes zero.

The number 10 is written as 10. A natural number p is denoted as

$$p = a_n\, 10^n + a_{n-1}\, 10^{n-1} + \ldots + a_1\, 10^1 + a_0 \qquad (1)$$

where n is a number from the extended series of natural number, a_n is one of the numbers

1, 2, 3, ... 8, 9 and each $a_0, a_1, a_2, \ldots a_{n-1}$ is one of the numbers 0, 1, 2, ... 7, 8, 9.

If the number exceeds 9 then it is written in the from given by (1).

The notation of natural number also depends on the principle of the place values of digits, for example we write 4503 as 4503 = $4.10^3 + 5.10^2 + 0.10 + 3$ on this principle.

$p = \overline{a_n\, a_{n-1}\, a_{n-2} \dots a_2\, a_1\, a_0}$

The bar given above means that the digits are not the product of the numbers $a_n, a_{n-1}, \dots a_1\, a_0$.

Thus $p = \overline{a_n\, a_{n-1}\, a_{n-2} \dots a_2\, a_1\, a_0}$

$= a_n\, 10^n + a_{n-1}\, 10^{n-1} + \dots + a_1\, 10^1 + a_0$ (2)

(iii) *Criteria for divisibility*: We always remember that zero can be divided by any natural number and any natural number can be divided by unity before we start to study the criteria for divisibility. In this context we have the following theorems with explanations and proofs.

(1) Prove that the necessary and sufficient condition that the natural number $p = \overline{a_n\, a_{n-1} \dots a_2\, a_1\, a_0}$ is divisible by 2 is its last digit a_0 is divisible by 2.

Proof: *The condition is sufficient:* Let a_0 be divisible by 2. Now we put

$p = \lambda + \mu$ (3)

where $\lambda = (a_n\, 10^{n-1} + a_{n-1}\, 10^{n-2} + \dots + a_1)\, 10$

and $h = a_0$

We see that each term of (3) in R.H.S. is divisible by 2 and hence the entire sum p is divisible by 2.

The condition is necessary: Now we have to prove if p is divisible by 2 then a_0 is also divisible by 2.

We have from (3)

$a_0 = p - [a_n\, 10^{n-1} + a_{n-1}\, 10^{n-2} + \dots + a_1].10$

each term of the subtrahend is divisible by, 2.

The minuend p is divisible by 2 by hypothesis.

Thus the difference a_0 is also divisible by 2.

(2) The necessary and sufficient condition for the natural number $p = \overline{a_n\, a_{n-1} \dots a_2\, a_1\, a_0}$ to be divisible by 4 is that the number $\overline{a_1\, a_0}$ be divisible by 4.

Proof: *The condition is sufficient:*

Assume $p = \lambda + \mu$ (4)

If $\overline{a_1\, a_0}$ be divisible by 4, then we have to prove p is also divisible by 4.

In the equation (4)

$\lambda = 10^2\,[a_n\, 10^{n-2} + a_{n-1}\, 10^{n-3} + ... + a_2]$

and $\mu = \overline{a_1\, a_0}$

Each term of (4) is divisible by 4 $\therefore$ p is divisible by 4.

The condition is necessary: Now we shall prove that if p is divisible by 4 then $\overline{a_1\, a_0}$ is divisible by 4. We write

$\overline{a_1\, a_0} = p - 10^2\,[a_n\, 10^{n-2} + a_{n-1}\, 10^{n-3} + ... + a_2]$

Each term of the difference is divisible by 4 hence $\overline{a_1\, a_0}$ is divisible by 4.

(3) The necessary and sufficient condition for the natural number $p = \overline{a_n\, a_{n-1} \cdots a_2\, a_1\, a_0}$ to be divisible by 9 is that the sum of all the digits of the natural number p is divisible by 9.

Proof: *The condition is sufficient:* Let the sum of the digits of p be divisible by 9. We have $p = a_n\, 10^n + a_n\, 10^{n-1} + ... + a_1\, 10 + a_0$.

We can express

$10^m = \overline{\underbrace{999...99}_{m \text{ times}}}$

Assume $p = \lambda + \mu$ (v)

where $\lambda = a_n \overline{\underbrace{999...99}_{n \text{ times}}} + a_{n-1} \overline{\underbrace{999...99}_{(n-1) \text{ times}}}$

$+ ...\, a_2\, \overline{99} + a_1\, 9$

and $\mu = a_n + a_{n-1} + ... + a_0$

Each term on the R.H.S. of (5) is divisible by 9 since the sum of the digits $\mu = a_n + a_{n-1} + ... + a_n$ is divisible by 9 by hypothesis and λ is obviously divisible by 9 and hence p is divisible by 9.

The condition is necessary: Let p be divisible by 9 then

$a_n + a_{n-1} + ... + a_1 + a_0$

$$= p - \left[a_n \underbrace{\overline{99...999}}_{n \text{ times}} + a_{n-1} \underbrace{\overline{99...999}}_{n-1 \text{ times}} + ... a_2 \underbrace{\overline{99}}_{2 \text{ times}} + a_1 9 \right]$$

R.H.S. is divisible by 9

$\therefore a_n + a_{n-1} + ... + a_1$ two is divisible by 9.

We can also prove the theorem for any natural number $p = \overline{a_n\, a_{n-1} ... a_2\, a_1\, a_0}$ to be even it is necessary and sufficient that the digits a_0 of p be an even number.

3.5 STRUCTURE OF NATURAL NUMBERS

We have (i) $1 \in N$ (ii) $1 \in N \Rightarrow 1^+ \in N$ (iii) $1^+ \in N \Rightarrow (1^+)^+ \in N$ and so on. Thus $N = \{1, 1^+, (1^+)^+, ...\}$

i.e. N = {1, 2, 3, 4 ...}. We now state some laws with proofs.

(A) *Closure law:* If m, n be the natural numbers, then $m + n \in N \; \forall \; m, n \in N$.

Assume $P(n)$: $m + n \in N$, where m is any natural number $n \in N$ and $P(n)$ is a statement (i) for $n = 1$, $P(1) = m + 1 \in N$ is true since $m + 1 = m + \in M$ and $m \in N \Rightarrow m^+ \in N$

(ii) For $n = r$ assume

$P(r)$: $m + r \in N$ is true, then

$m + r \in N \Rightarrow (m + r)^+ \in N$

$\Rightarrow \quad m + r^+ \in N \; [\therefore (m + r)^+ = m + r^+]$

$\Rightarrow \quad m + (r + 1) \in N$

$\Rightarrow \quad P(r + 1)$ is true.

Hence in accordance with the first principle of mathematical induction closure law is true for every natural number.

Thus $m, n \in N \Rightarrow m + n \in N$.

(B) *Associative law of addition:* For each triple of natural numbers l, m, n we have

$$(l + m) + n = l + (m + n)$$

Proof: Let l and m be the definite natural numbers and $P(n)$: $(l + m) + n = l + (m + n)$ is a statement.

(i) For $n = 1$ we have

$P(1): (l + m) + 1 = (l + m)^+ = l + m^+ = l + (m + 1)$

$\therefore$ $P(1): (l + m) + 1 = l + (m + 1)$ is true for $n = 1$.

(ii) Assume now that $P(r): (l + m) + r = l + (m + r)$ is true for $n = r$

$$(l + m) + r = l + (m + r)$$

$\Rightarrow$ $[(l + m) + r]^+ = [l + (m + r)]^+$

$\Rightarrow$ $(l + m) + r^+ = l + (m + r)^+$

$\Rightarrow$ $(l + m) + r^+ = l + (m + r^+)$

$\Rightarrow$ $P(r^+)$ is true

$\therefore$ $P(n): (l + m) + n = l + (m + n)$ is true.

(C) *Commutative law of addition:* For every pair of natural numbers m, n we have

$m + n = n + m$

Proof: Let $A = \{m: m + 1 = 1 + m \ \forall\ m \in N\}$

$\therefore$ $1 \in A$ as $1 + 1 = 1 + 1$

If $m \in A$ then $m^{+1} + 1 = (m + 1) + 1$

$\Rightarrow$ $m^+ + 1 = (m + 1)^+ = (1 + m)^+$ as $m \in A$.

$\Rightarrow$ $m^+ + 1 = 1 + m^+ \ \therefore\ m \in A \Rightarrow m + \in A$

$\therefore$ $A = N$ (By axiom of induction)

$\therefore$ $m + 1 = 1 + m \ \forall\ m \in N$

Again assume $B = \{n: m + n = n + m \ \forall\ m \in N\}$

Since $m + 1 = 1 + m \ \forall\ m \in N \ \therefore\ 1 \in B$

If $n \in B$ then $m + n^+ = m + (n + 1) = m + (1 + n)$

$= (m + 1) + n = n + (m + 1) = n + (1 + m)$

$= (n + 1) + m = n^+ + m \ \therefore\ n \in B$

$\Rightarrow$ $n^+ \in B \ \therefore\ B = N$

Hence $m + n = n + m \ \forall\ m, n \in N$.

(D) *Cancellation law of addition:* If l, m, n be natural numbers such that $l + n = m + n$ then $l = m$.

Proof: We assume A to be the set of all $n \in N$ such that $l + n = m + n \Rightarrow l = m \ \forall\ l, m \in N$, then

$l + 1 = m + 1 \ \forall\ l, m \in N \Rightarrow l^+ = m^+ \Rightarrow l = m \ \therefore\ 1 \in A$.

Again if $n \in A$, then $l + n^+ = m + n^+$

$\Rightarrow$ $(l + n)^+ = (m + n)^+ \Rightarrow l + n = m + n$

$\therefore$ $l + n = m + n \Rightarrow l = m$ as $n \in A$

$\therefore$ $n \in A \Rightarrow n^+ \in A$

$\therefore$ By the axiom of induction $A = N$

Thus $l + n = m + n \Rightarrow l = m \ \forall \ l, m, n \in N$

This is known as right cancellation law of addition.

We can prove in a similar way

$$n + l = n + m \Rightarrow l = m \ \forall \ l, m, n, \in N$$

Which we know as the left cancellation law of addition.

(E) *Non-existence of identity for addition in N.*

There does not exist any identity element for addition in the set of natural number N.

i.e. $m + n \neq m \ \forall \ m, n \in N$.

Let $n \in N$ and $A = \{p \in N: p + n \neq p \ \forall \ n \in N\}$

Now $1 + n = n + 1 = n^+ \neq 1$ (from Peano's axioms – 3)

$\therefore$ From $A = \{p \in N : p + n \neq p \ \forall \ n \in N\}$

We have $1 \in A$

If $p \in A$, then $p + n \neq p \ \forall \ n \in N$

Also from cumulative law

$$p^+ + n = n + p^+ = (n + p)^+$$

or $\quad p^+ + n = (p + n)^+$

Again $\quad p + n \neq p \Rightarrow (p + n)^+ \neq p^+$

$\Rightarrow \quad p^+ + n \neq p^+$

$\therefore \quad p \in A \Rightarrow p^+ \in A$

Hence $A = N$ by mathematical induction,

$\therefore \quad m + n \neq m \ \forall \ m, n \in N$.

(F) We now state few theorems without proof. They are as follows:

(i) If l, m, n are three natural numbers then

$$n \neq m \Rightarrow l + n \neq l + m$$

(ii) If l, m be any two natural numbers, then only one of the following possibilities holds:

(i) $l = m$ (ii) $l = m + x$, where $x \in N$ (iii) $m = l + y$, where $y \in N$.

(G) *Subtraction in the set of natural numbers:*

If $m, n \in N$ and $\exists \ p \in N$ such that

$m = n + p$ then p is obtained by subtracting n from m

i.e. $\quad p = m - n$

$\therefore \ m = n + p \Rightarrow p = m - n$ and p exists in the set of natural numbers iff $m > n$ and hence subtraction is not defined always.

3.6 MULTIPLICATION ON THE SET OF NATURAL NUMBERS AND LAWS RELATED TO IT

Multiplication on the set of natural numbers is defined by

(i) $l.\ 1 = 1.\ l = l$ for all l belonging to N, where 1 is the natural element for multiplication.

(ii) $l.\ m^+ = l.\ m + l$, where l and m are natural numbers. Following laws in the set of natural number hold good.

(A) *Closure law*: $l.\ m \in N\ \forall\ l, m \in N$

Proof: For any definite natural number assume that the statement $P(m)$: $l.\ m \in N\ \forall\ m \in N$.

(i) For $m = 1$, $P(1)$: $l\ .\ 1 \in N$ is true,

since $l\ .\ 1 = l \in N$

(ii) For $m = r$, assume $P(r) : l\ .\ r \in N$ is true,

then $P(r): l\ .\ r \in N \Rightarrow l\ .\ r + l$ also belongs to N according to the closure law of addition on N.

$\Rightarrow \qquad l\, r^+ \in N \quad \Rightarrow P(r^+)$ is true

Thus $l\, n \in N\ \forall\ l, m \in N$.

(B) *Multiplicative identity:* $\forall\ m \in N, P(m): m\ .\ 1 = 1\ .\ m = m.$

Proof: (i) for $m = 1$

$P(1) = 1\ .\ 1 = 1\ .\ 1 = 1$ which is true.

(ii) Now for $m = r$ assume

$P(r) = r\ .\ 1 = 1\ .\ r = r$ is true.

Hence $P(r^+)$: $r^+ .\ 1 = r^+ = r + 1 = r\ .\ 1 + 1 = 1\ .\ r + 1 = 1\ .\ r^+$.

$\therefore\ P(r^+)$ is true.

Hence $P(n) = m\ .\ 1 = 1\ .\ m = m$ is true for all m.

(C) *L. Distributive law:* For $l, m, n \in N$ we have

$P(n): l\ .\ (m + n) = l\ .\ m + l\ .\ n.$

Proof: (i) Let $n = 1 \therefore P(1): l\,(m + 1) = l\, m^+$

$= l\ .\ m + l = l\ .\ m + l\ .\ 1 \therefore P\ (1)$ is true.

(ii) Now for $n = r$. Suppose

$P(r): l\,(m + r) = lm + lr$ is true, then

$$P(r^+) = l\,(m + r^+) = l\ .\ (m + r)^+$$
$$= l(m + r) + l = lm + lr + l\ .\ (\therefore P(r) \text{ is true})$$
$$= l\ .\ m + (lr + l) = l.\ m + lr^+$$

$\therefore P(r^+)$ is true.

$\therefore P(n): l\,(m + n) = lm + ln$ for all $n \in N$.

(D) *R. Distributive law:* Let the statement

$P_1(n): (l + m) . n = l . n + m . n \; \forall \; n \in N$.

Proof: (i) For $n = 1$, then

$P_1(1): (l + m) . = l . 1 + m. 1$ which is true.

(ii) Now for $n = r$ let.

$P_1(r) = (l + m) . r = l . r + m . r$ is true

Now $\quad P_1(r^+) = (l + m)\, r^+ = (l + m)\, r + l + m$

$= l . r + mr + l + m = (\therefore P(r)$ hold true)

$= l . r + l + mr + m = lr^+ + mr^+ \;\therefore P_1(r^+)$ is true.

$\therefore P_1(n): (l + m) . n = l . n + m . n$ for all $n \in N$.

(E) *Associative law:* We have to prove

$P(n): (l . m). n = l . (m . n) \; \forall \; n \in N$.

Proof: (i) For $n = 1$

$P(1) = (l . m) . 1 = l . m = l . (m . 1) \;\therefore P(1)$ is true.

(ii) Now for $n = r$ let

$P(r) = (l . m). r = l . (m . r)$ true

$\therefore \quad P(r^+) = (l . m). r^+ = (l . m)\, r + (l . m)$

$= l . (m . r) + l . m \; (\therefore P(r)$ is true)

$= l\,(mr + n)$

$= l\,(m . r^+) \qquad \therefore P(r^+)$ hold good.

$\therefore \quad P(n): (l . m) . n = l . (m . n) \; \forall \; n \in M$.

(F) *Commulative law:* We have to prove that $P(n): m . n = n . m$ $\forall \; n \in N$.

Proof: (i) For $n = 1$ we have

$P(1) = m . 1 = 1 . m = m$ (multiplicative identity) hence $P(1)$ is true.

(ii) Now for $n = r$ assume $P(r): mr = r . n$ is ture.

$\therefore \quad P(r^+) = mr^+ = mr + m = rm + m \; (\therefore P(r)$ is true)

$= r . m + m . 1 = (r + 1) . m$ [*R* distributive law]

$= r + m \qquad \therefore P(r^+)$ is true.

Thus the statement $P(n): m. n = n . m$ for all n holds true.

(G) *Cancellation law:* We have to prove that for definite natural number l, m the statement $P(n): l . n = m . n \Rightarrow l = m \; \forall \; n \in N$.

Proof: (i) For $n = 1$

$P(1)$: $l.\,1 = m.\,1 \Rightarrow l = m$. Thus $P(1)$ is ture

(ii) Now for $n = r$. Let

$P(r)$: $l\,.\,r = m\,.\,r \Rightarrow l = m$ is true.

$\therefore \quad P(r^+)$: $l\,.\,r^+ = m\,.\,r^+$

$\Rightarrow \quad lr + l = mr + m$

$\Rightarrow \quad l + l = m + m \quad (\because P(r)$ is true)

$\Rightarrow \quad l = m \quad \therefore P(r+)$ is true

Thus the statement $P(n)$: $l.\,n = mr \Rightarrow l = m$ is true for all $n \in N$.

3.7 UNIQUENESS ON NEUTRAL ELEMENT FOR MULTIPLICATION AND DIVISION IN *N*

Theorem: One and only one neutral element exists for multiplication in the set of natural numbers.

Proof: If possible let us suppose that there exist two neutral elements e_1 and e_2 for multiplication in N.

Then we have $e_1\, m = m\, e_1 = m\ \forall\ m \in M$ (i)

and $e_2\, m = m\, e_2 = m\ \forall\ m \in N$ (ii)

Now we put $m = e_2$ in (i) and $m = e_1$ in (ii) and

We get $e_1.\, e_2 = e_2.\, e_1 = e_2$ (iii)

and $e_2\, e_1 = e_1.\, e_2 = e_1$ (iv)

For (iii) and (iv) e_1 and e_2 are the same and hence the theorem.

Division in N: If $m, n \in N$ and there is $p \in N$ such that $m = np$ then p is obtained by dividing m by n and is written $p = \dfrac{m}{n}$.

Division is here defined $\forall$ values of $m, n \in N$. m is a multiple of n and n is a division of m.

Now we give a theorem on multiplication in N without proof whose statement is $m^p = n^p \Leftrightarrow m = n\ \forall\ m, n, p \in N$.

3.8 ISOMORPHIC SETS, MULTIPLICATIVE IDENTITY, ORDER RELATIONS IN *N* AND LAW OF TRICHOTOMY

Isomorphic sets: The set $\{1, 1^+, (1^+)^+, ...\}$ with the relation and operations on it differs from the set $\{1, 2, 3, ...\}$ with the relations and operations on it only in the symbols used and hence they are called isomorphic sets.

Multiplicative Identity: A multiplicative identity is that element which when multiplied to a natural number m gives the same number m.

Thus $m \,.\, n = m = m = m - 1$

$\therefore \quad e = 1$ by cancellation law

1 is both right and left multiplicative identity element in N.

Order relation: Followings are the order relation in the set of natural numbers:

(A) *Greater than "relation":* A natural number m is greater than the natural number n if $\exists$ a natural number p such that $m = n + p$.

(B) *Less than "relation":* A natural number m is less then the natural number n if $\exists$ a natural number p such that $n = m + p$.

$\therefore \quad m < n \Leftrightarrow n > m$

(C) *Less than or equal to "relation":* For natural number m and n this relation is denoted as $m \leq n \Rightarrow m < n \vee m = n$.

(D) *Greater than or equal to "relation":* For any two natural numbers m and n, $m \geq n \Rightarrow m > n$ or $m = n$.

Theorem 1: If $m, n, p \in N$ then

(i) $m > n, n > p \Rightarrow m > p$

(ii) $a < b, b < p \Rightarrow m < p$

i.e. the properties of transitivity exist in natural numbers.

Proof: (i) $m > n \Rightarrow m = n + x \;\forall\; x \in N$

$n > p \Rightarrow n = p + y \;\forall\; y \in N$

$\therefore \quad m = n + x = p + x + y$

$\Rightarrow m = p + K$ where $K = x + y$

$\therefore \quad m > p.$

(i) Do Yourself.

Theorem 2: If $m, n\ p \in N$ then

(i) $m > n \Rightarrow m + p > n + p$

(ii) $m < n \Rightarrow m + p < n + p$

Proof: (i) $m > n \Rightarrow m = n + x$

$\Rightarrow \quad m + p = (n + x) + p$

$\Rightarrow \quad m + p = n + (x + p) \Rightarrow m + p = n + (p + x)$

$\Rightarrow \quad m + p = (n + p) + x \Rightarrow m + p > n + p$

(ii) Do Yourself.

Theorem 3: If $m, n\ p \in N$ then

$$m > n \Rightarrow m \,.\, p > n \,.\, p.$$

Proof: $m > n \Rightarrow m = n + x$

$\Rightarrow \quad m \,.\, p = (n + x) \,.\, p$

$\Rightarrow \quad mp = np + px \Rightarrow mp = np + K$

$\Rightarrow \quad mp > np.$

Trichotomy law: This law states if $m, n \in N$ then only one of the following relations holds good

(i) $m > n$ (ii) $m = n$ and (iii) $m < n$.

Now we state some theorem on order relation without proofs.

Theorem 1: If there be any two natural numbers m and n, then (i) $m + n > m$ (ii) $m \geq 1$ (iii) $m > n \Rightarrow m \geq n + 1$ and (iv) $m < n + 1 \Rightarrow m \leq n$.

Theorem 2: If $m, n, p \in N$ then $m \leq n, n < p \Rightarrow m < p$.

3.9 CARDINAL NUMBERS, ORDINAL NUMBERS, COUNTABLE AND UNCOUNTABLE SETS AND WELL ORDERING PRINCIPLE

The sets A and B are equivalent if there is a mapping $F: A \to B$ which is bijective.

We denote equivalent sets by $A \sim B$. Equivalent sets have the same power i.e. they are equipotent.

Denumerable sets are equipotent to N i.e. there is one to one component between the set and the set of natural number N.

A set which is either finite or denumerable is said to be countable.

We use the term cardinal number in order to represent the property which the equipotent sets have in common. Sometimes we also use cardinal number to be the measure of number of points in sets. Equipotent sets have the same cardinal numbers.

Thus $A \sim B \Leftrightarrow |A| = |B|$ where $|A|$ and $|B|$ are respectively the cardinal numbers of the set A and B.

$A \sim B$ is read "A wiggle B". When the natural numbers are used to connect elements of a set they are sometimes called as ordinal numbers.

Well ordering principle: A set is said to satisfy the well ordering principle if it contains the first (or last) element. We define the first (or last) element in subsets of N as follows:

Let S be of any subsets of N and there is some $m \in S$ such that $m \leq n \; \forall \; n \in S$ then m is called a first (or last) element of S.

Now we give the statements of few theorems without proofs.

(i) If S be a proper subsets of N and m, n be the first element of S then $m = n$.

(ii) 1 is the first element of N.

(iii) If $m \in N$, then the set of all $n \in N$ is empty if $m < n < m^+$.

(iv) Every non-empty subset of natural numbers contains a first element.

3.10 SECOND PRINCIPLE OF INDUCTION

Let $P(n)$ be a statement for $n \in N$ and $\forall \; m \in N$ the truth of $P(1)$. $P(2)$ ... $P(m)$ simultaneously imply the truth of $P(m^+)$ then $P(n)$ is true, $\forall \; n \in N$.

We omit the proof of this theorem.

3.10 (A) THE GIST OF THE METHOD OF MATHEMATICAL INDUCTION

Firstly we prove that an assertion hold good for $n = 1$ (this is the basis of the induction), secondly we assume that the assertion is valid for $n = m$ (this is the hypothesis of the induction) and we prove in that case that the assertion holds true for $n = m + 1$ (this is the induction step).

EXERCISE 3(A) SIMPLE QUESTIONS

Prove by mathematical induction that, for all natural numbers $n \in N$.

1. $a + ar + ar^2 + \ldots + ar^{n-1} = \dfrac{a\left(r^{n-1}\right)}{r-1}, r > 1$ [U.P. 1989]

2. $1 + 2^2 + 3^2 + \ldots + n^2 = \dfrac{n(n+1)(2n+1)}{6}$ [U.P. 1990]

3. $1^3 + 2^3 + 3^3 + ... + n^3 = \frac{1}{4} n^2 (n^+)^2$ [U.P. 1990]

4. $2^1 + 2^2 + 2^3 + ... + 2^n = 2(2^{n-1})$ [U.P. 1986]

5. Use mathematical induction to prove: If n is any odd positive integer then $n(n^2 - 1)$ is divisible by = 24.

[I.I.T. 1983]

6. Use mathematical induction to prove:

If $a^1 = a, a^{r+1} = a^r . a$ then $(a\,b)^n = a^n\, b^n\, n \in N$.

7. Prove that $7^{2n} + 2^{3n-3}, 3^{n-1}$ is divisible by 25, $n \in N$.

[I.I.T. 1982]

[**Hint:** Let the statement be

$P(n)$: $7^{2n} + 2^{3n-3} . 3^{n-1}$.

(i) For $n = 1$, $P(1) = 7^2 + 2^0 . 3^0 = 49 + 1 = 50$.

Which clearly shows $P(1)$ is divisible by 25.

(ii) Now assume $P(m)$ is divisible by 25.

$\therefore\ 7^{2m} + 2^{3m-3} . 3^{m-1} = 25k, k \in N$

$$\begin{aligned}\therefore \quad P^{(m+1)} &= 7^{2(m+1)} + 2^{3(m+1)-3} . 3^{m+1-1}\\ &= 7^{2m} . 7^2 + 2^{3m-3} . 2^3\, 3^{\,m-1} . 3\\ &= 49 . 7^{2m} + (2^{3m-3} . 3^{m-1}). 24.\\ &= (50 - 1)\, 7^{2m} + (25 - 1)\, 2^{3m-3} . 3^{m-1}\\ &= 50 . 7^{2m} + 252^{3m-3} . 3^{m-1} - 7^{2m} - 2^{3m-3} . 3^{m-1}\\ &= 25\,[2 . 7^{2m} + 2^{3m-3} . 3^{m-1}] - 25k\end{aligned}$$

which is divisible by 25.

$\therefore$ $P(m + 1)$ is divisible by 25

$\therefore$ $P(n)$ is true $\forall\ n \in N$.]

8. Explain the method of mathematical induction and use it to show that $11^{n+2} + 12^{2n+1}$ where n is a natural number is divisible by 133. [Roorkee 1982]

[**Hint:** Let $P(n) = 11^{n+2} + 12^{2n+1}$.

(i) $$\begin{aligned}P(1) &= (11)^{1+2} + (12)^{2.1+1} = 11^3 + 12^3\\ &= 3059 = 133 \times 23\end{aligned}$$

$P(1)$ is true.

(ii) Now for $n = m$ assume

$P(m)$: $11^{m+2} + 12^{2m+1}$ is divisible by 133.

$\therefore \quad P(m+1)\ 11^{m+1+2} + 12^{2(m+1)+1}$

$$= 11^{m+2} . 11 + 12^{2m+1} . 144$$

$$= 11(11^{m+2} + 12^{2m+1}) + 133 . 12^{2m+1}$$

$$= 11(133k) + 133 . 12^{2m+1}$$

$\therefore \quad P(m+1)$ is divisible by 133.].

Answer to Exercise 3 (A) **Hints and Solutions**

1. Solution Putting $n = 1$ in both the sides of the given formula, we get $ar^{1-1} = \dfrac{a(r^1 - 1)}{r-1}$

i.e. $ar^0 = a . 1$ i.e. $a = 1$

$\therefore$ the formula is true for $n = 1$

Now assume that the formula is true for $n = m$

$$\therefore \quad a + ar + ... + ar^{m-1} = \frac{a(r^n - 1)}{r-1}.$$

Now for $n = m + 1$

L.H.S. $= a + ar + ar^2 + ... + ar^{m-1} + ar^m$

$$\text{R.H.S.} = \frac{a(r^m - 1)}{r-1} + ar^m = \frac{ar^m - a + ar^{m(r-1)}}{r-1}$$

$$= \frac{ar^m - a + ar^{m+1} - ar^m}{r-1} = \frac{a(r^{m+1} - 1)}{r-1}$$

Hence the formula is true for $n = m + 1$.

$\therefore$ the formula holds true for all $n \in N$.

2. Solution Putting $n = 1$ is both the sides of the given formula, we get $1^2 = \frac{1}{6}$ (1) (1 + 1) (2 . 2 + 1) = 1

$\therefore$ 1 = 1 which is true.

$\therefore$ the formula holds true for $n = 1$.

Assume that the formula holds good for $n = m$.

$$\therefore \quad 1 + 2^2 + 3^2 + ... + m^2 = \frac{1}{6}\ [m(m+1)(2m+1)]$$

Now for $n = m + 1$

$$\text{L.H.S.} = 1 + 2^2 + 3^2 + ... + m^2 + (m+1)^2$$

and $\quad \text{R.H.S.} = \frac{1}{6}\,[m(m+1)\,(2m+1)] + (m+1)^2$

$$= \frac{1}{6}\,(m+1)\,[m(2m+1) + 6(m+1)]$$

$$= \frac{1}{6}\,(m+1)\,[2m^2 + m + 6m + 6]$$

$$= \frac{1}{6}\,(m+1)\,[2m^2 + 7m + 6]$$

$$= \frac{1}{6}\,(m+1)\,[2m^2 + 4m + 3m + 6]$$

$$= \frac{1}{6}\,(m+1)\,[2m(m+2) + 3(m+2)]$$

$$= \frac{1}{6}\,(m+1)\,(m+2)\,[2(m+1) + 1]$$

$\therefore$ the formula holds good for $n = m + 1$

$\therefore$ $\forall\, n \in N$ the formula holds true.

3. Solution Setting $n = 1$ in both the sides of the given formula we get

$$1^3 = \frac{1}{4}(1)^2 \times (1+1)^2 = 1$$

i.e. $\quad 1 = 1$ which is true.

$\therefore$ The formula holds good for $n = m$

i.e. $1^3 + 2^3 + 3^3 + \ldots + m^3 = m^2(m+1)^2/4$

Now setting $n = m + 1$, we get

$$1^3 + 2^3 + 3^3 + \ldots + m^3 + (m+1)^3 = \frac{1}{4}\,m^2\,(m+1)^2 + (m+1)^3$$

$$= (m+1)^2\left[\frac{1}{4}m^2 + m + 1\right]$$

$$= \frac{1}{4}\,(m+1)^2\,(m^2 + 4m + 4) = \frac{1}{4}\,(m+1)^2\,(m+2)^2$$

hence the formula holds good for $n = m + 1$

i.e. the formula holds good for all $n \in N$.

4. Solution Setting $n = 1$ in both the sides of the given formula we get

$$2^1 = 2(2^1 - 1) \Rightarrow 2 = 2 \text{ which is true.}$$

Thus the given formula holds true for $n = 1$ and hence the formula is true for $n = m$

$\therefore \quad 2 + 2^2 + 2^3 + ... + 2^m = (2^m - 1).$

Now setting $n = m + 1$, we get

$2 + 2^2 + 2^3 + 2^m + 2^{m+1} = 2(2^m - 1) + 2^{m+1}$

$= 2^{m+1} - 2 + 2^{m+1} = 2\,2^{m+1} - 2 = 2(2^{m+1} - 1)$

5. Solution Since m is an odd positive integers we can set $n = 2^{m-1}$ where m is any positive integer.

Now $n(n^2 - 1) = (2m - 1)\,[(2m - 1)^2 - 1]$

$= (2m - 1)\,(2m - 1 + 1)\,(2m - 1 - 1)$

$= (2m - 1), 2m.\, 2\,(m - 1)$

$= 4m(m - 1)\,(2m - 1)$

Now we shall show for every $m \in N$

$4m(m - 1)\,(2m - 1)$ is divisible by 24.

First we set $m = 1$ and see that $4.1\,(1 - 1)\,(2\,.\,1 - 1) = 0$ which is divisible by 24.

Now we assume that $4m(m - 1)\,(2m - 1)$ is divisible by 24 for $m = k$

i.e. $4k(k - 1)\,(2k - 1)$ is divisible by 24.

Again setting $m = k + 1$ we see that

$4(k + 1)\,(k + 1 - 1)\,(2k + 2 - 1) = (4k + 4)\,(k)\,(2k + 1)$

$= (4k^2 + 4k)\,(2k + 1)$

$= 8k^3 + 8k^2 + 4k^2 + 4k = 8k^3 + 12k^2 + 4k$

$= 4k[2k^2 + 3k + 1]$

$= 4k[2k^2 - 3k + 1] + 24k^2$

$= 4k[(k - 1)\,(2k - 1)] + 24k^2$

which is divisible by 24. Hence proved.

6. Solution Setting $n = 1$ in both the sides

$(ab)^1 = a^1\, b^1 \Rightarrow ab = ab$ which is true.

Hence the formula holds true for $n = 1$.

Now assume, the formula holds true for $n = k$

$\therefore \quad (ab)^k = a^k b^k$

Setting again $n = k + 1$ we get

$$(ab)^{k+1} = (ab)^k . (ab) = (a^k b^k)(ab)$$
$$= a^k (b^k b) a = (a^k a) b^{k+1} = a^{k+1} b^{k+1}$$

hence the formula holds true for $n = k + 1$.

7. Solution Already given is the question.

8. Solution Already given is the question.

EXERCISE 3 (B) SOME MORE IMPORTANT PROBLEMS WITH MODEL SOLUTIONS

1. Use mathematical induction to prove that $2 . 7^n + 3 . 5^{n-5}$ is divisible by 24 for all $n > 0$ [I.I.T. 1985]
2. Prove that $x(x^{n-1} - n a^{n-1}) + a^n(n-1)$ is divisible by $(x-a)^2$ for all positive integers n greaten than 1. [I.I.T. 1977]
3. If p be a natural number then prove that $p^{n+1} + (p + 1)^{2n-1}$ is divisible by $p^2 + p + 1$ for every positive inter n. [I.I.T. 1984]
4. If $n > 1$ prove that

   (i) $\underline{|n} < \left(\frac{n+1}{2}\right)^n$ (ii) $\frac{\underline{|2n}}{(\underline{|n})^2} > \frac{4n}{2n+1}$ [I.I.T. 1981]
5. Prove by mathematical induction that $\frac{\underline{|2n}}{2^{2n}(\underline{|n})^2} \le \frac{1}{(3n+1)^{\frac{1}{2}}}$ [I.I.T. 1987]
6. Use mathematical induction to prove that $\sum_{k=0}^{n} k^2 \, {}^nC_k =$ $n(n+1) 2^{n-1}$ for $n \ge 1$ [I.I.T. 1986]
7. Let $u_1 = 1$, $u_2 = 1$ and $u_{n+2} = u_{n+1} + u_n$ for $n \ge 1$. Use mathematical induction to show that

   $$u_n = \frac{1}{\sqrt{5}}\left[\left(\frac{1+\sqrt{5}}{2}\right)^n - \left(\frac{1-\sqrt{5}}{2}\right)^n\right]$$ [I.I.T. 1981]

8. Using mathematical induction to prove that

$${}^{m}c_{o} \cdot {}^{n}c_{k} + {}^{m}c_{1} \cdot {}^{n}c_{k-1} + \ldots + {}^{m}c_{k}\ {}^{n}c_{o} = {}^{m+n}c_{k} \quad \text{[I.I.T. 1989]}$$

9. Using mathematical induction or otherwise prove that for any non-negative integers *m*, *n r* and *k*

$$\sum_{m=0}^{k} (n-m) \frac{\lfloor r+m}{\lfloor m} = \frac{\lfloor r+k+1}{\lfloor k} = \left[\frac{n}{r+1} - \frac{k}{r+2}\right]$$

[I.I.T. 1991]

10. For all positive integers *n*, prove that $\frac{n^7}{7} + \frac{n^5}{5} + \frac{2n^3}{3} - \frac{n}{105}$ is an integer. [I.I.T. 1990]

EXERCISE 3 (B)
ANSWER TO SOME MORE IMPORTANT PROBLEMS HINTS AND SOLUTIONS

1. **Solution :** Let the assertion be

$P(n) = 2 \cdot 7^n + 3 \cdot 5^n - 5$. For $n = 1$, this assertion take the form $P(1) = 2.7^1 + 3.5^1 - 5 = 14 + 15 - 5 = 24$ which is divisible by 24 hence the basis of mathematical induction holds good. Now we assume that the hypothesis of induction holds true for $n = m$,

$\therefore \quad P(m) = 2 . 7^m + 3 . 5^m - 5$ is divisible by 24.

Setting now the induction step as

$n = m + 1$ we have

$$P(m + 1) = 2.\ 7^{m+1} + 3.\ 5^{m+1} - 5$$

$\therefore \quad P(m + 1) - P(m)$

$$= [2.\ 7^m.\ 7 + 3.\ 5^m.\ 5 - 5] - [2.\ 7^m + 3.\ 5^m - 5]$$
$$= 14.7^m + 15.\ 5^m - 5 - 2.\ 7^m - 3.\ 5^m + 5$$
$$= 12.\ 7^m + 12.\ 5^m = 12(7^m + 5^m),$$

where $m \in N$.

But 7^m and 5^m both are odds hence $7^m + 5^m$ is even. Let $7^m + 5^m$ be $2k$, then $P(m + 1) - P(m) = 12.\ 2k = 24\,k$, where $k \in N$.

$\therefore \quad P(m + 1) = P(m) + 24k$ which is divisible by 24 hence $P(m + 1)$ is also true.

2. **Solution:** Let the assertion by

$$P(n) = x(x^{n-1} - n\,a^{n-1}) + a^n(n-1).$$

For $\quad n = 2$ assertion takes the form

$$P(2) = x(x-2a) + a^2\,(2-1) = x^2 - 2ax + a^2$$
$$= (x-a)^2$$

Therefore $P(2)$ holds good. Thus the basis of mathematical induction holds good.

Now we assume that the hypothesis of induction holds good for $n = m$

$\therefore \quad P(m) = x(x^{m-1} - ma^{m-1}) + a^m(m-1)$ is true.

This $P(m)$ can be written as

$$P(m) = x^m - mxa^{m-1} + a^m \cdot m - a^m$$
$$= (x-a)^2 f(x)$$

$$\therefore \quad x^m = mxa^{m-1} + a^m - ma^m + (x-a)^2 f(x).$$

Setting now the induction step as $n = m + 1$ we have

$$P(m+1) = x\,[x^m - (m+1)\,a^m] + m \cdot a^{m+1}$$

Substituting the value of x^m we get

$$P(m+1) = x\,[mxa^{m-1} + a^m - ma^m + (x-a)^2 f(x)]$$
$$- (m+1)\,xa^m + ma^{m+1}$$
$$= x^2\,ma^{m-1} + x \cdot a^m - mxa^m + x(x-a)^2 f(x)$$
$$- (m+1)\,x\,a^m + ma^{m+1}$$
$$= x^2\,m\,a^{m-1} + xa^m - mxa^m + x(x-a)^2 f(x)$$
$$+ ma^{m+1} - xa^m - mxa^m$$
$$= x^2ma^{m-1} - 2mxa^m + ma^{m+1} + x(x-a)^2 f(x)$$
$$= ma^{m-1}\,[x^2 - 2ax + a^2] + x(x-a)^2 f(x)$$
$$= (x-a)^2\,[ma^{m-1} + xf(x)]$$

which is divisible by $(x-a)^2$.

Hence $P(m+1)$ is also true.

3. **Solution:** For $n = 1$

$$P(1) = p^{1+1} + (p+1)^{2-1} = p^2 + p + 1$$

Which is divisible by $p^2 + p + 1$ and hence the basis of mathematical induction is established.

Now we assume that the hypothesis of mathematical induction holds true for $n = m$ and therefore

$\therefore \quad P(m) = p^{m+1} + (p+1)^{2m-1}$ is true.

i.e. $P(m) = p^{m+1} + (p+1)^{2m-1} = K(p^2 + p + 1) \qquad (1)$

Setting now the induction step as $n = m + 1$ we have

$$\begin{aligned}
P(m+1) &= p^{m+2} + (p+1)^{2m+1} \\
&= p^{m+2} + (p+1)^{2m-1}(p+1)^2 \\
&= p^{m+2} + [K(p^2+p+1) - p^{m+1}](p+1)^2 \\
&= p^{m+2} + K(p^2+p+1)(p+1)^2 - p^{m+1}(p+1)^2 \\
&= p^{m+1}[p - (p+1)^2] + K(p^2+p+1)(p+1)^2 \\
&= p^{m+1}[p - p^2 - 2p - 1] + K(p^2+p+1)(p+1)^2 \\
&= p^{m+1}[-p^2 - p - 1] + K(p^2+p+1)(p+1)^2 \\
&= (p^2+p+1)[K(p+1)^2 - p^{m+1}]
\end{aligned}$$

which is divisible by $p^2 + p + 1$.

Hence $P(m + 1)$ is also true.

4. Solution: (i): for $n = 2$

L.H.S. = $\lfloor\underline{2} = 2$

R.H.S. is $\left(\dfrac{2+1}{2}\right)^2 = \dfrac{9}{4}$.

Clearly $2 < \dfrac{9}{4}$ hence $\lfloor\underline{n} < \left(\dfrac{n+1}{2}\right)^2$ is true.

For $n = 2$.

New for $n = m$ we assume

$$\lfloor\underline{m} < \left(\frac{m+1}{2}\right)^m \text{ is true.} \qquad (1)$$

We have to prove now $\lfloor\underline{m+1} < \left(\dfrac{m+1+1}{2}\right)^{m+1}$

$$\text{i.e. } \lfloor\underline{m+1} < \left(\frac{m+2}{2}\right)^{m+1} \qquad (2)$$

From (1) $\lfloor\underline{m} < \left(\dfrac{m+1}{2}\right)^m$

$$\therefore \quad (m+1)\lfloor\underline{m} < (m+1)\left(\frac{m+1}{2}\right)^m$$

$$\Rightarrow \qquad \underline{|m+1} < \frac{(m+1)^{m+1}}{2m}$$

We have $\dfrac{(m+2)^{m+1}}{2^{m+1}} - \dfrac{(m+1)^{m+1}}{2^m}$

$$= \frac{(m+1+1)^{m+1}}{2^{m+1}} - \frac{(m+1)^{m+1}}{2^m}$$

$$= \frac{(m+1)^{m+1}\left[1+\dfrac{1}{m+1}\right]^{m+1} - 2(m+1)^{m+1}}{2^{m+1}}$$

$$= \frac{(m+1)^{m+1}}{2^{m+1}}\left\{\left(1+\frac{1}{1+m}\right)^{m+1} - 2\right\}$$

Which is positive when $1+\left(\dfrac{1}{1+m}\right)^{m+1} > 2$

i.e. $1 + (m+1)\ \dfrac{1}{(m+1)} + \ldots > 2$

This inequality is true clearly

$$\therefore \qquad \frac{(m+2)^{m+1}}{2^{m+1}} > \frac{(m+1)^{m+1}}{2m} \tag{3}$$

For (2) and (3) the result follows.

(ii) For $n = 2$

L.H.S. $= \dfrac{\underline{|4}}{\{\underline{|2}\}^2} = 6.$

R.H.S. $= \dfrac{4\times 2}{5} = \dfrac{8}{5}. \qquad \therefore > \dfrac{8}{5}$

$\therefore$ The inequality $\dfrac{\underline{|2n}}{\{\underline{|n}\}^2} > \dfrac{4n}{2n+1}$ holds true.

Now we assume for $n = m$ the inequality

$$\frac{\lfloor 2m}{\{\lfloor m\}^2} > \frac{4m}{2m+1} \text{ is true} \tag{1}$$

We now proceed to prove $\dfrac{\lfloor 2(m+1)}{\{\lfloor m+1\}^2} > \dfrac{4(m+1)}{2(m+1)+1}$

i.e. $\dfrac{(2m+2)(2m+1)\lfloor 2m}{(m+1)^2\,\{\lfloor m\}^2} > \dfrac{4m+4}{2m+3}$

But $\dfrac{(2m+2)(2m+1)\,4m}{(m+1)^2\,(2m+1)} < \dfrac{(2m+2)(2m+1)\lfloor 2m}{\{\lfloor m+1\}^2}$ (2)

($\therefore$ (1) holds good)

We can write $\dfrac{(2m+2)(2m+1)\,4m}{(m+1)^2\,(2m+1)} - \dfrac{4m+4}{2m+3}$

$$= \frac{12m^2+16m^2-4}{(2m+3)(m+1)} \text{ after simplification.}$$

This is greater than 0 as $m \geq 2$.

$$\therefore \quad \frac{(2m+2)(2m+1)4m}{(m+1)^2\,(2m+1)} > \frac{4m+4}{2m+3} \tag{3}$$

From (2) and (3) the result follows.

5. Solution: For $n = 1$, the L.H.S. of $\dfrac{\lfloor 2n}{2^{2n}\,(\lfloor n)^2} \leq \dfrac{1}{(3n+1)^{1/2}}$ is $\dfrac{1}{2}$

and R.H.S. is also $\dfrac{1}{2}$ and hence the inequality holds true for $n = 1$.

We now assume that the inequality holds good for $n = m$

i.e. $\dfrac{\lfloor 2m}{2^{2m}\,(\lfloor m)^2} \leq \dfrac{1}{(3m+1)^{1/2}}$ (1)

We now proceed to prove the inequality for $n = m + 1$

i.e. $$\frac{\lfloor 2m+2}{2^{2m+2}(\lfloor m+1)^2} \le \frac{1}{(3m+4)^{1/2}} \quad (2)$$

i.e. $$\frac{(2m+2)(2m+1)\lfloor 2m}{2^{2m+2}(\lfloor m+1)^2} \le \frac{1}{(3m+4)^{1/2}}$$

i.e. $$\frac{2(m+1)(2m+1)\lfloor 2m}{4(m+1)^2(\lfloor m)^2\, 2^{2m}} \le \frac{1}{(3m+4)^{1/2}}$$

i.e. $$\frac{(2m+1)}{2(m+1)} \cdot \frac{1}{(3m+1)^{1/2}} \le \frac{1}{(3m+4)^{1/2}} \quad (3)$$

If (3) holds true, then

$\dfrac{(2m+1)^2}{4(m+1)^2} \cdot \dfrac{1}{(3m+1)} \le \dfrac{1}{(3m+4)}$ which when simplified gives

$3m\,[-4m-3] + 4\,(3m^2 + 2m) \le 0$

i.e. $-m \le 0$ $\quad\Rightarrow m \ge 0$ which is true hence (2) holds good.

6. **Solution:** For $n = 1$, L.H.S. is $\sum_{k=0}^{1} k^2 \cdot {}^1c_k$

$$= 0 \cdot {}^1c_0 + 1^2 - {}^1c_1 = 1$$

R.H.S. $= 1\,(1+1)\,2^{1-2} = \dfrac{2}{2} = 1.$

Hence the given equality holds good for $n = 1$.

Now we assume, the above inequality holds true for $n = m$

i.e. $$\sum_{k=0}^{m} k^2 \cdot {}^mc_k \cdot = m(m+1)2^{m-1} \quad (1)$$

We have then to prove for $n = m + 1$, the equality

$\sum_{k=0}^{m+1} k^2 \cdot {}^{m+1}c_k = (m+1)\,(m+2)2^{m-1}$ also holds true.

We have $$\sum_{k=0}^{m+1} k^2 \cdot {}^{m+1}c_k = \sum_{k=0}^{m+1} k^2 \left[{}^{m}c_k + {}^{m}c_{k-1} \right]$$

$$= \sum_{k=0}^{m+1} k^2 \cdot {}^{m}c_k + \sum_{k=0}^{m+1} k^2 \cdot {}^{m}c_{k-1}$$

$$= \sum_{k=0}^{m} k^2 \cdot {}^{m}c_k + \sum_{k=1}^{m+1} k^2 \cdot {}^{m}c_{k-1} \tag{2}$$

Since $\sum_{k=0}^{m+1} k^2 \cdot {}^{m}c_k$ for $k = m + 1$ is meaningless and

$\sum_{k=0}^{m+1} k^2 \cdot {}^{m}c_{k-1}$ for $k = 0$ is also meaningless.

Now $\sum_{k=1}^{m+1} k^2 \cdot {}^{m}c_{k-1}$

$$= [1^2 \cdot {}^{m}c_0 + 2^2 \cdot {}^{m}c_1 + 3^2 \cdot {}^{m}c_2 + \ldots$$

$+(m+1)^2\, {}^{m}c_m]$ and $\sum_{k=0}^{m} (k+1)^2\, {}^{m}c_k$

$$= [1^2 \cdot {}^{m}c_0 + 2^2 \cdot {}^{m}c_1 + \ldots + (m+1)^2\, {}^{m}c_m]$$

$$\therefore \quad \sum_{k=1}^{m+1} k^2 \cdot {}^{m}c_{k-1} = \sum_{k=0}^{m} (k+1)^2 \cdot {}^{m}c_k$$

and (2) reduces to

$$\sum_{k=0}^{m+1} k^2 \cdot {}^{m+1}c_k = \sum_{k=0}^{m} k^2 \cdot {}^{m}c_k + \sum_{k=0}^{m} (k+1)^2 \cdot {}^{m}c_k$$

$$= \sum_{k=0}^{m} \left(2k^2 + 2k + 1\right) \cdot {}^{m}c_k$$

$$= 2\sum_{k=0}^{m} k^2\, {}^{m}c_k + 2\sum_{k=0}^{m} k \cdot {}^{m}c_k + \sum_{k=0}^{m} {}^{m}c_k \tag{3}$$

In order to obtain the value of $\sum_{k=0}^{m} k \cdot {}^{m}c_k$

We differentiate the relation $(1+x)^n = c_0 + c_1 x + c_2 x^2 + ... + c_n x^3$ and obtain

$n(1+x)^{n-1} = 0 + c_1 + 2 \cdot c_2 x + 3 \cdot c_3 x^2 + ... + n \cdot c_n x^{n-1}$

$$= \sum_{r=0}^{n} r \cdot c_r \, x^{r-1} \tag{4}$$

Put $x = 1$ the (4) and obtain

$$n \cdot 2^{n-1} = \sum_{r=0}^{n} r \cdot c_r.$$

$$\therefore \quad m \cdot 2^{m-1} = \sum_{k=0}^{m} k \cdot {}^{m}c_k \tag{v}$$

Thus (3) becomes $\sum_{k=0}^{m+1} k^2 \cdot {}^{m+1}c_k$

$$\begin{aligned}
&= 2 \cdot m(m+1)\, 2^{m-2} + 2m \cdot 2^{m-1} + 2^m \\
&= m(m+1)\, 2^{m-1} + 2 \cdot m \cdot 2^{m-1} + 2^m \\
&= 2^{m-1}[m(m+1) + 2m + 2] \\
&= 2^{m-1}[m(m+1) + 2(m+1)] \\
&= 2^{m-1}(m+1)(m+2)
\end{aligned}$$

7. Solution: We have $u_n = \frac{1}{\sqrt{5}}\left[\left(\frac{1+\sqrt{5}}{2}\right)^n - \left(\frac{1-\sqrt{5}}{2}\right)^n\right]$

For $\quad n = 1$

L.H.S. $= u_1 = 1$

R.H.S. $= \frac{1}{\sqrt{5}}\left[\left(\frac{1+\sqrt{5}}{2}\right) - \left(\frac{1-\sqrt{5}}{2}\right)\right] = 1$

For $\quad n = 2$

L.H.S. $= u_2 = 1$.

and R.H.S. = 1. So the equality holds true for $n = 1$ and $n = 2$.

Now we assume the equality holds true for $n = m$

$$\therefore \quad u_m = \frac{1}{\sqrt{5}}\left[\left(\frac{1+\sqrt{5}}{2}\right)^m - \left(\frac{1-\sqrt{5}}{2}\right)^m\right] \tag{1}$$

We shall prove now for $n = m + 1$ the equality holds true.

$$\text{i.e } u_{m+1} = \frac{1}{\sqrt{5}}\left[\left(\frac{1+\sqrt{5}}{2}\right)^{m+1} - \left(\frac{1-\sqrt{5}}{2}\right)^{m+1}\right]$$

We are given $u_{m+1} = u_m + u_{m-1}$

$$\therefore \quad u_{m+1} = \frac{1}{\sqrt{5}}\left[\left(\frac{1+\sqrt{5}}{2}\right)^{m} - \left(\frac{1-\sqrt{5}}{2}\right)^{m}\right]$$

$$+ \frac{1}{\sqrt{5}}\left[\left(\frac{1+\sqrt{5}}{2}\right)^{m-1} - \left(\frac{1-\sqrt{5}}{2}\right)^{m-1}\right]$$

$$= \frac{1}{\sqrt{5}}\left[\left(\frac{1+\sqrt{5}}{2}\right)^{m-1}\left\{\frac{1+\sqrt{5}}{2}+1\right\} - \left(\frac{1-\sqrt{5}}{2}\right)^{m-1}\left\{\frac{1-\sqrt{5}}{2}+1\right\}\right]$$

$$= \frac{1}{\sqrt{5}}\left[\left(\frac{1+\sqrt{5}}{2}\right)^{m-1}\left(\frac{6+2\sqrt{5}}{4}\right) - \left(\frac{1-\sqrt{5}}{2}\right)^{m-1}\left(\frac{6-2\sqrt{5}}{4}\right)\right]$$

$$= \frac{1}{\sqrt{5}}\left[\left(\frac{1+\sqrt{5}}{2}\right)^{m-1}\left(\frac{1+\sqrt{5}}{2}\right)^{2} - \left(\frac{1-\sqrt{5}}{2}\right)^{m-1}\left(\frac{1-\sqrt{5}}{2}\right)^{2}\right]$$

$$= \frac{1}{\sqrt{5}}\left[\left(\frac{1+\sqrt{5}}{2}\right)^{m+1} - \left(\frac{1-\sqrt{5}}{2}\right)^{m+1}\right]$$

8. **Solution :** For $m = n = 1, k = 1$, since k is a positive integer less than in equal to m and n

$\therefore$ L.H.S. $= {}^1c_0 \cdot {}^1c_1 + {}^1c_1\, {}^1c_0 = 1 + 1 = 2$

R.H.S. $= {}^{1+1}c_1 = {}^2c_1 = 2$

So the equality holds true for $m = n = 1$

Now we assume that the equality holds true for any fixed positive integers m and n

i.e. ${}^mc_0\,{}^nc_k + {}^mc_1\,{}^nc_{k-1} + {}^mc_2\,{}^nc_{k-2} + \ldots + {}^mc_k\,{}^nc_o = {}^{m+n}c_k$. (1)

We shall now prove that the equality holds true for $m + 1$ and $n + 1$. We have now

$$^{m+1}C_0\,^{n+1}C_k + ^{m+1}C_1\,^{n+1}C_{k-1} + \ldots + ^{m+1}C_k\,^{n+1}C_0$$

$$= 1\,[^nC_k + ^nC_{k-1}] + [^mC_0 + ^mC_1]\,[^nC_{k-1} + ^nC_{k-2}]$$

$$+ \ldots + [^mC_k + ^mC_{k-1}]\,.\,1$$

$$[^nC_{k-1} + ^mC_1 \cdot ^nC_{k-2} + ^mC_2 \cdot ^nC_{k-3} + \ldots + ^mC_{k-1}\,^nC_0]$$

$$+ [^nC_k + ^mC_1\,^nC_{k-1} + ^mC_2\,^nC_{k-2} + \ldots + ^mC_k]$$

$$+ [^mC_0\,^nC_{k-2} + ^mC_1\,^nC_{k-3} + \ldots + ^mC_{k-2}\,^nC_0]$$

$$+ [^mC_0\,^nC_{k-1} + ^mC_1\,^nC_{k-2} + \ldots + ^mC_{k-1}]$$

$$= [^mC_0\,^nC_{k-1} + ^mC_1\,^nC_{k-2} + \ldots + ^mC_{k-1}\,^nC_0]$$

$$+ [^mC_0\,^nC_k + ^mC_1\,^nC_{k-1} + \ldots + ^mC_k\,^nC_0]$$

$$+ [^mC_0\,^nC_{k-2} + ^mC_1\,^nC_{k-3} + \ldots + ^mC_{k-2}\,^nC_0]$$

$$+ [^mC_0\,^nC_{k-1} + ^mC_1\,^nC_{k-2} + \ldots + ^mC_{k-1}\,^nC_0]$$

$$= ^{m+n}C_{k-1} + ^{m+n}C_k + ^{m+n}C_{k-2} + ^{m+n}C_{k-1}$$

$$= ^{m+n+1}C_{k-1} + ^{m+n+1}C_k$$

$$= ^{m+n+2}C_k.$$

Hence the theorem for $m + n$ and $n + 1$ holds true.

9. **Solution:** Setting $k = 1$ we get two terms in

$$\sum_{m=0}^{k} (n - m)\frac{\lfloor r + m}{\lfloor m} \quad \text{i.e. } m = 0 \text{ and } m = 1$$

$$\therefore \qquad \text{L.H.S.} = (n - 0)\frac{\lfloor r + 0}{\lfloor 0} + (n - 1)\frac{\lfloor r + 1}{\lfloor 1}$$

$$= n\lfloor r + n\lfloor r + 1 - \lfloor r + 1$$

$$= \lfloor r\,[n + n(r + 1) - (r + 1)]$$

$$= \lfloor r\,[n(r + 2) - (r + 1)]$$

$$\text{R.H.S.} = \frac{\lfloor r + 1 + 1}{\lfloor 1}\left[\frac{n}{r+1} - \frac{1}{r+2}\right]$$

$$= \frac{\lfloor r + 2\,[n(r+2) - (r+1)]}{(r+1)(r+2)}$$

$$= \frac{(r+2)(r+1)\,|\underline{r}\,[n(r+2)-(r+1)]}{(r+1)\,(r+2)}$$

$$= |\underline{r}\;[n(r+2)-(r+1)]$$

Hence the equality holds true for $k = 1$.

Assume now that the equality holds true for $k = t$

$$\therefore \quad \sum_{m=0}^{t}(n-m)\frac{|\underline{r+m}}{|\underline{m}} = \frac{|\underline{r+t+1}}{|\underline{t}}\left[\frac{n}{r+1}-\frac{t}{r+2}\right] \qquad (1)$$

We prove then the equality holds true for $k = t + 1$

i.e. $$\sum_{m=0}^{t+1}(n-m)\frac{|\underline{r+m}}{|\underline{m}}$$

$$= \frac{|\underline{r+t+2}}{|\underline{t+1}}\left[\frac{n}{r+1}-\frac{t+1}{r+2}\right].$$

Adding $\dfrac{(n-t-1)|\underline{r+t+1}}{|\underline{t+1}}$ both the sides in (1) we

get $$\sum_{m=0}^{t+1}\frac{(n-m)|\underline{n+m}}{|\underline{m}}$$

$$= \frac{|\underline{r+t+1}}{|\underline{t}}\left[\frac{n}{r+1}-\frac{t}{r+2}\right]+\frac{(n-t-1)|\underline{n+t+1}}{|\underline{t+1}}$$

$$= \frac{|\underline{r+t+1}}{|\underline{t+1}}\left[\frac{n(t+1)}{r+1}-\frac{t(t+1)}{r+2}-\frac{(n-t-1)}{1}\right]$$

$$= \frac{|\underline{r+t+1}}{|\underline{t+1}}\left[\frac{(t+1)n}{r+1}+n-\frac{t(t+1)}{r+2}-t-1\right]$$

$$= \frac{|\underline{r+t+1}}{|\underline{t+1}}\left[n\left\{\frac{t+1}{r+1}+1\right\}-t\left\{\frac{t+1}{r+2}+1\right\}-1\right]$$

$$= \frac{|\underline{r+t+1}}{|\underline{t+1}}\left[n\left\{\frac{t+1+r+1}{r+1}\right\}-t\left\{\frac{t+1+r+2}{r+2}\right\}-1\right]$$

$$= \frac{\underline{|r+t+1}}{\underline{|t+1}}\left[n\left\{\frac{r+t+2}{r+1}\right\}-t\left\{\frac{r+t+2}{r+2}\right\}-\left\{\frac{t}{r+2}+1\right\}\right]$$

$$= \frac{\underline{|r+t+1}}{\underline{|t+1}}\left[n\left\{\frac{r+t+2}{r+1}\right\}-t\left\{\frac{r+t+2}{r+2}\right\}-\left\{\frac{t+r+2}{r+2}\right\}\right]$$

$$= \frac{\underline{|r+t+2}}{\underline{|t+1}}\left[\frac{n}{r+1}-\frac{t}{r+2}-\frac{1}{r+2}\right]$$

$$= \frac{\underline{|r+t+2}}{\underline{|t+1}}\left[\frac{n}{r+1}-\frac{t+1}{r+2}\right]$$

10. Solution: Let $P(n) = \frac{n^7}{7}+\frac{n^5}{5}+\frac{2n^3}{3}-\frac{n}{105}$

For $\quad n = 1$

$$P(1) = \frac{1}{7}+\frac{1}{5}+\frac{2}{3}-\frac{1}{105} = \frac{15+21+70-1}{105}$$

$$= \frac{106-1}{105} = 1 \text{ which is an integer.}$$

$\therefore \quad P(1)$ holds true.

We now assume

$$P(k) = \frac{k^7}{7}+\frac{k^5}{5}+\frac{2k^3}{3}-\frac{k}{105} \text{ holds true.}$$

We prove now the induction step

i.e. $P(k+1) = \frac{(k+1)^7}{7}+\frac{(k+1)^5}{2}+\frac{2(k+1)^3}{3}-\frac{k+1}{105}$ is an integer.

$$\frac{(k+1)^7}{7} = \frac{1}{7}\,[{}^7c_0 k^7 + {}^7c_1 k^6 + {}^7c_2 k^5 + {}^7c_3 k^4 + {}^7c_4 k^3 + {}^7c_5 k^2 + {}^7c_6 k + {}^7c_7]$$

$$\frac{(k+1)^5}{5} = \frac{1}{5}\,[{}^5c_0 k^5 + {}^5c_1 k^4 + {}^5c_2 k^3 + {}^5c_3 k^2 + {}^5c_4 k + {}^5c_5]$$

$$\frac{2}{3}(k+1)^3 = \frac{2}{3}[{}^3c_0\, k^3 + {}^3c_1\, k^2 + {}^3c_2\, k + {}^3c_3]$$

$$\frac{(k+1)}{105} = \frac{k}{105} + \frac{1}{105}$$

Adding we get

$$P(k+1) = \frac{k^7}{7} + \frac{k^5}{5} + \frac{2k^3}{3} - \frac{k}{105} + \frac{1}{7}\text{ (multiple of 7)} + \frac{1}{7}$$

$$+ \frac{1}{5}\text{ (multiple of 5)} + \frac{1}{5}$$

$$+ \frac{2}{3}\text{ (multiple of 3)} + \frac{2}{3} - \frac{1}{105}$$

$$= \text{Integer} + \frac{1}{7} + \frac{1}{5} + \frac{2}{3} - \frac{1}{105}$$

$$= \text{integer.}$$

PROBLEMS AND EXERCISES (C)

Prove the following identities and inequalities by induction method:

1. $1 + 2 + 3 + \ldots + n = \dfrac{n(n+1)}{2}$
2. $1.\,2 + 2.\,3 + 3.\,4 + \ldots + n\,(n+1) = \dfrac{n(n+1)(n+2)}{3}$
3. $\dfrac{1}{1\cdot 2} + \dfrac{1}{2\cdot 3} + \dfrac{1}{3\cdot 4} + \ldots + \dfrac{1}{n(n+1)} = \dfrac{n}{n+1}$
4. $1^2 + 2^2 + 3^2 + \ldots + n^2 = \dfrac{n(n+1)(2n+1)}{6}$
5. $2^2 + 4^2 + 8^2 + \ldots + (2n)^2 = \dfrac{2n(n+1)(2n+1)}{3}$
6. $1.\,2 + 2.\,3 + 3.\,4 + \ldots + n\,(n+1) = \dfrac{n(n+1)(n+2)}{3}$

7. $1^2 + 3^2 + 5^2 + ... + (2n-1)^2 = \dfrac{n(2n-1)(2n+1)}{3}$

8. $1^3 + 2^3 + 3^3 + ... + n^3 = \left[\dfrac{n(n+1)}{2}\right]^2$

9. $3 + 3^2 + 3^3 + ... + 3^n \; \dfrac{3(3^n-1)}{2}$

10. $\dfrac{1}{2\cdot 3} + \dfrac{1}{3\cdot 4} + \dfrac{1}{4\cdot 5} + ... + \dfrac{1}{(n+1)(n+2)} = \dfrac{n}{2(n+2)}$

11. $\dfrac{1}{1\cdot 3\cdot 5} + \dfrac{2}{3\cdot 5\cdot 7} + \dfrac{3}{5\cdot 7\cdot 9} + ... + \dfrac{n}{(2n-1)(2n+1)(2n+3)}$

12. $\dfrac{1}{1^2} + \dfrac{1}{2^2} + \dfrac{1}{3^2} + ... + \dfrac{1}{n^2} \leq 2$

13. $\dfrac{1}{1} + \dfrac{1}{1\cdot 2} + \dfrac{1}{1\cdot 2\cdot 3} + ... \dfrac{1}{\lfloor n} < 2$

14. $\lfloor n > \left(\dfrac{n}{3}\right)^n$

15. $(1 + a)^n > 1 + na$, where $a > -1$; $a \neq 0$ and $n > 1$

16. (i) $2^n > n^2$ for $n \geq 5$

(ii) $\lfloor n > 2^{n-1}$ for $n \geq 3$

17. $\cos\alpha \cos 2\alpha \cos 4\alpha \cos 8\alpha \ldots \cos 2^n\alpha = \dfrac{\sin 2^{n+1}\alpha}{2^{n+1}\sin\alpha}$

[**Hint:** The equality holds true for $n = 1$

as $\cos\alpha = \dfrac{\sin 2\alpha}{2\sin\alpha} = \cos\alpha$.

Thus the equality holds true for $n = m$

i.e. $\cos\alpha \cos 2\alpha \cos 4\alpha \ldots \cos 2^m\alpha = \dfrac{\sin 2^{m+1}\alpha}{2^{m+1}\sin\alpha}$ (1)

We shall now prove that the equality holds true for $n = m + 1$.
Multiplying both sides by $\cos 2^{m+1}\alpha$ in (1) we get
$\cos\alpha \cos 2\alpha \cos 4\alpha \ldots \cos 2^m\alpha \cos 2^{m+1}\alpha$

$$= \frac{\sin 2^{m+1}\alpha}{2^{m+1}\sin\alpha} \cdot \cos 2^{m+1}\alpha$$

$$= \frac{2\sin 2^{m+1}\alpha \cos 2^{m+1}\alpha}{2\cdot 2^{m+1}\sin\alpha} = \frac{2\sin 2^{m+2}\alpha}{2^{m+2}\sin\alpha}\Bigg]$$

18. (i) Prove that $n^3 + 11^n$ is divisible by 6.
(ii) Prove that $4^n + 15^{n-1}$ is divisible by 9.

19. (i) Prove that $n^5 - n$ is divisible by 30.
(ii) Prove that $6n^5 + 15n^4 + 10n^3 - n$ is divisible by 30.
(iii) Prove that $n^5 - 5n^3 + 60n^2 - 56n$ is multiple of 120 for $n > 1$.

20. (i) Prove that $8n^3 + 40n$ is divisible by 48
(ii) Prove that $5^{n+1}. 4^{n+1} + 4^{n+1}. 4^{n+1} - 3^{n+1} - 1$ is divisible by 323.

21. (i) $\frac{1}{\lfloor n} \le \frac{1}{2^{n-1}}$

(ii) $(\lfloor n)^2 < \left[\frac{(n+1)(2n+1)}{6}\right]^n$

22. Prove that $[\cos\theta + i\sin\theta]^n = \cos n\theta + i\sin n\theta$.

23. (i) Prove that $a^n - b^n$ is always divisible by $a - b$
(ii)Prove that $x^n - y^n$ is divisibe by $x + y$ when n is even.
[**Hint:** (i) For $n = 1$, P(i) is true as $a^1 - b^1$ is divisible by $a - b$.

$\therefore P(m)$ is assume to be true, i.e. $\frac{a^m - b^m}{a - b} = k$

i.e. $a^m = b^m + k(a - b)$ (1)
We shall now prove $P(m + 1)$ is true.
i.e. $a^{m+1} - b^{m+1}$ is divisible by $a - b$.

We write

$$a^{m+1} - b^{m+1} = a^m\, a - b^m.\, b$$
$$= a\,[b^m + k(a-b)] - b^m\, b \text{ from (1)}$$
$$= b^m(a-b) + ak(a-b)$$
$$= (a-b)\,(b^m + ak) \text{ which is divisible by } a-b.$$

Hence $P(m+1)$ is true.

(ii) When $n = 2$

$x^n - y^n = x^2 - y^2$ which is divisible by $x + y$.

$\therefore$ $P(2)$ is true.

$\therefore$ $P(m)$ is true

i.e. $x^m - y^m$ is divisible by $x + y$.

i.e. $x^m - y^m = (x+y)\, f(x, y)$ (1)

where $f(x, y)$ is polynomial of degree m – 1.

We shall now prove the induction step

i.e. $P(m+2)$ holds true.

i.e. $x^{m+2} - y^{m+2}$ is divisible by $x + y$.

We write $x^{m+2} - y^{m+2}$

$$= x^m \cdot x^2 - y^m \cdot y^2$$
$$= [y^m + (x+y)\, f(x, y)]\, x^2 - y^m \cdot y^2$$
$$= y^m\,(x^2 - y^2) + (x+y) \cdot x^2 f(xy)$$
$$= (x+y)\,[y^m(x-y) + x^2 f(x, y)]$$

which is divisible by x + y.

$\therefore$ $P(m+2)$ is correct.

24. (i) For n > 1 prove that $\underline{|n} < \left(\dfrac{n+1}{2}\right)^n$

(ii) For n > 2 prove that $\underline{|n} > 2^{n-1}$

(iii) For n > 2 prove that $2^n \cdot \underline{|n} < n^n$.

25. Prove that for positive integer n the inequality $|\sin nx| \le n\,|\sin x|$ holds true.

26. Prove that for natural number k the equality

$$\sin\frac{\pi}{3} + \sin\frac{2\pi}{3} + \ldots + \sin\frac{k\pi}{3} = 2\sin\frac{k\pi}{6} \cdot \sin\frac{k+1}{6}\pi \text{ holds true.}$$

27. Prove that for every positive a and b and for natural values n the inequality $(a + b)^n \leq 2^n (a^m + b^m)$ holds good.

28. For positive integers n and k prove that

$^{n+1}c_0 - {}^{n+1}c_1 + {}^{n+1}c_2 + \ldots + (-1)^k\, {}^{n+1}c_k$

$= (-1)^k\, {}^nc_k$ holds true where $^mc_0 = 1$ for all m and $^pc_q = 0$ if $q > p$.

29. (i) Prove that $\lfloor 2n < \left(\dfrac{2n+1}{2}\right)^{2n}$

(ii) Prove that the sum of n terms of a geometric progression is $S_1 = \dfrac{a\left(r^n - 1\right)}{r-1}$.

(iii) Prove that for $n > 1$ the relation $\lfloor n = 1.\ 2.\ 3 \ldots n$ holds true.

30. Prove that at any time the total number of persons on the earth who shake hands an odd number of times is even.

[**Hint**: We first assign to each hand shake a number n in natural order i.e. $n = 1, 2, 3 \ldots$.

Then our assertion becomes equivalent to the following: "For every n, after a hand shake with number n, the number of people who have made an odd number of handshakes is even." This assertion clearly depends on n and will be proved by induction. At our convenience we frame two groups of people, group A and group B.

Group A contains those people who have made handshakes an odd number of time and rest people are included in group B.

After the handshake with number $n = 1$, we have two people of group A i.e. an even number of people. Thus the statement holds true for $n = 1$.

Hence the statement holds true for $n = k$ i.e. the number of people of group A is even with number $n = k$.

We shall now prove the statement for $n = k + 1$ i.e. the number of people of group A is even with number $n = k + 1$.

Here there are three conditions: the handshake number $(k + 1)$ will take place between

(i) two people of group A (ii) two people of group B.

(iii) one person of group A and one person of group B.

In the first condition two persons of group A odd one handshake to their odd number of handshakes and becomes the persons of group B.

In the second condition two persons of group B become the persons of group A. In the third condition a person of group A becomes a person of group B and a person of group B becomes a person of group A.

Thus, the number of people of group A either decreases by two, or increases by two or remains unaltered.

In any circumstance the number remains even and the proof is completed.]

31. Prove that for any n the positive numbers $x_1, x_2 \ldots x_n$ which satisfy the conditions $x_1 x_2 \ldots x_n = 1$ the relation $x_1 + x_2 + \ldots + x_n \geq n$ holds true.

[Hint: For $n = 1$ we see that

$x_1 = 1$ since $x_1 x_2 \ldots x_n = 1$

Hence the relation $x_1 + x_2 + \ldots + x_n \geq n$ for $n = 1$ holds true.

We now assume that the relation

$x_1 + x_2 + \ldots + x_n \geq n$ holds good for $n = k$

i.e $x_1 + x_2 + \ldots + x_k \geq k$ (1)

We now proceed to prove that the relation (1) holds true for $n = k + 1$.

If all the numbers $x_1 x_2 \ldots x_k x_{k+1}$ one equal to unity then their algebraic sum is equal to $k + 1$ and then $x_1 + x_2 + \ldots + x_k + x_{k+1} = k + 1$ holds true.

If there is at least one number different from unity among the numbers $x_1 x_2 \ldots x_k, x_{k+1}$ then there is necessarily one more number which is even equal to unity and if one number is larger than 1, then other is definitely smaller than one. For our convenience we assume that $x_k > 1$ and $x_{k+1} < 1$. The product of k numbers of $x_1 x_2 \ldots x_{k-1} x_k x_{k+1}$ is equal to unity since $x_1 x_2 \ldots x_k = 1$ holds true.

$\therefore \quad x_1 + x_2 + ... + x_{k-1} + x_k x_{k+1} \geq k$

$\Rightarrow \quad x_1 + x_2 + ... + x_k x_{k+1} + x_k + x_{k+1} \geq k + x_k + x_{k+1}$

$\Rightarrow \quad x_1 + x_2 + ... + x_{k+1} \geq k + 1 + x_k + x_{k+1} - x_k x_{k+1} - 1$

$\Rightarrow \quad x_1 + x_2 + ... + x_{k+1} \geq (k + 1) + (1 - x_{k+1}) (x_{k-1})$

$\Rightarrow \quad x_1 + x_2 + ... + x_{k+1} \geq k + 1$

Thus (1) is satisfied for $n = k + 1$.]

32. (i) Prove that $v_n = 2^n + 1$ if we are given $v_{n+1} = 3v_n - 2 v_{n-1}$ and $v_0 = 2$ and $v_1 = 3$.

(ii) Prove that $v_n = 2^n - 1$ if we are given $v_{n+1} = 3v_n - 2 v_{n-1}$ and $v_0 = 0$ and $v_1 = 1$.

33. For whole number n prove that

$$\frac{a_n - \sqrt{A}}{a_n + \sqrt{A}} = \left[\frac{a_1 - \sqrt{A}}{a_1 + \sqrt{A}}\right]^{2n-1}$$

34. The terms x_0, x_1, x_2 ... are connected by the equality

$$x_n = \frac{\alpha x_{n-1} + \beta}{\gamma x_{n-1} + \delta}$$

prove that $x_n = \dfrac{x_0}{2nx_0 + 1}$

35. If p is a prime number, prove that $n^p - n$ is divisible by p when n is a natural number greater than 1.

36. Prove that n distinct straight lines drawn in a plane through a point divide the plane into $2n$ parts.

37. For the natural number $\overline{a_n a_{n-1} ... a_1 a_o}$ to be divisible by 5, it is necessary and sufficient that either $a_0 = 0$ or $a_0 = 5$.

38. For the natural number $\overline{a_n a_{n-1} ... a_1 a_o}$ to be divisible by 8 it is necessary and sufficient that $a_2\ a_1\ a_0$ be divisible by 8 where $n \geq 2$.

39. A natural number is divisible by 11 if and only if the difference between the sum of its digits occupying the even places is divisible by 11.

40. If $n \geq 2$ prove that $9\,2\sqrt{n} > 1 + \frac{1}{\sqrt{2}} + \frac{1}{\sqrt{3}} + ... + \frac{1}{\sqrt{n}}$

41. If $n \geq 2$ Prove that $1 + \frac{1}{2} + \frac{1}{3} + ... \frac{1}{2^n - 1} < n$

42. If $n \geq 3$ and $n \in N$ prove that $2^n > 2\,n+1$.

3.11 INTEGERS

We know that operation of subtraction is not always defined in the set of natural numbers and hence for solving problems in equation, mathematicians extended the set of natural numbers. Thus, the entire class of integers consists of all the natural numbers, all the negative numbers and zero and is written as,

$$I = \{0, \pm 1, \pm 2, \pm 3 \; ....\}.$$

3.12 CONSTRUCTION OF INTEGERS: AXIOMATIC APPROACH

If a and b be two natural numbers then

(i) $a - b$ is positive if $a > b$

(ii) $a - b$ is negative if $a < b$

(iii) $a - b$ is zero if $a = b$.

(i) Let (a, b) be an ordered pair of natural numbers and $a > b$ then $a - b = 2, x \in N$.

If $(a, b) \Rightarrow (a - b)$ then $x = (a, b)$ represents a positive integer.

Thus all the ordered pairs (4, 3), (5, 4), (6, 5) represent the same integer i.e. 1.

$\therefore$ There exist a relation $4 + 5 = 3 + 6$ in (4, 3) and (6, 5).

In general (a, b) and (c, d) represent the same positive integer if $(a, b)\ R\ (c, d) \Leftrightarrow a + b = b + c$.

(ii) If (a, b) be a positive integer then $a - b = x$ or $b - a = -x$.

Thus the ordered pair (b, a) represents a negative integer.

In general if $a < b$ and $c < d$ then

$(a, b)\ R\ (c, d) \Leftrightarrow a + d = b + c$

(iii) In the ordered pair (a, b) if $a = b$ then $a - b = 0$ and hence $(a, a), (b, b), (c, c), (3, 3), (4, 4)$ all represent zero.

3.13 PROPERTIES OF INTEGERS

1. The operation of subtraction in integers obeys closure law.
2. The operations of addition and multiplication in integers obey (A) closure law (B) commutative law (C) Associative law and (D) Cancellation law.
3. Zero is the additive identity in the integers. One is the multiplicative identity in the integers.
4. The additive inverse of an arbitrary integer a is $-a$.
   An integer has one and only one additive inverse.
5. The operation of multiplication in integers is distributive on addition and substraction i.e.

   $a \times (b + c) = a \times b + a \times c$

   $a \times (b - c) = a \times b - a \times c$

3.14 EQUIVALENCE RELATION

By virtue of axiomatic approach we conclude that an ordered pair always represent an integer (positive, negative or zero) and hence the set I can be obtained from the set of natural numbers N. We have the following theorem.

Theorem 1: If $N \times N = \{(a, b) : a, b \in N\}$ and $(a, b), (c, d) \in N \times N$ then the relation R is an equivalence relation in $N \times N$, where $(a, b)\ R\ (c, d) \Leftrightarrow a + d = b + c$

Proof: (i) Since $a + b = b + a$

$\therefore (a, b)\ R\ (c, d)$ and hence R is reflexive.

(ii) Let $(a, b), (c, d) \in N \times N$

and $(a, b)\ R\ (c, d) \Rightarrow a + d = b + c$

$\Rightarrow \quad b + c = a + d \Rightarrow c + b = d + a$ (commutative law)

$\Rightarrow \quad (c, d)\ R\ (a, b)$

$\therefore \quad R$ is symmetric.

(iii) Let $(a, b), (c, d)\ (e, f) \in N \times N$ then $(a, b)\ R\ (c, d)$

$\Rightarrow \quad a + d = b + c$ and $(c, d)\ R\ (e, f) \Rightarrow (c + f) = d + e$

$\Rightarrow \quad (a + d) + (c + f) = (b + c) + (d + e)$

$\Rightarrow \quad (a + f) + (c + d) = (b + e) + (c + d)$

$\Rightarrow \quad (a + f) + (b + e) \Rightarrow (a + f) + (e + b)$

$\Rightarrow \quad (a, b)\ R\ (e, f)$

Hence R is transitive and as a result of which R is an equivalence relation is $N \times N$.

Note: From Article 2.20 (v) chapter 2(c) it is known to us that an equivalence relation partitions the set into disjoint classes known as equivalence classes such that any two members of difference classes are non-equivalent where as those of the same classes are equivalent.

If (a, b) is an element of the equivalence classes then the latter is denoted by $[a, b]$ or $\overline{(a, b)}$. $[a, b]$ is the set of all the ordered pairs $(c, d) \in N \times N$. Which are connected with (a, b) by the equivalence relation R.

i.e. $[a, b] = \{(c, d) : (c, d)\ R\ (a, b)\}$.

This equivalence class $[a, b]$ represents one and only one integer x $(a - b = x)$ where x may be positive, negative or zero.

Thus $x = [a, b]$

also
$$1 = [2, 1] = \{(2, 1), (3, 2), (4, 3) \ldots\}$$
$$2 = [3, 1] = \{(3, 1), (4, 2), (5, 3) \ldots\}$$
$$-1 = [1, 2] = \{(1, 2), (2, 3), (3, 4) \ldots\}$$
$$0 = [1, 1] = \{(1, 1), (2, 2), (3, 3) \ldots\}$$

3.15 DEFINITION OF INTEGERS

(i) **Definition of Integers:**

Let (a, b) be an element of $N \times N$ then the equivalence class $[a, b] = \{(c, d) : (c, d)\ R\ (a, b)\ \forall\ c, d \in N\}$ is called an integer where $(a, b)\ R\ (c, d) \Leftrightarrow a + d = b + c$.

(ii) **Set of Integers:**

The set of all the equivalence classes of $N \times N$ defined by R $[(a, b)\ R\ (c, d) \Rightarrow a + d = b + c]$ is known as the set of integers and is denoted by I.

In symbol $x \in I \Leftrightarrow x = [a, b] : a, b \in N$.

Theorem Two integers $[a, b]$ and $[c, d]$ be equal if $a + d = b + c$

Proof: $[a, b] = [c + d] \Rightarrow [a, b]\ R\ [c, d]$

$\Leftrightarrow (a, b)\ R\ (c, d) \Leftrightarrow a + d = b + c.$

3.16 ADDITION OF INTEGERS

(i) **Addition of Integers:**

Let $x = [a, b]$ and $y = [c, d]$

then $x + y = [a, b] + [c, d] = [a + c, b + d]$

Theorems: For any three integers $x, y, z \in I$

1. Closure law hold, true i.e. $x, y \in I \Rightarrow x + y \in I$.
2. Commutative law holds true i.e. $x + y = y + x$.
3. Associative law holds true i.e. $(x + y) + z = x + (y + z)$.
4. Additive identity exists i.e.

   $x + 0 = 0 + x = x \ \forall \ x$.
5. Additive inverse exists i.e.

   $x + (-x) = 0 \ \forall \ x$
6. Cancellation law holds true, i.e.

   $x + x = y + z \Rightarrow x = y$.

Proof 1: Let $x = [a, b], y = [c, d]$

where $a, b, c, d \in N$

then $\quad x + y = [a, b] + [c, d] = [a + c, b + d]$

$\quad = [p, q] \in I; p = a + c \in N$

and $\quad q = b + d \in N$ (closure law in N).

2. $\quad x + y = [a + c, b + d]$ (Addition of integers)

$\quad = [c + a, d + b]$ (commutative law in N)

$\quad = [c, d] + [a, b]$

$\quad = y + x$.

3. If $x = [a, b], y = [c, d]$ and $x = [e, f]$

then $(x + y) + z = ([a, b] + [c, d]) + [e, f]$

$\quad = ([a + c, b + d] + [e, f])$

$\quad = [(a + c) + e, (b + d) + f]$

$\quad = [a + (c + e), b + (d + f)]$

Associative law is addition

$\quad = [a, b] + [c + e, d + f]$

$\quad = [a, b] + ([c, d] + [e, f])$

$\quad = x + (y + z)$

4. If $x = [a, b]$ and $0 = [n, n]$

then $\quad x + 0 = [a, b] + [n, n]$

$$= [a + n, b + n] = [a, b] = x$$

$$= [n + a, n + b] = [n, n] + [a, b] = 0 + x = x.$$

From all $x \in I$ zero is called the additive identity which belongs to I.

5. If $x = [a, b]$ then $-x = [b, a]$

and $\quad x + (-x) = [a, b] + [b, a]$

$$= [a + b, b + a] = [a + b, a + b]$$

$$= [n, n], n = a + b \in N = 0$$

$-x \in I$ is known as additive inverse $\forall\ x \in I$.

6. If $x = [a, b], y = [c, d], z = [e, f]$

then $\quad x + z = y + z$

$\Rightarrow \quad [a, b] + [e, f] = [c + d] + [e + f]$

$\Rightarrow \quad [a + e, b + f] = [c + e, d + f]$

$\Rightarrow \quad (a + e) + (d + f) = (b + f) + (c + e)$

$\Rightarrow \quad (a + d) + (e + f) = (c + b) + (e + f)$

$\Rightarrow \quad a + d = c + b = b + c$

$\Rightarrow \quad [\mathrm{a, b}] = [\mathrm{c, d}]$

$\Rightarrow \quad x = y.$

3.17 SUBTRACTION OF INTEGERS

If $x = [a, b]$ and $y = [c, d]$ then $-y = [d, c]$

Where $x, y \in I$

$$x - y = x + (-y) = [a, b] + [d + c]$$

$$= [a + d, b + c].$$

Similarly $\quad y - x = [b + c, a + d]$

Note: Subtraction is not an independent operation rather it is an addition of special type in which commutative law and associative law are not obeyed.

3.18 MULTIPLICATION OF INTEGERS

If $x = [a, b]$ and $y = [c, d]$

$\therefore \quad x, y = [a, b] \cdot [c, d]$

$$= [ac + bd, ad + bc]$$

3.19 THEOREMS

For any there integers $x, y, z \in I$

1. $x, y \in I \Rightarrow x.y \in I$ (Closure law)
2. $x.y = y.x$ (Commutative law)
3. $(x.y).z = x.(y.z)$ (Associative law)
4. $x.1 = 1.x \quad \forall\, x \in I$ (Multiplicative identity)
5. $x.(y + z) = x.y+x.z$ (Distributive law)
6. $x.0 = 0.x = 0\ \forall\, x \in I$
7. $x.y = 0 \Rightarrow x = 0$ or $y = 0\ \forall\, x, y \in I$
8. $x.\, z = y.z \Rightarrow x = y\ (z \neq 0)$ (Cancellation law)

Proof: 1. If $x = [a, b]$ and $y = [c, d]$

then $x.y = [a, b].\,[c, d]$

$= [ac + bd, ad + bc]$

$= [p, q]$ where $p = ac + bd \in N$

and $q = ad + bc \in N$

2. We have $x.y = [ac + bd, ad + bc]$

$= [ca +ab, cb + da]$

[By the commutative law of additive and multiplication is N]

$= [cd].[a.b] = y.x$

3. If $x = [a, b]$, $y = [c, d]$ and $z = [e, f]$

then $(x.y).z = ([a, b][c, d].\,[e.f])$

$= [ac + bd, ad + bc].[ef]$

$= [(ac + bd)e + (ad + bc)f, (ac + bd)f + b(df + ce)]$

$= [ace + bde + adf + bcf, acf + bdf + ade + bce)]$

$= [a(ce + df) + b(de + cf), a(cf + de) + b(df + ce)]$

$= [a, b].[ce + df, cf + de = [a, b]([c, d].\,[ef])$

$= x.\,(y.z)$

4. If $x = [a, b]$ and $1 = [a + 1, 1]$

then $x.1 = [a, b].[1 + 1, 1] = [a.(1 + 1) + b.1.\,a.1 + b(1 + 1)]$

$= [a + a + b, a + b + b] = [a, b] = x$

(Def. of equality of integers)

$= [1 + 1, 1][a, b]$

$\therefore \quad x.1 = 1.x = x.$

Note: [1 + 1, 1] or [2, 1] is the multiplicative identity is I.

5. If $x = [a, b], y = [c, d]$ and $z\ [e, f]$

then $x.(y + z) = [a, b]. ([c, d] + [e, f])$

$= [a, b][c + e, d + f]$

$= [a\ (c + e) + b(d + f), a(d + f) + b(c + e)]$

$= [ac + ae + bd + bf, ad + af + bc + be]$

$= [(ac + bd) + (ae + bf), (ad + bc) + (af + be)]$

$= [ac + bd, ad + be] + [ae + bf, af + be]$

$= [a, b].[c, d] + [a, b]. [e, f]$

$= xy + xz.$

6. If $x = [a, b]$ and $0 = [1, 1]$ then $x.0 = [a, b]. [1, 1]$

$= a.1 + b.1, a.1 + b.1]$

$= [a + b, a + b] = [n, n]$ where $a + b = n \in N$

$= [1, 1]= 0 = [1, 1].[a, b]$

7. (i) If $x = [a, b]$ and $y = [c, d]$ $\quad a, b, c, d \in N$

When $y = 0, x.y = x.0 = 0$ which holds true.

When $y \neq 0, [c, d] \neq 0$ i.e. $c \neq d$.

The following eases arise here:

(i) $c > d$ i.e. $c = d + p \quad p \in N$

(ii) $c > d$ i.e. $d = e + q \quad q \in N$

where $c = d + p.\ xy = 0 \Rightarrow [a, b]\ [c.d] = 0$

which we can write $[a, b][c, d] = 0 = [1, 1]$

$\Rightarrow \quad [ac + bd, ad + bc] = [1, 1]$

Now substituting $c = d + p$

$a(d + p) + bd = ad + b(d + p)$

$\Rightarrow \quad ad +ap + bd = ad + bd + bp$

$\Rightarrow \quad ap = bp$ (using cancellation law in addition)

$\Rightarrow \quad a = b$

i.e. $\quad [a, b] = [1, 1] = 0 = x$

By substituting $d = c + q$, we can prove $x\ .\ y = 0 \Rightarrow x = 0$.

7.(ii) Let N denoted the set of all natural numbers and R be the relation on $N \times N$ defined by $(a, b)\ R\ (c, d) \Leftrightarrow ad\ (b + c) = bc(a + d)$ check weather R is an equivalence relation on $N \times N$.

(Roorkee 1995)

Solution: $(a, b) \in N \times N \Rightarrow a, b \in N$

where (a, b) is an arbitrary element of $N \times N$.

We have $(a + b) = (b + a)$ by commutivity of addition and $ab = ba$ by commutivity of addition multiplication

Thus $ab(b + a) = ba(a + b)$

$\therefore \quad (a, b)\ R\ (a, b)\ \forall\ (a, b) \in N \times N$

So R is reflexive on $N \times N$

Symmetry let $(a, b), (c, d) \Rightarrow N \times N$ be such that $(a, b)\ R\ (c, d)$

$\therefore \quad ad(b + c) = bc(a + d)$

$\Rightarrow \quad cb(b + a) = da\ (c + b)$

$\Rightarrow (c, d)\ R\ (a, b)$ by commutivity of addition and multiplication

$\therefore$ R is symmetric on $N \times N$

Transitivity let $(a, b), (c, d), (e, f) \in N \times N$

$\therefore\ (a, b)\ R\ (c, d) \Rightarrow ad(b + c) = bc\ (a + d)$

$$\Rightarrow \quad \frac{b+c}{bc} = \frac{a+d}{ad} \quad \Rightarrow \quad \frac{1}{b} + \frac{1}{c} = \frac{1}{a} + \frac{1}{d}. \qquad \text{(A)}$$

and $\quad (c, d)\ R\ (e, f) \quad \Rightarrow \quad cf\ (d + e) = de\ (c + f)$

$$\Rightarrow \quad \frac{d+e}{de} = \frac{c+f}{cf} \quad \Rightarrow \quad \frac{1}{d} + \frac{1}{e} = \frac{1}{c} + \frac{1}{f} \qquad \text{(B)}$$

Adding (A) and (B) we get

$$\frac{1}{b} + \frac{1}{c} + \frac{1}{d} + \frac{1}{e} = \frac{1}{a} + \frac{1}{d} + \frac{1}{c} + \frac{1}{f}$$

$$\Rightarrow \quad \frac{1}{b} + \frac{1}{e} = \frac{1}{a} + \frac{1}{f}$$

$$\Rightarrow \quad \frac{b+e}{be} = \frac{a+f}{af} \Rightarrow af(b + e) = be\ (a + f)$$

$\Rightarrow (a, b)\ R\ (e. f)$

Thus $(a, b)\ R\ (c, d)$ and $(c, d)\ R\ (e, f) \Rightarrow (a, b)\ R\ (e, f)$

$\therefore$ R is transitive on $N \times N$, as a result of which R is an equivalence relation on $N \times N$.

(iii) Let R be a relation on the set of all lines in a plane defined by $(L_1\ L_2) \in R \Leftrightarrow L_1$ is parallel to L_2. Show that R is an equivalence relation.

Solution: For each line $L \in l$ we have $L \mid\mid L \in R \; \forall \; L \in l$

$\Rightarrow R$ is reflexive. Now $L_1, L_2 \in l$ such that $(L_1, L_2) \in R$ then $L_1 \mid\mid L_2 \Rightarrow L_2 \mid\mid L_1 \Rightarrow (L_2 L_1) \in R$.

$\therefore R$ is symmetric.

Also $L_1 L_2 L_3 \in l$ such that $(L_1 L_2) \in R, (L_2 L_3) \in R$

$\therefore (L_1 L_2) \in R$ and $(L_2 L_3) \in R \Rightarrow L_1 \mid\mid L_2$ and $L_2 \mid\mid L_3 \Rightarrow L_1 \mid\mid L_3$

$\Rightarrow (L_1 L_3) \in R \therefore R$ is transitive.

$\therefore R$ is equivalence relation on l.

8. $[x + (-y)].z = xz + (-y)z$

$= yz + (-y)z)$ $\quad (\because xz = yz)$

$= [y + (-y)].z = 0 \,.\, z = 0$

$\therefore \quad [c + (-y)] \,.\, z = 0$

But $z \neq 0$

$\therefore \quad [x + (-y)].z = 0 \Rightarrow x + (-y) = 0$

$\Rightarrow \quad x + (-y) = y + (-y) = 0$

$\therefore \quad x = y$

$\therefore \quad xz = yz \Rightarrow x = y$

3.20 ORDER RELATION IN I

If x and y be two integers the $x - y$ is positive when $x > y$ and $x - y$ is negative when $x < y$

$\therefore \quad x > y \Leftrightarrow y < x$

(ii) $x > y \Rightarrow x + z > y + z$

(iii) $x > y, z > 0 \Rightarrow xz > yz$

(iv) $x > y, y > z \Rightarrow x > z$

(v) (Trichotomy law): For every $x, y \in I$ there is a law viz:

(A) $x = y$, (B) $x > y$ (C) $x < y$.

3.21 ISOMORPHISM OF ALGEBRAIC STRUCTURES

A set with one or more binary operations 3 on a set A which satisfies certain condition is an algebraic structure. Let there be two algebraic structures. (A, o) and (A', o') where o and o' are respectively binary operation is the sets A and A' if f: $A \rightarrow A'$

$$f(aob) = f(a)\, o'\, f(b)$$

where $[a, b \in A, f(a), f(b) \in A']$ is one-one and onto then A and A' are said to be isomorphic with each other. In symbol we write $A \cong A'$. A binary operation 'o' on a non-empty set A is a mapping of $A \times A$ into A.

Theorem: Show that the structures $(N, +, \cdot, >)$ and (I+, +, $\cdot$, >) are isomorphic.

Proof: (a) *One-one and onto mapping.*

Let $f: N \rightarrow I^+$ is a mapping

where $x \in N, f(x) = [n + 1, 1]$ $[n + 1, 1] \in I^+$

Now $\forall\, n \in N, f(n) = [n + 1, 1]$ and $[n + 1, 1]$ is positive i.e. $f(x) \in I^+$ i.e. f is well defined.

Again $m, n \in N$

$$f(m) = f(x) \in [m + 1, 1] = [n + 1, 1]$$

$\Rightarrow \quad m + 1 + 1 = 1 + 1 + n \Rightarrow m = n$

$\therefore \quad f$ is one-one

Let $a \in N$ be an element such that $f(a) = p$ for arbitrary $p \in I^+$, $[m, n] = p, m > n$ and $mn \in N$.

If $m > n$ we can write

$$m = n + a, a \in N$$

on $\quad 1 + m = 1 + n + a$ ...(1)

$\therefore \quad f(a) = [a + 1, 1] = [m, n] = p$

Thus $f: W \rightarrow I^+$ is one-one and onto.

(b) *Isomorphism:*

(i) $(N, +) \cong (1^+, +)$

i.e. $\forall\, m, n \in N\, f(m + n) = f(m) + f(n)$

Since $f(m) + f(n)$

$$\begin{aligned} &= [m + 1, 1] + [n + 1, 1] \\ &= [m + n + 2, 2] \\ &= [m + n + 1, 1] \\ &= f(m + n) \end{aligned}$$

(ii) $(N, \cdot) \cong (I^+, \cdot)$

i.e. $\quad f(m), f(n) = f(m.n)$

Since $\quad f(m).f(n) = [m + 1, 1].[n + 1, 1]$

$$\begin{aligned} &= [(m + 1)(n + 1) + 1, (m + 1) + (n + 1)] \\ &= [mn + m + n + 1 + 1, m + n + 1 + 1] \end{aligned}$$

$$= [(mn + 1) + (m + n + 1), 1 + (m + n + 1)]$$
$$= [mn + 1, 1] = f(m\,n)$$

(iii) $(N, > \cong (I^+, >))$

i.e. $f(m) > f(n) \Leftrightarrow m > n$

Since $f(m) > f(n) \Leftrightarrow [m + 1, 1] > [n + 1, 1]$

$\Leftrightarrow \quad [m + 1, 1] - [n + 1, 1] > 0$

$\Leftrightarrow \quad [m + 1, 1] + [1, n + 1] > 0$

$\Leftrightarrow \quad [m + 2, n + 2] > 0$

$\Leftrightarrow \quad (m + 2) - (n + 2) > 0$

$\Leftrightarrow \quad m > n.$

3.22 THEOREM

If $x, y, z \in I$ prove that

(i) $(x + z) - (y + z) = x - y$

(ii) $(x - z) + (y - z) = x - z$ [U.P.B. 1978]

(iii) $(x + z) - (y + z) = x - y$ [U.P.B. 1980, 1982]

(iv) $(x + z) - (y + z) = x - y$ [U.P.B. 1976, 1982, 1984]

(v) $(x + z) - (y + z) = x - y$ [U.P.B. 1978, 1983, 1984]

Proof: Let $x = [a, b]$; $y = [c, d]$ and $z = (e, f)$

(i) $(x + z) - (y - z)$

$$= ([a, b] + [e, f]) - ([c, d] + [e, f])$$
$$= [a + e, b + f] - [c + e, d + f]$$
$$= [a + e, b + f] + [d + f, c + e]$$
$$= [a + e + d + f, b + f + c + e]$$
$$= [a + d + e + f, b + c + e + f]$$
$$= [a + b, b + c] = [a, b] + [dc]$$

(cancellation law in addition)

$$= [a, b] - [c, d] = x - y$$

(ii) $(x - y) + (y - z)$

$$= \{x + (-y)\} + \{y + (-z)\}$$
$$= ([a, b] + [d + c] + [c, d] + [f, e])$$
$$= [a + d, b + c] + [c + f, d + e]$$
$$= [a + d + c + f, b + c + d + e]$$
$$= [a + f + c + d, b + e + c + d]$$

$$= [a+f, b+e] = [a, b] + [f+e]$$
$$= [a, b] - [e, f] = x - y$$

(iii) $(-x) + (-y) = [b, a] + [d, c]$
$$= [b+d, a+c] \qquad ...(A)$$

But $x + y = [a, b] + [c, d] = [a+c, b+d]$

$\therefore \quad -(x+y) = [b+d, a+c] \qquad ...(B)$

From (A) and (B) the result follows

(iv) $(-x) \cdot (-y) = [b, a] \cdot [d, c]$
$$= [bd + ac, bc + ad]$$
$$= [ac + bd, ad + bc]$$
(commutative law in addition)
$$= [a, b] \cdot [c, d] = x \cdot y$$

(v) $(-x)y = [b, a][c, d] = [bc + ad, bd + ac]$
$$x(-y) = [a, b]\,[d, c] = [ad + bc, ac + bd]$$
$$x \cdot y = [a, b][c, d] = [ac + bd, ad + bc]$$
$$-(x \cdot y)\,[ad + bc, ac + bd]$$

Thus $\quad (-x)\,y = x\,(-y) = -(x \cdot y)$

3.23 DIVISION WITH REMAINDER

To divide an integer a by *a* natural number m with a remainder means to find two integers q and r such that the relation $a = mq + r$ holds true where r satisfies the condition $0 \leq r < m$. If $r = 0$ then we can say that the integer a is exactly divisible by the natural number m.

Theorem: If a be an integer and m a natural number, then there is a unique pair of integers q and r which satisfies the conditions.

$$a = mq + r \text{ and } 0 \leq r < m.$$

We omit the proof of this theorem. We shall use the following prepositions:

(A) 1. If a divides a product c and is prime to b. Then it will divide the factor c.

2. If a is prime and it divides a product $bcd...$, then a must divide one of the factor of the product.

3. If a is prime to each of b and c then it is also prime to the product bc.

4. If a and b are prime to each other, then every positive integral power of a is also prime to every positive integral power of b.

We now state some general theorem without explanations and proofs:

(B) 1. The number of primes is infinite.

2. No rational algebraical formula can represent prime numbers only. In other words, no general formula for the primes has been presented as yet.

3. A number can be resolved into prime factors is only one way.

(C) We now state some theorems with explanations and proofs.

1. Prove that the number of divisions of an composite number $N = a^p b^q c^r$ .... where a, b, c are different prime numbers and p, q, r .... are positive integers is given by the formula $(p + 1)(q + 1)(r + 1)$ ..... which includes both unity and number itself as division.

Proof: We have $N = a^p b^q c^r$ ..... In order to obtain the formula for the number of divisions of N we consider the following expression $(1 + a + a^2 + ... + a^p)(1 + b + b^2 + ... + b^q)(1 + c + c^2 + ... + c^r)$ .....

We see that each term of the product in the aforesaid expression is a division of the given number N. There does not exist any other number which may divide N.

Thus the no. of divisions is $(p + 1)(q + 1)(r + 1)$ ....

(Since the number of terms is each bracket or parentheses exceeds the highest power of primes by one.)

1 is a term of the product and the number $N = a^p b^q c^r$ .... is also a term of the product and hence they are included in $(p + 1)(q + 1)(r + 1)$ ....

2. Prove that the numebr of ways in which the number $N = a^p b^q c^r$ .... (where N is a composite number, a, b, c, ... are different prime numbers and p, q, r ... are positive integers) can be resolved into two factors is given by $\frac{1}{2}(p + 1)(q + 1)(r + 1)$ ..... N is not a perfect square and at least one of the p, q, r ... is an odd number.

3. Prove that the no. of ways in which the numebr $N = a^p b^q c^r$ .... (N is a perfect square) can be resolved into two factor is

$$\frac{1}{2}\{(p+1)(q+1)(r+1) \ldots + 1\}$$

We omit the proofs of (2) and (3).

3.24 IMPORTANT THEOREM

(1) To find the number of ways in which a composite number $N = a^p b^q c^r$ .... can be resolved into two factor which are prime to each other.

Suppose $N = a^p b^q c^r$ .... and let the two factors be F_1 and F_2 then one of F_1 and F_2 contains a^p, otherwise some power of a be in F_1 and some in F_2 and as a result of which two factors F_1 and F_2 can never be prime to each other. The same logic exists for a^p and c^r i.e. b^q occurs in one of F_1 and F_2.

The number of ways in which the product abc ..... can be resolved into two factors is given by $\frac{1}{2}[(1+1)(1+1)(1+1) \ldots]$

$\frac{1}{2}[2^n] = 2^{n-1}$, where n is the numebr of different primes in N.

2. To find the sum of the division of a numebr.

Suppose $N = a^p b^q c^r$ ....

Each term of the product $(1 + a + a^2 + \ldots + a^p)(1 + b + b^2 + \ldots + b^q)(1 + c + c^2 + \ldots + c^r)$ .... is a division of N and hence the sum is

$$\frac{a^{p+1}-1}{a-1} \cdot \frac{b^{q+1}-1}{b-1} \cdot \frac{c^{r+1}-1}{c-1}$$

3. To find the highest power of prime number a which is contained in $\underline{|n}$.

Denote the greatest integer contained in $\frac{n}{a}, \frac{n}{a^2}, \frac{n}{a^3}$..... by

$I\left(\frac{n}{a}\right), I\left(\frac{n}{a^2}\right), I\left(\frac{n}{a^3}\right)$.....

Now among the numebrs 1, 2, 3, ... n there exist

$I\left(\frac{n}{a}\right)$ which contain a at least once vizi a, $2a$, $3a$ ...

Similarly there exist $I\left(\frac{n}{a^2}\right)$ Which contain a^2 at least among the numbers 1, 2, 3 .... n and so on.

Hence the highest power of a contained in 1, 2, 3 .... n. i.e.

is $\lfloor n$ is $I\left(\frac{n}{a}\right)+I\left(\frac{n}{a^2}\right)+I\left(\frac{n}{a^3}\right)+\ldots$

4. **Fermat's Theorem:** If n is a prime number and N is prime to n, then prove that $N^{n-1}-1$ is a multiple of n.

Proof: In order to prove Fermat's Theorem we have to prove a theorem which states:

"If n is a prime number prove that $(a + b + c + d + ...)^n = a^n + b^n + c^n + d^n + ... + M(n)$

where the symbol $M(n)$ represents a multiple of n.

Substitute β for $b + c + d +$ ..... in $(a + b + c + d + ...)^n$ and obtain lets L.H.S. as

$$(a + \beta)^n = a^n + \beta^n + M(n)$$

Again $\beta n = (b + c + d + ...)^n = (b + y)^n$

$$= b^n + y^n + M(n)$$

Proceeding in this way? we obtain the result is R.H.S. as

$a^n + b^n + c^n + d^n + ... + M(n)$

Thus we have

$$(a + b + c + d + ...)^n = a^n + b^n + c^n + d^n + ... + M(n) \quad ...(1)$$

Put $a = b = c = d = ... = 1$ and assume that they are N in numbers, then

$$N^n = N + M(n) \quad \text{[from (1)]}$$

$\Rightarrow \quad N^n - N = M(n) \quad \Rightarrow N(N^{n-1} - 1) = M(n)$

Since N is prime to n hence $N^{n-1} - 1$ is a multiple of n. Thus we prove the Fermat's theorem.

Note: n is prime $\quad \therefore n - 1$ is even, except when $n = 2$

$\therefore \quad N^{n-1} - 1 = M(n)$

$$\Rightarrow \quad \left(N\frac{n-1}{2}\right)^2 - (1)^2 = M(n)$$

$$\Rightarrow \quad \left(N\frac{n-1}{2}+1\right)\left(N\frac{n-1}{2}+1\right) = M(n)$$

Hence either $N\frac{n-1}{2}+1$ or $N\frac{n-1}{2}-1$ is a multiple of n.

When $N\frac{n-1}{2}+1 = K_n$, then $N\frac{n-1}{2} = K_n - 1$.

When $N\frac{n-1}{2}-1 = K_n$ then $N\frac{n-1}{2} = K_n - 1$

$$\therefore \quad N\frac{n-1}{2} = K_n \pm 1$$

Note: While proving fermat's theorem we saw $N^n - N = M(n)$, whether N is prime to n or not this result $N^n - N = M(n)$ is found more valuable than fermat's theorem in solving problems.

Some worked out problems:

If n is odd prove that $n^5 - n$ is divisible by 240.

Solution: We have $n^5 - n = n(n^4 - 1) = (n-1) \cdot n. (n+1)(n^2+1)$

Since n is odd therefore $(n-1)$ and $(n+1)$ are even.

$(n-1)\ n+1)$ are three consecutive numbers hence one of them is divisible by 3. Among the even numbers $(n-1)(n+1)$ one of them is divisible by 2 and other by 4 as they are consecutive even numbers.

Thus $(n-1). n. (n+1)$ is divisible by $2 \cdot 3 \cdot 4$ i.e. by 24.

In $n^5 - n$ since 5 is a prime number

$\therefore \quad n^5 - n \qquad \therefore n^5 - n = M(5)$

$\therefore \quad n^5 - n = (n-1) \cdot n\ (n+1) \cdot (n^2+1)$ is divisible by 5 also.

Since n is odd $\therefore n^2 + 1$ is even hence $n^2 + 1$ is divisible by 2

$\therefore \quad n^5 - n$ is divisible by $2 \cdot 3 \cdot 4 \cdot 5 \cdot 2 = 240$.

2. If x and y are positive and if $x - y = 2k$ where $k = 0, 1, 2, 3$; prove that $x^2 - y^2$ is a multiple of 4.

Solution: We have $x^2 - y^2 = (x - y)(x + y)$

$$= 2k(x + x - 2k) \ [\therefore x - y = 2k]$$

$\Rightarrow x^2y^2 = 4k(x - k)$ which is a multiple of 4.

3. If $4x - y$ is a multiple of 3, show that $4x^2 + 7xy - 2y^2$ is divisible by 9.

Solution: Put $4x - y = 3k$

$$\therefore \quad 4x^2 + 7xy - 2y$$
$$= 4x^2 + 8xy - xy - 2y$$
$$= 4x(x + 2y) - y(x + 2y)$$
$$= (4x - y)(x + 2y)$$
$$= 3k[x + 2(4x - 3k)] = 3k[9x - 6k]$$
$$= 9k(3x - 2k) \text{ which is divisible by 9.}$$

4. Prove that $n(n + 1)(n + 5)$ is a multiple of 6.

Solution: The expression $n(n + 1)(n + 5)$ can be written as

$$n(n + 1)(n + 5) = n(n + 1)[n + 2 + 3]$$
$$= n(n + 1)(n + 2) + 3n(n + 1)$$

Now n, $(n + 1)$, $(n + 2)$ are three consecutive number and hence one of them is divisible by 3.

If n is odd then $(x + 1)$ is even and $(x + 2)$ is odd

In this case $(n + 1)$ is divisible by 2.

$\therefore \quad n(n + 1)(n + 2)$ is divisible by 6.

$3n(n + 1)$ is also divisible by 6.

$\therefore \quad n(n + 1)(x + 5) = n(n + 1)(n + 2) + 3n(n + 1)$ is a multiple of 6.

If n is even then $n + 2$ is also even and $(n + 1)$ is odd. In this case $n(n + 1)(n + 2)$ and $3n(n + 1)$ one also divisible by 6.

$\therefore \quad n(n + 1)(n + 5) = M(6)$.

5. Prove that 8th power of any number is of the form $17n$ or 17 ± 1.

Solution: If N is not prime to 17 then

$$N^8 = 17n \qquad \text{...(1)}$$

If N is prime to 17 then according to Fermat's theorem

$$N^{16} - 1 = M(17)$$

$\Rightarrow (N^8 - 1)(N^8 + 1) = M(17)$

$$\Rightarrow \qquad N^8 = M(17) + 1$$

or $$N^8 = M(17) - 1$$

$$\therefore \qquad N^8 = 17n \pm 1 \text{ Proved.}$$

6. If n, $n + 2$ and $n + 4$ are primes find n.

Solution: One out of the three consecutive number n, $n + 1$, $n + 2$ must by divisible by 3. Thus either $n = 3$ or $n + 1$ is divisible by 3. The latter condition is not proper as $n + 4 = n + 1 + 3$ can never be prime since $n + 1$ is divisible by 3.

7. In how many ways can the number 7056 be resolved into two factors

Solution: $7056 = (4 \times 21)^2$ which is a perfect square and hence the number of ways in which the number $N = 7056$ can be resolved into two factors is given by the

Formula $\frac{1}{2}\{(p + 1)(q + 1)(r + 1) \ldots + 1\}$

Here $N = 7056 = (4 \times 21)^2 = 2^4 \times 3^2 \times 7^2$

$\therefore$ the required number is $\frac{1}{2}\{(4 + 1)(2 + 1)(2 + 1) + 1\}$

$$= \frac{1}{2}\{5 \times 3 \times 3 + 1\} = 23.$$

8. Find the no. of divisible in 420.

Solution: $420 = 2^2 \times 3 \times 5 \times 7$

$\therefore$ No. of divisible in 420 is $(2 + 1)(1 + 1)(1 + 1)(1 + 1)$

$$= 3 \cdot 2 \cdot 2 \cdot 2 = 24$$

24 includes the unity and the number itself. If the unity is left then the factors of 420 be 23.

9. Find the number of divisors of 2520. Also compute their sum.

Solution: We have $2520 = 2^3 \times 3^2 \times 5 \times 7$ and therefore the number of divisors of 2520 is $(3 + 1)(2 + 1)(1 + 1)(1 + 1)$ i.e. $4 \cdot 3 \cdot 2 \cdot 2$ i.e. 48.

In order to compute the sum of the divisors of 2520 we frame an expression as follows:

$$(1 + 2 + 2^2 + 3^2)(1 + 3 + 3^2)(1 + 5)(1 + 7).$$

Each term of the product of this expression is a divisor of $N = 2520$.

The sum of this divisors is therefore

$$\frac{2^4-1}{2-1} \cdot \frac{3^3-1}{3-1} \cdot (1+5)(1+7)$$

$$= 15 \cdot 13 \cdot 8 \cdot 6 = 9360$$

The sum also be computed as $\frac{2^4-1}{2-1} \cdot \frac{3^3-1}{3-1} \cdot \frac{7^2-1}{7-1} \cdot \frac{5^2-1}{5-1}$

$$= 15 \cdot \frac{26}{2} \cdot \frac{48}{6} \cdot \frac{24}{4} = 15 \cdot 13 \cdot 8 \cdot 6 = 9360$$

10. Show that $n^5 - n$ is divisible by 30.

Solution: In $n^5 - n$ we see 5 is prime and hence $n^5 - n = M(5)$ i.e. $n^5 - n$ is a multiple of 5.

Now $n^5 - n = n(n^4 - 1) = n(n + 1)(n - 1)(n^2 + 1)$ $n(n + 1)(n - 1)$ is always divisible by $3 \cdot 2$ i.e. by 6 if n is even or odd.

$\therefore n^5 - n$ is divisible by $6 \times 5 = 30$.

11. How many zeros are there of the end at the product of all natural numbers from 1 to 1962 inclusive.

Solution: Let $N = 1 \cdot 2 \cdot 3 \cdot 4 \ldots 1961 \cdot 1962$

$$= 2^a \times 3^b \times 5^c$$

Each pair of prime factors 2 and 5 generate one zero in N since $2 \times 5 = 10$.

Now we proceed to compute the values of a and c.

The value of c is the integral quotient of $\frac{1962}{5}$ + integral quotient of $\frac{1962}{5^2}$ + the integral quotient of $\frac{1962}{5^3}$ + the integral quotient of $\frac{1962}{5^4}$. [See Art. 3.24 (3)]

Thus $c = 39^2 + 78 + 15 + 3 = 488$

The value of a is similarly the sum of the integral quotient of

$$\frac{1962}{2}, \frac{1962}{2^2}, \frac{1962}{2^3}, \frac{1962}{2^4}, \frac{1962}{2^5}, \frac{1962}{2^6}, \frac{1962}{2^7}, \frac{1962}{2^8}, \frac{1962}{2^9}, \frac{1962}{2^{10}}$$

Thus $a = 981 + 490 + 245 + 122 + 61 + 30 + 15 + 7 + 3 + 1 = 1955$

Hence we conclude that only 488 pairs of the primes 2 and 5 generate zero.

Thus N ends in 488 zero.

12. Find the last digit of $3^{3^{4n}}$

Solution: 3^{4^n} can be written as

$$3^{4n} = [3^4]^n = (81)^n = (80+1)^n$$
$$= c_0 80^n + c_1 80^{n-1} + c_2 80^{n-2} + \dots + c_{n-1} 80 + 1$$
$$= 4\,[4^{n-1} 20^n + n.\, 4^{n-2}.\, 20^{n-1} + \dots c_{n-1}.\, 20] + 1$$
$$= 4m + 1, \text{ where } m \text{ is a positive integer.}$$

Thus $$3^{3^{4n}} = 3^{4m+1} = 3^{4m}.\, 3$$
$$= (81)^m.\, 3$$

Any power of 81 gives 1 in the but which when multiplied by 3 gives three in the last.

13. Find the last digit of $9^{(9^9)}$.

Solution: We know that even power of 9 can be expressed in the term of 81 as

$$9^{2n} = (81)^n = 81.\, 81 \dots .81$$

where 81 has been written n times. This shows that is 9^{2n} the last digit is 1. Every odd power of 9 has 9 as its last digit and hence $9^{(9^9)}$ has 9 as its last digit as 9^{9^9} is an odd power of 9 i.e. 9^{81}.

14. If $N = \underline{|1962}$, find the sum of

$$\frac{1}{\log_2^N} + \frac{1}{\log_3^N} + \frac{1}{\log_4^N} + \dots + \frac{1}{\log_{1962}^N}.$$

Substituting $\log_2 N = x$ we have

$$2x = N \Rightarrow x \log 2 = \log N \Rightarrow \frac{1}{x} = \frac{1}{\log_2 N} = \frac{\log 2}{\log N}$$

$$\text{Hence } \frac{1}{\log_2 N} + \frac{1}{\log_3 N} + \frac{1}{\log_4 N} + \dots + \frac{1}{\log_{1962} N}$$

$$= \frac{\log 2}{\log N} + \frac{\log 3}{\log N} + \frac{\log 4}{\log N} + \ldots \frac{\log \lfloor 1962}{\log N}$$

$$= \frac{\log(2 \cdot 3 \cdot 4 \ldots 1962)}{\log N} = \frac{\log \lfloor 1962}{\log \lfloor 1962} = 1$$

15. Find the number of integers from 1 to 100 which are divisible by 2 or 5.

Solution: No. of integers from 1 to 100 divisible by 2 is 2, 4, 6 ... 100 = 50 i.e. [100 = 2 + $(n - 1)$. 2]

No of integers form 1 to 100 divisible by 5 is 5, 10, 15 ... 100 = 20 i.e. [100 = 5 + $(n - 1)$. 5]

No. of integers from 1 to 100 divisible by 2 and 5 is 10, 20 ... 100 = 10

∴ Required no. is 50 + 20 – 10 = 60.

16. Prove that $\underbrace{111\ldots1}_{2n \text{ times}} - \underbrace{222\ldots2}_{n \text{ times}}$ is the square of an integer for any natural number n.

Solution: $\underbrace{111\ldots1}_{2n \text{ times}} - \underbrace{222\ldots2}_{n \text{ times}}$

$$= \frac{1}{9}[\underbrace{999\ldots9}_{2n \text{ times}}] - \frac{2}{9}[\underbrace{999\ldots9}_{n \text{ times}}]$$

$$= \frac{1}{9}[10^{2n} - 1] - \frac{2}{9}[10^n - 1]$$

(Since $9 = 10 - 1$; $99 = 10^2 - 1$; $999 = 10^3 - 1$ ... and so on)

$$= \frac{1}{9}[10^{2n} - 1 - 2 \cdot 10^n + 2]$$

$$= \frac{1}{9}[10^{2n} - 2 \cdot 10^n + 1] = \frac{1}{9}[10^n - 1]^2$$

$$= \left(\frac{10^n - 1}{3}\right)^2 = \left[\underbrace{999\ldots9}_{n \text{ times}}\Big/3\right]^2$$

$$= \left[\underbrace{333\ldots3}_{n \text{ times}}\right]^2 \text{ square of an integer.}$$

3.25 RATIONAL NUMBERS

For making the division possible always in the set of natural numbers we introduce new numbers called fractions (parts of natural numbers). We extend the set of natural numbers when we make subtraction always possible in it. A fraction is also defined as an ordered pair of integers (p, q) of the form p/q when $p, q \in I$ and $q \neq 0$. If $p < q$, then p/q is a proper fraction and if $p > q$ then it is an improper fraction. The idea of different number was formed under the influence of needs.

We define the set of rational numbers as follows: "Numbers of the form p/q, where q is a natural number and p is an integer form a set of rational number".

Rational numbers are usually denoted by Q. The set of rational number contains the natural numbers, all the positive fractions and zero and also all the negative integers *l* fractions. We can write every rational number either as a finite decimal or as an infinite decimal with an indefinitely repeating finite group of digits, both types of decimals being referred to as periodic decimals. An irrational number is expressed as a non-terminating non-periodic decimal fraction. π, e, $\sqrt{2}, \sqrt{3}, \sqrt{5}$ ... are the examples of irrational numbers.

We express the set of rational numbers as

$$Q = \{x: x = p/q; p, q \in I, \text{ and } q \neq 0\}.$$

1. Construction of Rational Numbers and Axiomatic Approach:

We frame two sets I and I_0. I is the set of integers and I_0 the set of non-zero integers. The product $I \times I_0$ is the set of pairs of integers (p, q) where $q \neq 0$. We define now the binary relation R in the set of $I \times I_0$ as $(p, q)\ R\ (m, n)$ if and only if $pn = qm$ $[p, m \in I$ and $q, n \in I_0]$.

2. Binary Relation R in the Set of $I \times I_0$ is an Equivalence Relation:

(i) *Symmetry:* $(p, q)\ R\ (m, n) \Rightarrow pn = qm \Rightarrow mq = np \Rightarrow (m, n)\ R\ (p, q)$. Thus we see that R is symmetric.

(ii) *Reflexivity:* $(p, q)\ R\ (p, q)$ since $pq = pq$

hence R is reflexive.

(iii) *Transitivity:* $(p, q)\ R\ (m, n)$ and $(m, n)\ R\ (r, s)$

$\Rightarrow \quad p\,n = q\,m$ and $m\,s = nr$.

Multiplying these two $pmns = qmnr$

$\Rightarrow \quad (p\,s)\,(m\,n) = (q\,r)\,(m\,n)$

$\Rightarrow \quad p\,s = q\,r$ if $r \neq 0$

$\Rightarrow (p, q)\ R\ (r, s)$ hence R is transitive. From (i) (ii) and (iii) we conclude that R is an equivalence relation and hence it separates the set into disjoint classes. The class whose members are equivalent to (p, q) is denoted by p/q and equivalence classes like $[p, q]$ represent the rational numbers $x = p/q$.

We now define a rational number as follows:

If $(q, p) \in I \times I_0$ then the equivalence class $[p, q]$ $= \{(m, n); n \neq 0: (m, n)\ R\ (p, q)\}$ is a rational number where $(p, q)\ R, (m, n) \Rightarrow pn = qm$.

If x be an element of the set of rational numbers Q, then $x \in Q \Rightarrow x = [p, q], p \in I$ and $q \in I_0$.

Thus $\frac{2}{1} \in Q = [4, 2] = \{(4, 2), (8, 4), (-4, -2), (-8, -4) \ldots\}$

In general $[p, q] = \{(px, qx): x \in I_0\}$.

Equality of Two Rational Number:

Two rational numbers $[p, q]$ and $[m, n]$ are equal when $(p, q)\ R\ (m, n)$ i.e. $pn = qm$.

4. The General Laws of Addition and Multiplication of Rational Number:

(i) *Closure law:* The addition and multiplication of two rational numbers are rational numbers.

(ii) *Commutative law:* This law also holds good in addition and multiplication of rational numbers.

(iii) *Associative law:* The associative law holds good in addition and multiplication of rational numbers.

(iv) There in an additive identity $\frac{0}{1}$ or 0 in Q. There in also an additive inverse $\frac{-p}{q}$ of $\frac{p}{q}$ in Q.

(v) There is a multiplicative identity $\frac{1}{1}$ or 1 in Q.

There is also a multiplicative inverse x^{-1} of $x \in Q$ in the set of rational numbers.

Some worked out examples and theorems

Example 1. If $x, y, z \in Q$ prove that

(A) $x + y = y + x$

(B) $x + (y + z) = (x + y) + z$

(C) $x + z = y + z \Rightarrow x = y$ and $z + x = z + y \Rightarrow x = y$.

Solution: Let $x = \frac{p}{q}$; $y = \frac{m}{n}$ and $z = \frac{r}{s}$

(A) $$x + y = \frac{p}{q} + \frac{m}{n} = \frac{pn + qm}{qn} = \frac{mq + np}{nq} \frac{m}{n} + \frac{p}{q} = y + x$$

(B) $$x + (y + z) = \frac{p}{q} + \left(\frac{m}{r} + \frac{r}{s}\right) = \frac{p}{q} + \left(\frac{ms + rn}{ns}\right)$$

$$= \frac{pns + msq + rnq}{qns} = \left(\frac{pns + msq}{qns}\right) + \frac{rnq}{qns}$$

$$= \left(\frac{p}{q} + \frac{m}{n}\right) + \frac{r}{s} \ (x + y) + z.$$

(C) Do yourself.

Theorem 1. Prove that the additive inverse of any element $x \in Q$ is unique.

Proof: Let there be two additive inverses x_1 and x_2 of an element $x \in Q$, where $x_1 \in Q$ and $x_2 \in Q$, then

$$x + x_1 = 0 \text{ and } x + x_2 = 0$$

Now we write $x_1 = x_1 + 0 = x_1 + (x + x_2)$ ($\therefore x + x_2 = 0$)

$\therefore$ $$x_1 = (x_1 + x) + x_2 = (x + x_1) + x_2$$

$$= 0 + x_2 \ (\therefore x + x_1 = 0) = x_2$$

Thus, the additive inverses x_1 and x_2 are the same and as a result of which we are bound to conclude that the additive inverse of any element is unique.

Example 2. If $x, y, z \in Q$ prove that

(A) $x \cdot y = y \cdot x$

(B) $x \cdot (y \cdot z) = (x \cdot y) \cdot z$

(C) $x \cdot z = y \cdot z \Rightarrow x = y$ and $z \cdot x = z \cdot y$.

$\Rightarrow \quad x = y$ where $z \neq 0$.

Proof: Let $x = \frac{p}{q}, y = \frac{m}{n}$ and $z = \frac{r}{s}$

Where $p, q, m, n, r, s \in I$.

(A) $x \cdot y = \frac{p}{q} \cdot \frac{m}{n} = \frac{pm}{q \cdot n} = \frac{mp}{nq} = \frac{m}{n} \cdot \frac{p}{q} = y \cdot x$

(B) $x \cdot (y \cdot z) = \frac{p}{q} \cdot \left(\frac{m}{n} \cdot \frac{r}{s}\right) = \frac{p}{q}\left(\frac{mr}{ns}\right)$

$$= \frac{pmr}{qns} = \frac{pm}{qn} \cdot \frac{r}{s} = \left(\frac{p}{q} \cdot \frac{m}{n}\right) \cdot \frac{r}{s} = (x \cdot y).\ z.$$

(C) Do yourself.

Theorem 2. The multiplicative inverse of any element $x \in Q$ is unique where $x \neq 0$.

Proof: Let there be two multiplicative inverses x_1 and x_2 of any element $x \in Q$ where x_1 and $x_2 \in Q$, then

$x \cdot x_1 = 1_Q$ and $x \cdot x_2 = 1_Q$

where 1_Q is the identity for multiplication.

Now $x_1 = x_1 \cdot 1_Q = x_1 \cdot (x \cdot x_2) = (x_1 \cdot x) \cdot x_2$

$= 1_Q\, x_2 = x_2$

Hence the multiplicative inverse of any element $x \in Q$ is unique.

Example 3. If $x_1\ y_1\ z \in Q$, then

(A) $x \cdot (y + z) = x \cdot y + x \cdot z$

(B) $(y + z).\ x = y.\ x + x.\ z$

Proof: Let $x = \frac{p}{q}, y = \frac{m}{n}$ and $z = \frac{r}{s}$

where $p, q, m, n, r, s \in I$.

(A) $$x.(y+z)=\frac{p}{q}\cdot\left(\frac{m}{n}+\frac{r}{s}\right)=\frac{p}{q}\left(\frac{ms+rn}{ns}\right)$$

$$=\frac{pms+prn}{qns}=\frac{pqms+pqrn}{qnqs}$$

$$=\frac{pqms}{qnqs}+\frac{pqrn}{qnqs}=\frac{pm}{qn}+\frac{pr}{qs}\left(\frac{p}{q}\cdot\frac{m}{n}\right)+\left(\frac{p}{q}\cdot\frac{r}{s}\right)$$

$$=x\cdot y+x\cdot z.$$

(B) Do yourself.

3.26 (I) ADDITION AND MULTIPLICATION OF RATIONAL NUMBERS

The sum over the set Q of rational numbers is defined as

$$x+y=\frac{p}{q}+\frac{m}{n}=\frac{pn+qm}{qn}\quad[pn+qm, qn]$$

where $x=[p,q]$ and $y=[m,n]$

This operation on the set Q is well defined.

The product over the set Q of rational numbers is defined as

$$xy=\frac{p}{q}\cdot\frac{m}{n}=\frac{pm}{qn}\quad[pm, qn]$$

where $x=[p,q]$ and $y=[m,n]$

This operation or the set Q is well defined.

(II) SUBTRACTION AND DIVISION OF RATIONAL NUMBERS

If x and y are two rational numbers then $x-y=x+(-y)$ $=[p,q]+[-m,n]=[pn-qm, qn]$

Note: y denotes the additive inverse of y.

$x\div y=x\,y^{-1}$ where y^{-1} denotes the multiplicative inverse of y.

It is important to mention have that these operations are neither associative nor commutative but the product is distributive with respect to subtraction. We can define the division in rational number also as: — A rational number p/q is said to be divisible by $\frac{m}{n}$ if there is a rational number $\frac{r}{s}$ such that $\frac{p}{q} = \frac{m}{n} \cdot \frac{r}{s}$.

This definition gives $\frac{r}{s} = \frac{pn}{qm}$ where q and $m \neq 0$ i.e. rational number $\frac{p}{q}$ is divisible by a non-zero rational number $\frac{m}{n}$ and the quotient $\frac{r}{s}$ is a rational number.

3.27 ZERO, POSITIVE AND NEGATIVE RATIONAL NUMBERS

(i) The rational number $(0, q)$ such that $q \neq 0$ is defined as rational zero and is denoted by 0_Q where $0 \in I$. This rational number may also be denoted as equivalence clause $[0, q]$, $q \in 0_Q$.

Thus [0, 1], [0, 2], [0, 3], [0, –2] are the examples of rational number zero.

(ii) Let $x = [p, q] \neq 0$ be a rational number ($p \neq 0$ and $q \neq 0$) then $[a, b]$ is positive or negative according as

$ab > 0$ or $ab < 0$

Theorem: The sum and the product of two rational numbers are always positive.

Proof: Let $x = [p, q]$ and $y = [m, n]$ be the positive rational numbers and hence $pq > 0$ and $mn > 0$ and therefore $x + y = [p, q] + [m, n] = [pn + qm, qn]$.

But the rational number $[pn + qm, qn] = [qn(pn + qm), q^n n^2]$ $= [pqn^2 + mnq^2, q^2 n^2]$ is a clearly greater than zero since $pq > 0$, $mn > 0$, $n^2 > 0$, $q^2 > 0$ and $q^2 n^2 > 0$.

$\therefore x + y = [pn + qm, qn] > 0$.

Now $x \cdot y = [p, q] \cdot [m, n] = [pm, qn]$.

But $(pm)(qn) = (pq)(mn) > 0$

$\therefore x \cdot y > 0$.

3.28 ORDER RELATION IS THE SET OF RATIONAL NUMBERS

Let x and y be two rational numbers, the

(i) $x > y \Rightarrow x - y$ is positive

i.e. $[p, q] > [m, n] \Leftrightarrow pn > qm$

(ii) $x < y \Leftrightarrow x - y$ is negative i.e.

$[p, q] < [m, n] \Leftrightarrow pn < qm$

Clearly $x > y \Leftrightarrow y < x$.

Theorem I. If p/q is a rational number then prove that either $\frac{p}{q} > 0$ or $\frac{p}{q} = 0$ or $\frac{p}{q} < 0$ i.e. only one of these holds true.

Proof: If p/q is a non zero rational number then either $pq > 0$ or $pq < 0$

i.e. $\frac{p}{q} > 0$ or $\frac{p}{q} < 0$.

If p/q is zero then the proof is obvious.

Law of Tricthotomy, only one of the followings holds good.

(i) $x = y$ (ii) $x > y$ (iii) $x < y$.

In addition: $x > y \Rightarrow x + z > y + z$

$x < y \Rightarrow x + z < y + z$.

$x > y \Rightarrow > 0 \Rightarrow xz > yz$.

Transitivity: $x > y, y > z \Rightarrow x > z$

$x < y, y < z \Rightarrow x < z$

Theorem II: Between two different rational numbers, there lies another rational number.

Proof: Let p and q be two rational numbers and $p > q$ then $p > q \Rightarrow p + p > p + q$

$$\Rightarrow \quad p > \frac{p+q}{2} \tag{1}$$

Again $p > q \Rightarrow p + q > q + q \Rightarrow \frac{p+q}{2} > q$ (2)

From (1) and (2) $p > \frac{p+q}{2} > b$.

Which completes the proof.

Theorem III. If $x, y \in Q$, prove that

$$(xy)^{-1} = y^{-1}\, x^{-1}$$

Proof: Let $x = [p, q]$ and $y = [m, n]$

then $\quad xy = [p, q]\,[m, n] = [pm, qn]$

Now $\quad xy = [pm, qn] \Rightarrow (xy)^{-1} = [nq, mp]$

$\Rightarrow \quad (xy)^{-1} = [n, m]\,[q, p] = y^{-1}\, x^{-1}$

Theorem IV. If x and y are positive rational numbers prove that $x < y \Rightarrow x^{-1} > y^{-1}$

Proof: Let $x = [p, q]$ and $y = [m, n]$ be two positive rational numbers, then

$p \cdot q > 0$ and $m \cdot n > 0$.

Again $x < y$ and hence $pn < qm$ $\quad \left[\therefore \dfrac{p}{q} < \dfrac{m}{n}\right]$

Now $\quad x^{-1} = [p, q];\ y^{-1} = [n, m]$

and $\quad x < y \Rightarrow pn < qm \Rightarrow qm > pn$

$$\Rightarrow \quad \frac{q}{p} > \frac{n}{m} \Rightarrow [q, p] > [n, m]$$

$$\Rightarrow \quad x^{-1} > y^{-1}$$

3.29 (I) ALGEBRAIC SYSTEMS OR ALGEBRAIC STRUCTURES

A set with one or more binary operations over the set A when satisfies certain given laws, viz; commutative, associative or distributive is called an algebraic structure or system.

(II) ISOMORPHISM

Mathematics Dictionary by Robert C. James and Edwin F. Beckonbeck defines "Isomorphism" to be a one to one correspondence of a set A with a set B (the sets A and B are then said to be equinumerable, equipotent or equivalent). If operations such as multiplication addition or multiplication be scalars are defined for A and B it is required that these correspond between A and B in the ways described as follows: If A and B are groups (or semi groups) with the operation denoted by •, and x corresponds to x^* and y to y^* then $x \cdot y$ must correspond to x^*, y^*. An isomorphism of a set with itself is an automorphism.

A system consisting of a non-empty set A of elements a, b, c etc. With an operation 0 is said to be a group if the following postulates are satisfied: closure property, associativity, existence of identity, and existence of inverse.

(III) IMBEDDING OF INTEGERS

If the rational number q is defined such that

$$q = [a, 1] = \left[\frac{a}{1}\right]$$

where $a \in I$ then q is known as rational integers and the set of rational integers is denoted by Q_1.

Thus $$Q_1 = \{[a, 1]: a \in I\}$$

$$= \left\{\ldots \frac{-3}{1}, \frac{-2}{1}, \frac{-1}{1}, 0, \frac{1}{1}, \frac{2}{1}, \frac{3}{1} \ldots\right\}$$

Theorem: Prove that the algebraic structures

$(I, +, \cdot, >)$ and $(Q_1, +, \cdot, >)$ are isomorphic ($I \cong Q_1$) i.e. the mapping

$f: I \to Q_1$ where $f(a) = [a, 1]$, $a \in I$ is (i) one-one (ii) onto (iii) $f(a + b) = f(a) + f(b)$

(iv) $f(a \cdot b) = (a).f(b)$ and (5) $f(a) > f(b) \Leftrightarrow a > b$.

Proof: (i) $f(a) = f(b) \Rightarrow [a, 1] = [b, 1]$

$\Rightarrow a.\,1 = b.\,1 \Rightarrow a = b$

i.e. f is one-one.

(ii) $\forall\ [a, 1] \in Q_1\ \exists\ a \in I: f(a) = [a, 1]$

i.e. f is onto.

(iii) $$f(a) + f(b) = [a, 1] + [b, 1] = [a + b, 1]$$
$$= f(a + b)$$

(iv) $$f(a).f(b) = [a, 1].[b, 1] = [ab, 1]$$
$$= f(a.\,b)$$

(v) $f(a) > f(b) \Leftrightarrow [a, 1] > [b, 1]$

$$\Leftrightarrow \frac{a}{1} > \frac{b}{1} \Leftrightarrow a > b$$

$\therefore \quad (I, +, \cdot >) = (Q_1, +, \cdot, >)$

Thus we conclude that the set of integers and the set of rational integers are isomorphic i.e. they are same i.e. integers are imbedded in the rational numbers.

3.30 SOME WORKED OUT EXAMPLES

Example 1: Prove that log 5 is not a rational number.

Solution: Assume that log 5 is a rational number then we can write $\log 5 = \frac{m}{n}$

where $m, n \in I$ and are co-prime numbers.

$\therefore \qquad (10)^{\frac{m}{n}} = 5$

$\Rightarrow \qquad (10)^m = 5^n \Rightarrow 2^m \cdot 5^m = 5^n$

In L.H.S. 2 is a factor where as is R.H.S. 2 is not a factor.

Therefore this equality is impossible as it contradicts the uniqueness of presenting whole numbers in the form of prime factors. Thus our assumption is wrong and log 5 is not a rational numbers.

Example 2: Prove that $\sqrt{2}$ is not a rational number.

Solution: If possible let us assume that $\sqrt{2}$ is a rational number. If p and q are co-prime numbers, and $p_1\, q \in I$

Put $\sqrt{2} = \frac{p}{q} \ \therefore\ 2 = \frac{p^2}{q^2} \Rightarrow p^2 = 2q^2.$

Since R.H.S. is divisible by two $\therefore$ L.H.S. must be divisible by 2. Now p^2 is divisible by 2 only if p is divisible by 2.

Since p is divisible by two $\therefore\ p = 2k$

$\therefore \qquad p^2 = 2q^2 \Rightarrow 4k^2 = 2q^2$

$\therefore \qquad q^2 = 2k^2$

This relation shows q is divisible by 2 as R.H.S. is divisible by 2.

$\therefore \qquad q = 2m.$

Thus p and q have a common factor the number 2. We have thus a contradiction and this signifies that our assumption is false.

$\therefore \sqrt{2}$ is not a rational numbers.

Example 3: Prove that $\sqrt{3}$ is not a rational number.

Solution: Assume $\sqrt{3}$ is a rational number.

$$\therefore \qquad \sqrt{3} = \frac{p}{q} \text{ where } p, q \in I$$

and are co-prime numbers.

$$\therefore \qquad 3 = \frac{p^2}{q^2} \Rightarrow 3q^2 = p^2.$$

As L.H.S. is divisible by 3 i.e. R.H.S. is also divisible by 3. New p^2 is divisible by 3.

$\therefore$ p is divisible by 3. Thus p and q have a common factors 3. Thus we have a contradiction.

Example 4: If p is a prime number and $n > 1$ prove that $\sqrt[3]{p}$ is not a rational number.

Solution: Let $\sqrt[3]{p}$ be a rational numbers then $\sqrt[n]{p} = \frac{a}{b}$, where a and b are prime factors.

$$\therefore \quad (p)^{\frac{1}{n}} = \frac{a}{b} \Rightarrow = \frac{a^n}{b^n}$$

$$\therefore \quad p\,b^n = a^n. \tag{1}$$

L.H.S. of (1) is divisible by p hence R.H.S. is also divisible by p.

$\therefore$ a^n is divisible by p only if a is divisible by p.

$$\therefore a = pk.$$

Substituting this value is (1) we get

$$p\,b^n = p^n\,k^n \Rightarrow b^n = p^{n-1}\,k^n \tag{2}$$

R.H.S. of (2) is divisible by p hence b^n is also divisible by p. With similar logic we put $b = p\,\lambda$. Thus a and b have a common factor p which contradicts the uniqueness of expressing the whole number in the form of prime factors.

EXERCISE 3 (D) SIMPLE QUESTIONS

1. Describe Peano's postulates (Axioms) related to natural numbers. [Merrut B.Sc. 1982]

2. Show that distributive law of multiplication over addition holds good in the set of natural numbers.

[Gorakhpur B.Sc of 1972, 1974, 1976, 1978]

3. Define integers with the help of equivalence relation and show that the addition in integers is associative. [U.P. 1985]

4. Define rational number with the help of equivalence relation. [Ranchi B. Sc. 1976]

5. Prove that the commutative law in addition holds good for the set of rational numbers.

6. Prove that the cancellation law is addition holds good for the set of rational numbers.

7. Show that the equivalence class [0, 1] is an identity in the set of rational numbers.

8. Show that there is multiplicative inverse of any non-zero element is the set of rational numbers is unique.

[Gorakhpur B.Sc. 1976, 1978]

9. If x and y be two integers prove that

(i) $(-x)\, y = x(-y) = -(x\, y)$ [U. P. 1984, 1988]

(ii) $-(x + y) = (-x) + (-y)$ [U. P. 1980, 1982]

(iii) $x(y - z) = xy - xz$

(iv) $(x - y) + (y - z) = x - z$

(v) $(x + z) - (y + z) = x - y$ [U.P. 1981]

10. Prove that 3 is not the square of any rational number.

[U.P. 1988]

11. If $x_1\, y \in Q$, prove that $(x\, y)^{-1} = y^{-1}\, x^{-1}$

12. $xy = 0 \Rightarrow x = 0$ or $y = 0,\, x, y \in I$ [U.P.1982, 1984, 1987]

[**Hint:** $x = [a, b], y = [c, d]$)

$$x \cdot y = [ac + bd, bc + ad]$$

Now $x \cdot y = 0 \Rightarrow [ac + bd, bc + ad] = 0.$

$\Rightarrow ac + bd = be + ad$ (i)

Now if $a, b \in N$ then either $a = b$ or $a > b$

(i) $a = b$ $\therefore\ x = [a, a] = 0.$

(ii) $a > b$ $\therefore\ a = x + b \quad x \in N$

$\therefore$ from $ac + bd = bc + ad$. We have

$(x + b)\, c + bd = bc + (x + b).\, d.$

$\therefore \quad xc + bc + bd = bc + xd + bd.$

$\Rightarrow xc = xd. \Rightarrow c = d.$

$\therefore\ y = [c, c] = [d, d] = 0$

Similarly we can prove $y = 0$ when $a < b$ i.e. $a + x = b$.]

ANSWERS TO EXERCISE 3(D)

Hints and Solutions

1. **Ans:** see Art. 3.3 chapter 3
2. **Ans:** see Art. 3.6 (C) and (D) chapter 3
3. **Ans:** see Art. 3.14 and 3.15 and 3.16(3) chapter 3
4. **Ans:** see Art. 3.25 (2) chapter 3
5. **Ans:** see worked out example 1(A) after Article 3.25 chapter 3.
6. **Hint:** We have to prove

   (i) $x + z = y + z \Rightarrow x = y$ (Right Cancellation Law)

   (ii) $z + x = z + y \Rightarrow x = y$ (Left Cancellation Law)

   Proof (i) We have

$$x = x + 0 = x + \{z + (-z)\} = (x + z) + (-z)$$
$$= (y + z) + (-z) \qquad \therefore x + z = y + z$$
$$= y + 0 = y$$

   $\therefore \quad x + z = y + z \Rightarrow x = y$

   (ii) $x = 0 + x = \{(-z) + (z)\} + x$

   $= (-z) + (z + x) = -z + z + y \qquad \therefore z + x = z + y = 0 + y = y.$

   $\therefore \quad z + x = z + y \Rightarrow x = y.$

7. **Hint:** Since $[p \cdot q] + [0, 1] = [p \cdot 1 + 0 \cdot q, q \cdot 1]$

$$= [p, q] \text{ for every } p, q \text{ where } q \neq 0$$

   $\therefore$ [0, 1] is the identity for addition in the set of rational numbers.

8. **Ans:** See theorem 2 of some worked out examples and theorem after Art. 3.25.
9. **Hint:** Let $x = [p, q], y = [m, n]$ and $z = [r, s]$

   (i) $(-x)y = [q, p]\,[m, n]$

$$= [qm + pn, qn + pm] \qquad (1)$$
$$x(-y) = [p, q]\,[n, m] = [pn + qm, pm + qn] \qquad (2)$$
$$x \cdot y = [p, q]\,[m, n] = [pm + qn, pn + qm]$$
$$-(x \cdot y) = [pn + qm, pm + qn] \qquad (3)$$

From (1), (2) and (3)

$(-x)\,y = x(-y) = -(x \cdot y)$

(ii) $(-x) + (-y) = [q, p] + [n, m] = [q + n, p + m]$

$x + y = [p, q] + [m, n] = [p + m, q + n]$

and $-(x + y) = (q + n, p + m)$

$\therefore \quad -(x + y) = (-x) + (-y)$

(iii) $x(y - z) = [p, q]\,\{[m, n] - [r, s]\}$

$= [p, q]\{[m, n] + [s, r]\}$

$= [p, q]\,[m + s, n + r]$

$= [pm + ps + qn + qr, pn + pr + qm + qs]$

$xy - xz = [p, q]\,[m, n] - [p, q]\,[r, s]$

$= [pm + qn, pn + qm] - [pr + qs, ps + qr]$

$= [pm + qn, pn + qm] + [ps + qr, pr + qs]$

$= [pm + qn + ps + qr, pn + qm + pr + qs]$

$\therefore \quad x(y - z) = xy - xz.$

(iv) $(x - y) + (y - z) = [p, q] + [n, m] + [m, n] + [s, r]$

$= [p + n, q + m] + [m + s, n + r] = [p + m + n +$
$s, q + m + n + r]$

$= [p + s, q + r]$ (using cancellation law)

$= [p, q] + [s, r] = [p, q] - [r, s] = x - z$

(v) $(x + z) - (y + z) = \{[p, q] + [r, s]\} - \{[m, n] + [r, s]\}$

$= [p + r, q + s] - [m + r, n + s]$

$= [p + r, q + s] + [n + s, m + r]$

$= [p + r + n + s, q + s + m + r]$

$= [p + n, q + m]$ (using cancellation law)

$= [p, q] + [n, m] = [p, q] - [m, n]$

$= x - y.$

10. Ans: see worked out example 3 Art 3.30.

11. Ans: see theorem III Art. 3.28.

12. Ans: see the hints given in the question.

PROBLEMS AND EXERCISES 3 (E)

1. Prove that $\log_3 2$ is not a rational number
2. Prove that $xy = xz \Rightarrow y = z$ if $x \neq 0$ where $x, y, z \in Q$.

[**Hint:** $xy = xz \Rightarrow x^{-1}(xy) = x^{-1}(xz)$

$\therefore\ x^{-1}$ exists as $x \neq 0$

$\Rightarrow (x^{-1}\,x)\,y = (x^{-1}\,x)\,z$

or $\quad xy = xz$

$\Rightarrow \quad (1_Q)\,y = (1_Q)\,z$

$\therefore \quad x^{-1}\,x = 1_Q$

$\Rightarrow \quad y = z.$]

3. Prove that $\sqrt{5}$ is not a rational number.
4. Prove that $\log_4 18$ is not a rational number.
5. Prove that $\sqrt{2} + \sqrt{3}$ is not a rational number.
6. How many factors 5 are there is $\underline{|1980}$? **[Ans.** 493]
7. Show that $n^7 - n$ is divisible by 42.
8. Prove that every square number is of the form $5n$ or $5n \pm 1$.
9. If n is a prime greater than 3, prove that $n^2 - 1$ is a multiple of 24.
10. Find the number of divisors of 8064. **[Ans.** 48]
11. Prove that the number of divisors of 21600 is 72.
12. Find the sum of the divisors of 72. **[Ans.** 195]
13. Find the number of ways in which 72 can be resolved into two factors prime to each other. **[Ans.** 2]
14. If n is odd show that $n(n^2 - 1)$ is divisible by 24.
15. How many zeros are there at the end of the number? $\underline{|1000}$ [Canadian Math Olympiad] **[Ans.** 249]
16. Prove that the number $\log_2 7$ is not a rational number.
17. Prove that the sum of three successive powers of the number 3 is divisible by 13.
18. Prove that when the square of an odd number is divided by 8 the remainder is 1.
19. Find the sum

$$\frac{1}{\sqrt{1}+\sqrt{2}} + \frac{1}{\sqrt{2}+\sqrt{3}} + \frac{1}{\sqrt{3}+\sqrt{4}} + \ldots + \frac{1}{\sqrt{99}+\sqrt{100}}$$ **[Ans.** 9]

20. Find the sum $\frac{1}{20}+\frac{1}{30}+\frac{1}{42}+\frac{1}{56}+\frac{1}{72}+\frac{1}{90}+\frac{1}{100}\frac{1}{32}$

$\left[\textbf{Ans.}\frac{1}{6}\right]$

21. $x_1\ y \in I$ solve the equation $xy = x + y$. **[Ans.** $\{2, 2\}, \{0, 0\}$]

22. Prove that the product of four consecutive natural numbers cannot be the square of an integer.

[Canadian Math Olympiad]

23. Let a, b, c, d be four integers. Prove that the product of the six differences $(b-a)(c-a)(d-a)(d-c)(d-b)(c-b)$ is divisible by 12. [Canadian Math Olympiad]

[Hint: Let $P = (b-a)(c-a)(d-a)(d-c)(d-b)(c-d)$ (i)

If the product P is divisible by 12. Then it is also divisible by 4 and 3 both.

If an integer is divided by 4, the remainders are 0, 1, 2, 3. If two of the given integer a, b, c, d, fall into the same category i.e. have the same remainder when divided by 4, their difference is also divisible by 4. We see that factors in (i) include all such differences and therefore P is divisible by 4. (i) is also divisible by 4 even if the remainders are different in that case since the difference of the even numbers is even and the difference of odd numbers is also even. Here two of the integers a, b, c, d, are even and two are odd as the remainders are 0, 1, 2 and 3. Thus we arrive at a conclusive that is all cases P is divisible by 4.

When an integer is divided by 3 the remainders are 0, 1, and 2 and hence at least two of the integers a, b, c, and d fall into the same category i.e. they have the same remainder. The difference of such integers is always divisible by 3.

$\therefore$ P is divisible by 4×3 i.e. by 12.]

24. Prove that $\frac{3+\sqrt{6}}{\sqrt[5]{3}-\sqrt[2]{12}-\sqrt{32}+\sqrt{50}}$ is an irrational number $\sqrt{3}$.

25. When $\underline{|30}$ is computed it ends in '7' zeros. Find the digit that immediately precedes these zeros.

[**Hint:** A number N is generally denoted as $N = a^p\, b^q\, c^r \ldots$ where $a, b, c \ldots$ are different prime numbers and $p, q, r \ldots$ are positive integers.

We have to find the unit digit of $N = \dfrac{\underline{|30}}{10^7}$. We now determine the highest powers of the prime factors in $\underline{|30}$.

By 3.24 (3) the power of 2 in $\underline{|30}$ is

$$I\left[\frac{30}{2}\right] + I\left[\frac{30}{22}\right] + I\left[\frac{30}{23}\right] + I\left[\frac{30}{24}\right]$$

$$= 15 + 7 + 3 + 1 = 26.$$

The power of 3 in $\underline{|30}$ is

$$I\left[\frac{30}{3}\right] + I\left[\frac{30}{32}\right] + I\left[\frac{30}{33}\right]$$

$$= 10 + 3 + 1 = 14.$$

Similarly the power of 5 is 7, the power of 7 is 4, the power of 11 is 2, the power of 13 is 2, the power of 17 is 1, the power of 19 is 1, the power of 23 is 1 and that of 29 is 1

$$\therefore \quad N = \frac{\underline{|30}}{10^7} = \frac{2^{26} \cdot 3^{14} \cdot 5^7 \cdot 7^4 \cdot 11^2 \cdot 13^2 \cdot 17 \cdot 19 \cdot 23 \cdot 29}{10^7}$$

$= 2^{19}, 3^{14}, 7^4, 11^2, 13^2, 17, 19, 23, 29$

If the unit digit of N is x.

Then $N = x \pmod{10}$

Now $2^{19} = 2^6 \cdot 2^6 \cdot 2^6 \cdot 2 = 64 \times 64 \times 64 \times 2 = 524288 \equiv 8$ (mod 10)

$3^{14} = 3^4 \cdot 3^4 \cdot 3^4 \cdot 3^2 = 4782969 \equiv 9 \pmod{10}$

$7^4 = 2401 \equiv 1 \pmod{10}$; $11^2 = 121 \equiv 1 \pmod{10}$

$13^2 \equiv 9$ (mod); $17 \equiv 7 \pmod{10}$; $23 \equiv 3 \pmod{10}$

$29 \equiv 9 \pmod{10}$ and $19 \equiv 9 \pmod{10}$

$$\begin{aligned} \therefore \qquad N &= 8 \times 9 \times 1 \times 1 \times 9 \times 7 \times 3 \times 9 \times 9 \pmod{10} \\ &= 9^4 \times 8 \times 7 \times 3 \times 1^2 \pmod{10} \\ &\equiv 6561 \times 168 \pmod{10} \end{aligned}$$

$\equiv 1 \pmod{10} \times 8 \pmod{10}$

$\equiv 8 \pmod{10}$

Thus the digit that precedes 7 zeros is 8.]

26. Find remainder when 19^{92} is divided by 92

[International Mathematical Olympiad Problems 94]

[**Ans.** 49]

Solution: We have $19^2 \equiv -7 \pmod{92}$; $19^4 \equiv 49 \pmod{92}$

$$19^8 \equiv 2401 \pmod{92} \equiv 9 \pmod{92};$$

$$19^{16} \equiv 81 \pmod{92} = (92 - 11) \pmod{92}$$

$$\equiv 92 \pmod{92} - 11 \pmod{92}$$

$$\equiv 0 \pmod{92} - 11 \pmod{92} \equiv -11 \pmod{92}$$

$$19^{32} \equiv 6561 \pmod{92} \equiv 29 \pmod{92}$$

$$19^{64} \equiv 841 \pmod{92} \equiv 13 \pmod{92}$$

Now $\quad 19^{92} \equiv 19^{64+16+8+4} \equiv 19^{64} \cdot 19^{16} \cdot 19^{8} \cdot 19^{4}$

$$\equiv 13 \pmod{92}. (-11) \pmod{92}. 9 \pmod{92}. 49 \pmod{92}$$

$$\equiv 5733 \pmod{92}. (-11) \pmod{92}$$

$$\equiv 29 \pmod{92}. (-11) \pmod{92}$$

$$\equiv -319 \pmod{92} \equiv -43 \pmod{92}$$

$$\equiv 0\,(49 - 92) \pmod{92}$$

$$\equiv -(92 - 49) \pmod{92}$$

$$\equiv -92 \pmod{92} + 49 \pmod{92}$$

$$\equiv -0 \pmod{92} + 49 \pmod{92}$$

$\equiv 49 \pmod{92}$. Hence finished

Aliter: $19^{92} = (19^4)^{23}$. Since 23 is a prime number hence from the derivation of Fermat's theorem $(19^4)^{23} - 19^4$ is divisible by 23.

$$(19^4)^{23} \equiv 194 \pmod{92}$$

$$= 19^{92} \equiv (23 - 4)^4 \pmod{23} \equiv (-4)^4 \pmod{23}$$

$\therefore \quad [(a + b)^n \text{(mode)} = b^n \text{(mode)}]$

$$\equiv 256 \pmod{23} \equiv 3 \pmod{23}$$

$\therefore \quad 19^{92} = 23\lambda + 3$ for $\lambda \in I$.

Now as 19^{92} is odd λ must be even.

$\therefore \quad \lambda$ is either $4n$ or $4n + 2$, where $n \in I$.

$\therefore \quad 19^{92} = 92\lambda n + 3$ or $92\lambda n + 49$

If $19^{92} = 92\,\lambda\, n + 3$ then $19^{92} \equiv 3 \pmod 4$
and if $19^{92} = 92\,\lambda\, n + 49$ then $19^{92} \equiv 49 \pmod 4$

i.e. $\quad 19^{92} \equiv 1 \pmod 4$ (1)

$\therefore \quad 19^{92} \equiv 3$ or $1 \pmod 4$

Now we write $19^{92} = (20 - 1)^{92}$

$$\equiv (-1)^{92} \text{ (mod 20.)} \equiv 1 \pmod{20}$$
$$\equiv 1 \pmod 4$$

$\therefore \quad 19^{92} = 92\,\lambda\, n + 49$ form (1)

$\therefore \quad$ The remainder is 49.

27. A four digit number has the following properties:
(a) If is a perfect square (b) Its first two digits are equal (c) Its last two digits or equal. Find all such 4 digit numbers.

[International Mathematical Olympiad] [**Ans.** 7744]

Solution: Let x and y be respectively the first and the last digits of the required number where $0 \le x$ and $y \le 9$ and $x \ne 0$ then the number N be $1000x + 100x + 10y + y$ i.e.

$$N = 1100x + 11y = 11\,(100\,x + y).$$

Since N is a perfect square

$\therefore\ 100x + y = 11k^2$, where $k \in I$,

i.e. $N = 11^2\, k^2$ (1)

Thus we arrive at a conclusion that

$100x + y$ is divisible by 11.

Now 11 divides $100x + y$

$\therefore \quad 100x + y = 11\lambda$, where $\lambda \in I$

$$\Rightarrow \quad 99x + x + y = 11\lambda \Rightarrow 9x + \frac{x+y}{11} = \lambda$$

$\Rightarrow \quad$ 11 divides $x + y$. Since x and $y \ngtr 9$

$\therefore \quad x + y \ngtr 18$. Similarly $x + y \nless 0$

Now 11 divides $x + y$; $x + y \ngtr 18$ and $x + y \nless 0$ we arrive at a conclusion that

$$x + y = 11 \qquad \therefore\ k^2 = \frac{100x + y}{11}$$

$$= 9x + \frac{x+y}{11} = 9x + 1$$

From $x + y = 11$, we have $2 \le x$ and $y \le 9$

$\therefore x, y \in [2, 9]$

From [2, 9] only $x = 7$ gives that square value of $9x + 1$

$\therefore x + y = 11$ gives

$y = 4$. $\therefore N$ is 7744.

28. Let $m_1, m_2, m_3 \dots m_n$ be rearrangement of the numbers 1, 2, 3 ... n. Suppose that n is odd.

Prove that the product $(m_1 - 1)(m_2 - 2) \dots (m_3 - n)$ is an even integer. [International Mathematical Olympiad]

29. A sequence of positive integer is defined by $a_n = \left[n + \sqrt{n} \, \frac{1}{2} \right]$

$n \in N$. Find the positive integer which belong to the sequence. **[Ans. ϕ]**

MISCELLANEOUS EXERCISE

1. If $A = \{1, 2, 3\}$, $B = \{2, 4, 6, 8\}$ $C = \{3, 4, 5, 6\}$, compute $A \cup B$, $B \cap C$, $A - B$ and $A \cap (B \cap C)$.

Solution: $A \cup B$ is the set of all elements of A and B and hence $A \cup B = \{1, 2, 3, 4, 6, 8\}$

$B \cap C$ is the set of common elements of B and C and hence $B \cap C = \{4, 6\}$

$A - B$ is the set of all elements which are obtained by removing the elements of B from A

$\therefore A - B = \{1, 3\}$

$A \cap (B \cap C)$ is the set containing the elements common to A and $B \cap C$

$\therefore A \cap (B \cap C) \phi$

2. If $A = \{1, 2, 3\}$, $B = \{2, 3, 4\}$ $C = \{3, 4, 5, 6\}$, compute $A - B$, $B - C$, $C - A$, $A - (B - C)$ and $(A - B) - C$.

Solution: $A - B = \{1\}$

$$B - C = \{2\}, C - A = \{4, 5, 6\}$$

$$A - (B - C) = \{1, 2, 3\} - \{2\} = \{1, 3\}$$

$$(A - B) - C = \{1\} - \{3, 4, 5, 6\} = \{1\}$$

3. If $U = \{1, 2, 3, 4, 5, 6, 7, 8, 9\}$, $A = \{1, 2, 3, 4\}$

$B = \{2, 4, 6, 8\}$, $C = \{3, 4, 5, 6\}$, compute

$A', B', (A \cap B)', (A \cap C)'$ and $(B - C)'$

Solution: $A' = U - A = \{5, 6, 7, 8, 9\}$

$B' = U - B = \{1, 3, 5, 7, 9\}$

$(A \cup B)' = U - (A \cup B) = \{5, 7, 9\}$

$(A \cap C)' = U - (A \cap C) = \{1, 2, 5, 6, 7, 8, 9\}$

Since $A \cap C = \{3, 4\}$

$(B - C)' = U - (B - C) = \{1, 3, 4, 5, 6, 7, 9\}$

Since $B - C = \{2, 8\}$

4. If $A = \{2, 3, 4, 8, 10\}$, $B = \{3, 4, 5, 10, 12\}$,
$C = \{4, 5, 12, 14\}$ compute
$(A \cup B) \cap (A \cup C)$ and $(A \cap B) \cup (A \cap C)$

Solution: We have $A \cap B = \{2, 3, 4, 5, 8, 10, 12\}$

$A \cup C = \{2, 3, 4, 5, 6, 8, 10, 12, 14\}$

$A \cap B = \{3, 4, 10\}; A \cap C = (4)$

$\therefore \quad (A \cup B) \cap (A \cup C) = \{2, 3, 4, 5, 8, 10, 12\}$

$(A \cap B) \cup (A \cap C) = \{3, 4, 10\}$

5. $A = \{1, 2, 4, 5\}$, $B = \{2, 3, 5, 6\}$, $C = \{4, 5, 6, 7\}$
prove that (i) $A \cup (B \cap C) = (A \cup B) \cap (A \cup C)$
(ii) $A \cap (B \cup C) = (A \cap B) \cup (A \cap C)$

Solution: Do yourself.

6. If $A = \{1, 2\}$, $B = \{2, 3\}$, $C = \{3, 7\}$,
compute $(A \times B) \cup (A \times C)$ and $(A \times B) \cap (A \times C)$

Solution: $A \times B = \{(1, 2), (1, 3), (2, 2), (2, 3)\}$

$A \times C = \{(1, 3), (1, 7)\ (2, 3), (2, 7)\}$

$\therefore \quad$ (i) $(A \times B) \cup (A \times C) = \{(1, 2), (1, 3), (1, 7), (2, 2), (2, 3), (2, 7)\}$

(ii) $(A \times B) \cap (A \times C) = \{(1, 3), (2, 3)\}$

7. A class has 175 students. The following table shows the number of students studying one or more of the following subjects in this class:

Subject	*No. of students*	*Subject*	*No. of students*
Mathematics	100	Mathematics and Chemistry	28
Physics	70	Physics and Chemistry	23
Chemistry	46	Mathematics, Physics and Chemistry	18
Mathematics and Physics	30		

How many students are enrolled in Mathematics alone, Physics alone and Chemistry alone?

Are there students who have not offered any of these three subjects? [Roorkee 1984]

Solution: Please see the solution of Q. No. 23 of " Some More Important Problems—1" Exercise 2 C (ii).

8. A relation R in the set of naturnal numbers is defined as follows

(i) $a\ R\ b$ if "a divides b" prove that R is reflexive, transitive but not symmetric.

(ii) $a\ R\ b$ if 'a and b both are even' prove that R is symmetric and transitive but not reflexive.

(iii) $a\ R\ b$ if "$a + b$ is odd" prove that R is symmetric but not reflexive and transitive.

(iv) $a\ R\ b$ if '$(a - b)\ (a - 5b) = 0$' prove that R is reflexive but not symmetric and transitive.

(v) $a\ R\ b$ if $|a - b| < 4$ prove that R is reflexive and symmetric but not transitive.

Solution: (i) Since a divides a hence $a\ R\ a$ and therefore R is reflexive.

If a divides b then $a\ R\ b$ but $a\ R\ b \not\Rightarrow b\ R\ a$ hence R is not symmetric.

If $a\ R\ b$, $b\ R\ c$ then $a\ R\ c$ since a divides b, b divides c hence a divides c and therefore R is transitive.

(ii) $a\ R\ b$ if a and b are even but $a \not R\ a$ if a is odd and hence $\forall\ a \in s\ a\ R\ a$ is not true.

$\therefore$ R is not reflexive

$a\ R\ b \Rightarrow b\ R\ a$ hence R is symmetric.

Again $a\ R\ b$, $b\ R\ c \Rightarrow a\ R\ c$ hence R is transitive.

(iii) $a\ R\ a$ if $a + a$ is odd, but 29 is even hence R is not reflexive

$a\ R\ b \Rightarrow b\ R\ a \quad \therefore \quad a + b = b + a =$ odd.

Hence R is symmetric

$a\ R\ b, b\ R\ c \not\Rightarrow a\ R\ c$

$\therefore$ $a + b$ is an odd number, $b + c$ is an odd number this does not imply that $a + c$ in an odd number.

$\therefore$ R is not transitive.

(iv) $a\ R\ a$ if $(a-a)\ (a-5a) = 0$ i.e. if $0 = 0$
which is true hence R is reflexive
If $a\ R\ b$ then $(a-b)\ (a-5b) = 0$
If $b\ R\ a$ then $(b-a)\ (b-5a) = 0$
but $(a-b)\ (a-5b) \neq (b-a)\ (b-5a)$
$\therefore \quad a\ R\ b \not\Rightarrow b\ R\ a$ $\therefore$ R is not symmetric.
Similarly $a\ R\ b, b\ R\ c \not\Rightarrow a\ R\ c$
$\therefore\ (a-b)\ (a-5b) = 0, (b-c)\ (b-5c) = 0$
$\not\Rightarrow (a-c)\ (a-5c) = 0$
$\therefore \quad R$ is not transitive.

(v) $a\ R\ a$ if $|a-a| < 4$ which is true hence R is reflexive.

$$a\ R\ b \Rightarrow b\ R\ a \qquad \therefore |a-b| < 4 \Rightarrow |b-a| < 4$$

$\therefore \quad R$ is symmetric.
$a\ R\ b_1\ b\ R\ c \not\Rightarrow a\ R\ c$

$$\therefore \quad |a-b| < 4,\ |b-c| < 4$$

$$\text{but}\ |a-c| = |a-b+b-c| = |(a-b)+(b-c)|$$

$$\leq |a-b| + |b-c| < 4+4 < 8$$

$\therefore \quad a\ R\ b, b\ R\ c \not\Rightarrow a\ R\ c.$
$\therefore \quad R$ is not transitive.

9. If $f = \{(1,2), (3,5), (4,1)\}$
and $g = \{(2,3), (5,1)\ (1,3)\}$ are mappings.
Write down the components of $f\ o\ g$ and $g\ o\ f$.
Solution: $f\ o\ g(2) = f(3) = 5$ ($\because$ g transforms 2 into 3 and f transforms 3 into 5)
and $f\ o\ g(5) = f(1) = 2$ ($\because$ g transforms 5 into 1 and f transforms 1 into 5)
Also $f\ o\ g\ (1) = f(3) = 5$

$$\therefore \quad f\ o\ g = \{(2,5)\ (5,2), (1,5)\}$$

Similarly $g\ o\ f = \{(1,3), (3,1)\ (4,3)\}$

10. there are two mappings defined as

$$f(x) = 2x + 1 \text{ and } g(x) = x^2 - 2$$

compute the value of $g \, o \, f(x)$ and $f \, o \, g(x)$.

Solution: $(g \, o \, f)(x) = g[f(x)] = g(x^2 + 1)$

$$= (2x + 1)^2 - 2 = 4x^2 + 4x + 1 - 2$$

$$= 4x^2 + 4x - 1.$$

$$(f \, o \, g)(x) = f[g(x)] = f(x^2 - 2)$$

$$= 2(n^2 - 2) + 1 = 2x^2 - 4 + 1$$

$$= 2x^2 - 3$$

11. If $f: R \to R$ where $f(x) = 2x + 1$, compute

(i) $f(\{4\})$ $f(\{-1, 0, 1\})$

(ii) $f^{-1}\{4\}, f^{-1}\{0, 3\}$ and $f^{-1}\{-1, 0, 1\}$

Solution: If A is a set then

$f(A)$ implies the set of f images of the components of A. $\{4\} = A$ is a set where one element is 4.

(i) $\therefore f(n) = 2x + 1$ gives $f(4) = 2 \cdot 4 + 1 = 9$

$\therefore \quad f(\{4\}) = \{9\}.$

In $f(\{-1, 0, 1\}), A = \{-1, 0, 1\}$

$\therefore \quad f(-1) = 2(-1) + 1 = -1 \qquad \because \quad f(x) = 2x + 1$

$$f(0) = 2 \cdot 0 + 1 = 1$$

$$f(1) = 2 \cdot 1 = 3$$

$\therefore f(\{-1, 0, 1\}) = \{-1, 1, 3\}$

(ii) Let $f^{-1}(4) = y$ then $f(y) = 4$

$\Rightarrow \quad f(y) = 2y + 1 = 4 \Rightarrow y = 3/2$

$\therefore \quad f^{-1}\{4\} = \{y\} = \{3/2\}$

In $f^{-1}\{0, 3\}$ $A = \{0, 3\}$

$\therefore \quad f^{-1}(0) = y_1 \therefore f(y_1) = 0 \Rightarrow 2y_1 + 1 = 0$

$\therefore \quad y_1 = -1/2$

$f^{-1}(3) = y_2 \qquad \therefore f(y_2) = 3 \Rightarrow 2y_2 + 1 = 3$

$\therefore \quad y_2 = 1$

$$\therefore f^{-1}\{0, 3\} = \{y_1, y_2\} = \left[\frac{-1}{2}, 1\right]$$

In a similar fashion $f^{-1}\{-1, 0, 1\} = \left[-1\frac{1}{2}, 0\right]$

12. If $f(x) = \dfrac{x^2}{1+x^2}$, where x is a real numbers.

    Find the domain and range. Is the mapping one-one.

13. If $f: R \to R$ where $f(x) =$ is $(5x + 2)$, is the inverse mapping positive?

14. $A = R - \{3\}$ and $B = R - \{1\}$ and $f: A \to B$ where $f(x) = \dfrac{x-2}{x-3}$ $\forall$ $x \in A$ Is this mapping one-one.

PROBLEMS ASKED IN VARIOUS ENGINEERING

Entrance Examinations with Model Solutions

1. Let $f: R \to R$ be given by $f(x) = (x + 1)^2 - 1$, $x \geq -1$. Show that f is invertible. Also find the set $S = \{x: f(x) = f^{-1}(x)\}$ [I.I.T. 1995]

Solution: To prove $f(x)$ is invertible, it is sufficient to show that $f(x)$ is a bijection (i.e. one-one function).

First we show f is an injection (one-one function):

$x, y \in R$ satisfying $x \geq -1, y \geq -1$

We have $f(x) = f(y)$

$\Rightarrow \quad (x + 1)^2 - 1 = (y + 1)^2 - 1$

$\Rightarrow \quad x^2 + 2x = y^2 + 2y$

$\Rightarrow \quad x^2 - y^2 = -2\,(x - y)$

$\Rightarrow \quad (x + y)\,(x - y) + 2(x - y) = 0$

$\Rightarrow \quad (x - y)\,(x + y + z) = 0 \therefore x - y = 0$ or $x + y + z = 0$

$\therefore \quad x = y$ or $x = y = -1$

Thus $f(x) = f(y) \quad \Rightarrow x = y \; \forall \; x \geq -1$ and $y \geq -1$

$\therefore$ $f(x)$ is an injection.

Now we prove that f is a surjection (i.e. onto function)

for $y \geq -1$ then is $x = -1 + \sqrt{y+1} \geq -1$ such that $f(x) = y$

$\therefore f$ is a surjection

$\therefore f$ is a bijection

$$y = f(x) = (x + 1)^2 - 1 \Rightarrow x = -1 + \sqrt{y+1}$$

$\therefore \quad f^{-1}(y) = -1 + \sqrt{y^2+1} \Rightarrow f^{-1}(x) = -1 + \sqrt{x+1}$

Now $\quad f(x) = f^{-1}(x)$

$\therefore \quad (x+1)^2 - 1 = -1 + \sqrt{x+1}$

$\Rightarrow \quad \sqrt{x+1}\ [(x+1)^{3/2} - 1] = 0 \Rightarrow \sqrt{x+1} = 0$

or$(x+1)^{3/2} - 1 = 0$

$\Rightarrow \quad (x+1) = 0$ or $x + 1 = 1 \qquad \therefore x = 0$ or $x = -1$

$\therefore \quad S = \{x: f(x) = f^{-1}(x)\} = \{0, -1\}$.

2. Let f be an injective map with domain $\{x, y, z\}$ and range $\{1, 2, 3,\}$ such that exactly one of the following statements is correct and remaining are false, $f(x) = 1, f(y) \neq 1$ and $f(z) \neq 2$. Find $f^{-1}(1)$. [Roorkee 1996]

Solution: 1. When $f(x) = 1$ is true, then $f(y) = 1$ and $f(z) = 2$ are true.

This means x and y has the same image. Thus $f(x)$ is not injective.

$\therefore \quad f(x) = 1$ is not true.

2. If $f(y) \neq 0$ true then $f(x) \neq 1$ and $f(z) = 2$ are true.

$\therefore x, y$ both are not mapped to 1. Then both are associated to 3 or both are associated to 2 or one is mapped to 3 and other to 2.

i.e. $\quad f(x) = 3, f(y) = 2, f(y) = 3, f(x) = 2$

$\therefore f$ is not an injection $\qquad \therefore f(y) \neq 1$

3. If $f(z) \neq 2$ is true then $f(x) \neq 1$ and $f(y) = 1$ are true. But f is an injective map

$\therefore \quad f(y) = 1\ f(z) = 3$ and $f(x) = 2$

$\therefore \quad f^{-1}(1) = y$.

Mark the correct alternative(s) in the following:

3. If $f(x) = \sin^2 x + \sin^2\left(x + \frac{\pi}{3}\right) + \cos x \cos\left(x + \frac{\pi}{3}\right)$ and $g\left(\frac{5}{4}\right) = 1$ then $g\, o\, f(n) =$

(a) 1 (b) 0

(c) $\sin x$ (d) none of these [I.I.T. 1996]

Ans. (a)

Solution: $f(x)\ \sin^2 x + \sin^2\left(x+\frac{\pi}{3}\right) + \cos x \cos\left(x+\frac{\pi}{3}\right)$

$$= \frac{1-\cos 2x}{2} + \frac{1-\cos\left(2x+\frac{2\pi}{3}\right)}{2} + \frac{1}{2}\left[2\cos x\cos\left(x+\frac{\pi}{3}\right)\right]$$

$$= \frac{1}{2}\left[1-\cos 2x + 1 - \cos\left(2x+\frac{2\pi}{3}\right) + \cos\left(2x+\frac{\pi}{3}\right) + \cos\frac{\pi}{3}\right]$$

$$= \frac{1}{2}\left[\frac{5}{2} - 2\cos\left(2x+\frac{\pi}{3}\right)\cos\frac{\pi}{3} + \cos\left(2x+\frac{\pi}{3}\right)\right]$$

$$= \frac{5}{4}$$

$$\therefore \quad g \circ f(x) = g\left(\frac{5}{4}\right) = 1$$

4. If $f: R \to R$ is given by $f(x) = 3x - 5$ then $f^{-1}(x)$

(a) is given by $\frac{1}{3x-5}$

(b) is given by $\frac{x+5}{3}$

(c) does not exist because f is not one-one

(d) does not exist because f is not onto. [I.I.T. 1998]

Ans. (b)

Solution: $f: R \to R$ is one-one onto function so it is invertible.

$$f(x) = y \quad \Rightarrow y = 3x - 5$$

$$\Rightarrow \quad x = \frac{y+5}{3} \quad \Rightarrow \quad f^{-1}(y) = \frac{y+5}{3} \quad \Rightarrow \quad f^{-1}(x) = \frac{x+5}{3}$$

5. If $g(f(x)) = |\sin x|$ and $f(g(x)) = \left(\sin\sqrt{2}\right)^2$ then

(a) $f(x) = \sin^2 x,\ g(x) = \sqrt{x}$

(b) $f(x) = \sin x,\ g(x) = |x|$

(c) $f(x) = x^2$, $g(x) = \sin\sqrt{x}$

(d) f and g cannot be determined. [I.I.T. 1998]

Ans: (a)

Solution: $f(g(x)) = \left(\sin\sqrt{x}\right)^2$

$\Rightarrow \quad g(x) = \sqrt{x}$ and $f(x) = \sin^2 x$

In this case $g(f(x)) = g\,(\sin x)^2 = |\sin x|$

6. Let A be a set containing 10 distinct elements, the total number of distinct function from A to A is

(a) $\underline{|10}$ (b) 10^{10}

(c) 2^{10} (d) $2^{10} - 1$ [MLNR 1992]

Ans. (b).

Solution: The image of any given element in A can be assigned images in 10^{10} image

$\therefore$ Thus are 10^{10} distinct functions in $A \times A$.

7. Let f: $R \to R$ be defined by $f(x) = 3x - 4$.

Then $f^{-1}(x)$ is (a) $\dfrac{x+4}{3}$ (b) $\dfrac{x}{3} - 4$ (c) $3x + 4$ (d) none of these.

[MLNR 1993]

Ans. (a) **[Hint:** $y = f(x) = 3x - 4$

$$\therefore \quad x = \frac{y+4}{3} = f^{-1}(y)$$

$$\therefore \quad f^{-1}(x) = \frac{x+4}{3}\Bigg]$$

8. $f(x) = |\sin x|$ has an inverse if its domain is

(a) $[o, \pi]$ (b) $\left[0, \dfrac{\pi}{2}\right]$

(c) $\left[-\dfrac{\pi}{4}, \dfrac{\pi}{4}\right]$ (d) none of these

[EAMCET 1994]

Ans. (b).

Solution: $f(x) = |\sin x|$ is an injective if its domain is $\left[0, \frac{\pi}{2}\right]$.

$f(x)$ is surjective if its co-domain is [0, 1].

$\therefore$ $f(x) = |\sin x|$ is invertible if it is a function for $\left[0, \frac{\pi}{2}\right]$ to [0, 1].

9. Let S be a finite set containing n elements. Then the total number of binary operations on S is

(a) n^n (b) z^{n^2} (c) n^{n^2} (d) n^2.

[EAMCET 1992]

Ans. (c).

Solution: Binary operations on S in a function from $S \times S$ to S. Thus the total number of functions true $S \times S$ to S = n^{n^2}

10. Subtraction of integers is an operation that is (a) commutative and associative (b) not commutative but associative (c) neither commutative nor associative (d) commutative but not associative. [CET 1994]

Ans: (c) **Hint:** Do yourself.

A SUMMARY OF THE CITERIA FOR DIVISIBILITY AND A SHORT DESCRIPTION OF BINARY OPERATION

1. If a natural number n is a division of the natural numbers p and q then it is also a division of $p + q$.

   Example: 3 is a division of 6 and 9

   $\therefore$ 3 is a divisible of 6 + 9 i.e. of 15.

2. If a natural number n is a division of the natural numbers p and q and $p > q$ then the number n is also a division of $p - q$.

   Example: 5 is a division of 25 and 20 and 25 > 20

   $\therefore$ 5 is also a division of 25–20 i.e. of 5.

   Note: Zero can be divided by any natural number and any natural number can be divided by unity.

3. If the natural number $p = a_n a_{n-1} \ldots a_2 a_1 a_0$ is divisible by 2 then the last digit a_0 is divisible by 2.

Example: 2704 is divisible by 2 because the last digit 4 is divisible by 2.

4. If the natural number $p = a_n a_{n-1} \ldots a_2 a_1 a_0$ is divisible by 4 then $a_1 a_0$ is divisible by 4.

Example: 2704 is divisible by 4 because 04 is divisible by 4.

5. For the natural number $p = a_n a_{n-1} \ldots a_2 a_1 a_0$ to be divisible by 9, it is necessary and sufficient that sum of all digits of the number is divisible by 9.

6. A natural number is divisible by 3 if the sum of the individual digits of the number is divisible by 3.

Example: 612, 1032 are divisible by 3.

7. A natural number is divisible by 5 if the digit at the unit place of the number is either 0 or 5.

Example: 250, 3565 are divisible by 5.

8. A number is divisible by 6 if it is divisible by 2 and 3 both.

Example: 12, 18 are divisible by 6 because they are divisible by 2 and 3 both.

9. (i) The product of two natural number is divisible by 2.

$3 \times 4, 4 \times 5, 5 \times 6$ are divisible by 2.

If n is a natural number, then $n(n + 1)$ is divisible by 2.

(ii) The product of three consecutive natural number is divisible by 3 and 6 both.

$31 \times 32 \times 33$ and $43 \times 44 \times 45$ are divisible by 6, i.e. $n(n + 1)(n + 2)$ is divisible by 6 if n is a natural number.

10. A natural number is divisible by 8 if it is divisible by 4 and 2.

216 and 424 are divisible by 8.

The product of four consecutive natural numbers is divisible by 2, 3, 4, 8, 12 and 24.

11. A natural number is divisible by 10 if the digit in the unit place of the number is zero.

12. A natural number $a_n a_{n-1} \ldots a_4 a_3 a_2 a_1 a_0$ is divisible by 11 if $|a_0 - a_1 + a_2 + \ldots + (-1)^n a_n|$ is divisible by 11

or $|(a_0 + a_2 + a_4 + \ldots) - (a_1 + a_3 + a_5 + \ldots)|$ is divisible by 11 or a natural number is divisible by 11 if the difference of the sum of the alternate digits is zero or divisible by 11.

In 1771561 we have $= |(1 + 5 + 7 + 1) - (6 + 1 + 7)|$

$$= |14 - 14| = 0.$$

161051 we have $|(1 + 0 + 6) - (5 + 1 + 1)|$

$$= |7 - 7| = 0.$$

and hence 1771561 and 165051 are divisible by 11.

13. To show $x^3 + 17n$ is divisible by 6.

We write $n^3 + 17n = n^3 - n + 18n = n(n + 1)(n - 1) + 18n$ Which is divisible by 6 because $18n$ as well as $n(n + 1)(n - 1)$ are divisible individually by 6.

$n^3 + 3n^2 + 8n$ is divisible by 6 because $n^3 + 3n^2 + 8n = n^3 + 3n^2 + 2n + 6n = n(n + 1)(n + 2) + 6n$ are separately divisible by 6.

We can test $4^{2n+1} + 3^{n+2}$ to divisible by 13 as follows.

By mathematical induction we put $n = 1$ and see that $4^3 + 3^3$ is $14 + 27 = 91$ which is divisible by 13.

$\therefore$ For $n = m$

$4^{2m+1} + 3^{m+2}$ is divisible by 13.

We now test it for $m = m + 1$

$$4^{2(m+1)+1} + 3^{m+1+2}$$

$$= 4^{2m+3} + 3^{m+3} = 4^{2m+1}. 16 + 3. 3^{m+2}$$

$$= (13 + 3)\, 4^{2m+1} + 3. 3^{m+2}$$

$$= 13. 4^{2m+1} + 3. 4^{2m+1} + 3. 3^{m+2}$$

$$= 13 \cdot 4^{2m+1} + 3(4^{2m+1} \cdot 3^{m+2})$$

Which is divisible by 13.

14. Prime Number: It is the number which has two divisions unity and the number itself.

Example: The set of prime number of the first thirty numbers is {2, 3, 5, 7, 11, 13, 17, 19, 23, 29}.

15. A composite number is a number which has more than two divisions.

16. Coprime number: Numbers which have no other natural divisions in common except unity are said to be co-prime (2 and 5) and (7 and 15) are coprime number.

17. The least common multiple of two or several numbers is the least of natural numbers which is divisible by all the given numbers.

The least common multiple of 3 and 4 is 12.

18. The least common division of different natural number is unity.

The greatest common multiple of natural numbers does not exist.

19. The sum of three successive powers of 2 is divisible by 7.

Example: $2^n + 2^{n+1} + 2^{n+2} = 2^n [1 + 2 + 2^2] = 7.\ 2^n$ which is divisible by 7.

20. When a square of an odd number is divided by 8, the remainder is 1.

Example: $(2n + 1)^2 = 4n^2 + 4n + 1$

$= 4n\,(n + 1) + 1$

$n\,(n + 1)$ is divisible by 2 $\therefore$ $4n\,(n + 1)' + 1$ when divided by 8 gives 1 as its remainder.

1. Binary Operation: A binary operation or a non empty set S is a function of $S \times S$ into S. Binary composition or internal composition are also used in place of binary operation.

If o is an operation such that $a \in S, b \in S \Rightarrow a\,o\,b \in S$ then o is a binary operation on the set S.

Binary operation is also symbolised as 0, $\odot$, $\oplus$, T and $\perp$

Example: Let S be a set of rational number, then the function.

$o : S \times S \rightarrow S$ given by $a\,o\,b = a\,b$ is a binary operation or the set S because the product of two rational numbers is a rational number.

2. Few Binary Operations:

(i) Addition (+) of numbers

on the set of R of real numbers,

on the set of Q of rational numbers,

on the set of N of natural numbers and

on the set of C of complex numbers is a binary operation.

(ii) Multiplicative ($\times$) or the set R, Q, I, C and N is a binary operation:

where R = the set of real numbers
Q = the set of rational numbers
I = the set of integers.
C = the set of complex numbers
N = the set of natural numbers.

(iii) Substraction (–) is not a binary operation for the set of natural numbers.

(iv) Division (÷) is not a binary operation on the set of R, Q, I, C and N.

(v) Vector addition is a binary operation on the set of vectors.

(vi) Cross product of two co-prime vectors is not a binary operations as $\vec{a} \times \vec{b}$ does not lie in the plane of $\vec{a}$ and $\vec{b}$.

(vii) Dot product of two vectors is not a binary operation because $\vec{a} \cdot \vec{b}$ is not a vector.

3. **Some Rules of Binary Operation:**

(i) If $a \text{ o } b = b \text{ o } a \ \forall \ a, b \in S$ then the binary operation o on the set S is commutative.

(ii) If $(a \text{ o } b) \text{ o } c = a \text{ o } (b \text{ o } c) \ \forall \ a, b, c \in S$ then the binary operation o on the set S is associative.

(iii) If $a, b, c \in S$ and o is a binary operation on the set S then left cancellation law holds good if $a \text{ o } b = a \text{ o } c \Rightarrow b = c$ and right cancellation law holds good if $b \text{ o } a = c \text{ o } a \Rightarrow b = c$.

4. **Number System:** A set S is said to be a number system if two binary operations on S such that

(i) both the operations are commutative

(ii) both the operations are associative

(iii) one operation is distributive on the other.

Each element of the number system is called a number.

Example: $I = \{-3, -2, -1, 0\ 1, 2, 3 \ldots\}$ is a set of integers. This set I possesses two binary operations $(I + \cdot)$
i.e. addition and multiplication due to the fact that
both operation are commutative;
both operation are associative;
and multiplication is distributed or addition.

5. **Boolean Algebra:** This is a system of mathematical logic. It differs from ordinary algebra. In Boolean Algebra 1 + 1 = 1. There are only two values of variables viz 1 and 0.

It $A = \{x, y, z ...\}$ and two binary operations (+) and (·) be defined on A the system $(A, +, \cdot)$ is a Boolean Algebra on the condition that the followings hold good:

(i) $x + y = y + x$ and $x \cdot y = y \cdot x$ (Commutative Law)

(ii) $x + (y + z) = (x + y) + z$ and $x. (y \cdot z) = (x \cdot y). z$ (Associative Law)

(iii) $x. (y + z) = x \cdot y + x \cdot z$
and $x + (y \cdot z) = (x + y) \cdot (x + z)$ (Distributive Law)

(iv) There is identity elements 0 and 1 in A for the operations (+) and (·) respectively such that $\forall\ x \in A, x + 0 = 0 + x = x$ and $x \cdot 1 = 1 \cdot x = x$ (Existence of Identity).

(v) For each element $x \in A$ there is an inverse elements $x' \in A$ such that $x + x' = x' + x = 1$ the identity element of (·) and $x \cdot x' = x' \cdot x = 0$ the identity element of (+) (Existence of inverse).

Boolean algebra is applicable to statement is mathematical logic also propositions are denoted by the element $x_1\ y_1\ z$, V is replaced by (+) and Λ is replaced by (·).

Theorem: Prove that the algebra of proposition (p) is a Boolean algebra under the operations V and Λ.

Proof: Let $p, q, r \in P$ then

P_1: commutative law:

(i) $p \vee q = q \vee p$ i.e. $p + q = P + p$

(ii) $p \wedge q = q \wedge p$ i.e. $p. q = q. p$

P_2: Associative Law:

(i) $p \vee (q \vee r) = (p \vee q)\ \mathrm{V}\ r$ i.e. $p + (q + r) = (p + q) + r$

(ii) $p \wedge (q \vee r) = (p \wedge q)\ \Lambda\ r$ i.e. $p. (q. r) = (p. q). r$

P_3: Distributive Law:

(i) p

(i) $p \vee (q \wedge r) = (p \vee q)\ \Lambda\ (p \wedge r)$ i.e. $p. (q + r) = (p. q) + (q. r)$

(ii) $p \vee (q \wedge r) = (p \vee q) \vee (p \vee \mathrm{r})$ i.e. $p + (q. r) = (p + q). (p + r)$

P_4: Identity: There is the identity elements 0 (false) and

1 (true) in P. For the operations ($\vee$) and ($\wedge$) respectively so that all $p \in P$

$p + 0 = 0 + p = p$ and $p \cdot 1 = 1 \cdot p = p$

P_5 Inverse: For $p \in P$ there is an inverse element $\bar{p}$ (or $\sim p$) $\in p$ such that $p \vee \bar{p} = 1$ the identity of ($\cdot$) and $p \wedge \bar{p} = \bar{p} \wedge 0 =$ 0 the identity element of (+).

Thus the set P of proposition in a Boolean algebra under $\vee$ and $\wedge$ which are the operations.

Translation of one notation to another:

Sets	Statements	Boolean Algebra
$A \cup B$	$p \vee q$	$a + b$
$A \cap B$	$p \wedge q$	$a \cdot b$
A'	$\tilde{p}$ or $-p$	$-a$
Ω	t	1
ϕ	f	$\odot$
$A \cup A = A$	$p \vee p = p$	$a + a = a$
$A \cap A = A$	$p \wedge p = p$	$a \cdot a = a$
$A \cup A' = \Omega$	$p \vee \tilde{p} = 1$ (true)	$a + (-a) = 1$
$A \cap A' = \phi$	$p \wedge \tilde{p} = 0$ (false)	$a\,(-a) = 0$

6. Truth Table, Algebraic Operation and Electronic Switching Circuit:

The algebraic operations or variables are limited in Boolean Algebra and are defined as AND, OR, NOT. We write hence

If $p = 1$ then $p \neq 0$

If $p = 0$ then $p \neq 1$

The AND operation: It is denoted by the symbol• and operation can be written as p AND $q = p.\, q = p\, q = r$.

Truth Table

p	$q = r$
0	0 = 0
0	1 = 0
1	0 = 0
1	1 = 1

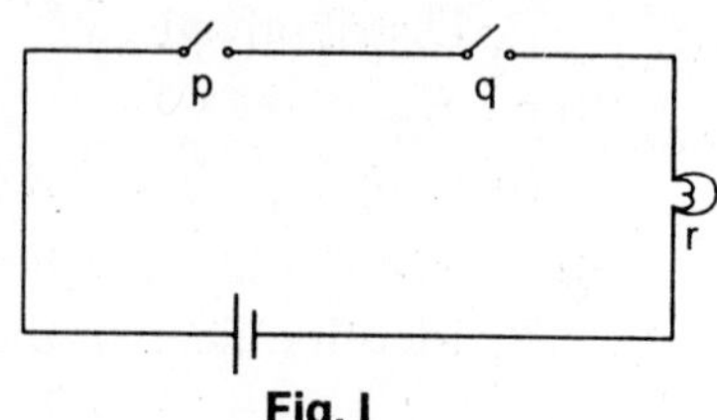

Fig. I

AND Gates: Electrical switching are used to denote.

AND Gates: Switches p and q are connected in series (Fig. I).

Lamp (r) glows only when switch p *AND* switch q are closed.

The OR operation: Here p or $q = p + q = r$

The Truth table is

$p + q = r$

$0 + 0 = 0$

$0 + 1 = 1$

$1 + 0 = 1$

$1 + 1 = 1$

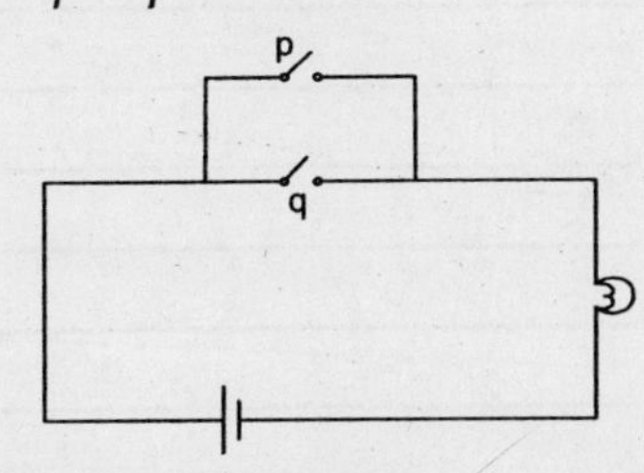

Fig. II

OR Gates: The OR Gates used in electronic circuit is shown in Fig. II. Such circuit produces an output when a signal is applied to any one or all its switches in its input circuit.

A General Truth Table

p	p	$\tilde{q}$	$p + \tilde{q}$
1	1	0	1
1	0	1	1
0	1	0	0
0	0	1	1

NOTES

NOTES

NOTES

NOTES

NOTES

NOTES

NOTES